PAYING FOR MEDICARE

SOCIAL INSTITUTIONS AND SOCIAL CHANGE
An Aldine de Gruyter Series of Texts and Monographs
EDITED BY
Michael Useem • James D. Wright

PAYING FOR MEDICARE
The Politics of Reform

RA
395
.A3
S66
1992

David G. Smith

ALDINE DE GRUYTER
New York

About the Author

David G. Smith is Professor of Political Science at Swarthmore College in
Pennsylvania. He received his Ph.D from Johns Hopkins University and
attended the London School of Economics. His primary teaching areas
are constitutional law and jurisprudence; health policy; American government and public policy. In these areas he has written numerous
journal articles.

ALDINE DE GRUYTER
A division of Walter de Gruyter, Inc.
200 Saw Mill River Road
Hawthorne, New York 10532

The paper used in this publication meets the minimum requirements of American National Standard for Information Sciences—Permanence of Paper for
Printed Library Materials, ANSI Z39.48-1984.

Library of Congress Cataloging-in-Publication Data
Smith, David G., 1926–
    Paying for medicare / David G. Smith.
        p.   cm. — (Social institutions and social change)
    Includes bibliographical references and index.
    ISBN 0-202-30393-4. — ISBN 0-202-30394-2 (pbk.)
    1. Medicare.   2. Hospitals—United States—Prospective payment.
3. Medical policy—United States.   I. Title.   II. Series.
RA395.A3S66   1992
338.4'33621'0973—dc20   91-29636
                                                                              CIP

Manufactured in the United States of America

10 9 8 7 6 5 4 3 2 1

Contents

Acknowledgments

The most agreeable parts of this enterprise were the interviews and the research, mostly done in Washington, D.C. and Baltimore. These activities depended on the help of many others, a fact that imposes the amiable obligation of acknowledging their contributions.

As a guest scholar at the Brookings Institution in 1987–88, I benefitted from use of their facilities. It was a happy and a profitable time, and I would like to express my thanks for the help and encouragement that I received from Brookings and from colleagues there, while absolving them of any responsibility for this book or its contents.

Without the contributions of many individuals who took time from their busy schedules, gave of their knowledge, and made available various materials and documents, this book could never have been written. It is impossible fully to acknowledge this debt, but I can say that I owe much and am profoundly grateful. Among those especially generous and helpful were: Peter Bouxsein, Allen Dobson, Marilyn J. Field, Paul B. Ginsburg, George D. Greenburg, H. Alan Hume, Larry Oday, Julien H. Pettengill, Lisa A. Potetz, Bruce Steinwald, and Donald A. Young.

I am happy to acknowledge separately and specially the contributions of Lynn Etheredge, who first suggested the topic of this book, helped in innumerable ways with the inquiry, read and criticized the manuscript, and offered friendly encouragement along the way.

This book is respectfully dedicated to those public servants, past and present, who worked so hard to make a better program of Medicare.

David G. Smith
Swarthmore College

1

Introduction

This book fills a gap in the health policy literature, by providing an account of the policy developments associated with the hospital prospective payment system and the Medicare fee schedule. Reform of hospital and physician payment is a topic that dominated Federal health politics for a decade. It merits reporting as such. The book is written with two additional objectives in mind. The first is to provide a description of Medicare hospital and physician payment that is sufficiently detailed to support a relatively sophisticated understanding. The second is to relate this description to the structure and processes of American government, and particularly to show how they shape, and may distort, the development of health policy.

The control of rising health care costs is a major problem of domestic policy in all advanced Western societies. This is so, in part, because these societies have aging populations, increasingly sophisticated medical technology, and high service expectations. Age correlates imperfectly, but older populations generally require more care. Medicine is technically progressive, requiring more capital and increasingly sophisticated labor. And quality generally costs money, whether for auto repairs, education, legal services, or medical care. However well the advanced countries of the West might control for excessive expenditures or charges, medical care inevitably costs more. So, in Canada, France, Germany, or Britain, as well as in the United States, mounting health care costs have been both perennial problems of public policy as well as top priority ones. Indeed, for these countries, health care costs have been among the most dynamic and intractable domestic budget items over the past decade.

Nevertheless, most other countries with which the United States compares itself, especially in the health and human services domain, have tackled health care costs, and especially the problem of rising public expenditures for hospital and physician services, with some measure of success. The tools they have used were not new or sophisticated, just the usual ones of negotiated fee schedules, franchising and certificate-of-need, use of co-pays, and the like. But they were used with a will and with effect, resulting in a dramatic slowing in the rate of inflation and the rising proportion of gross national product devoted to health care.

When it comes to health care cost inflation, the United States is in a class by itself. Total health care costs have already passed the $660 billion mark, well over half a trillion dollars a year. As a proportion of GNP, these costs reached 12.2% in 1990, a higher percentage than any other advanced Western country. As for the future, some of the gloomier projections are for 15% of GNP by the year 2000 and 20 to 25% by the year 2020. In the aggregate, health care eats up more and more of the nation's total resources and wealth; it is the fastest growing sector of the economy. This huge amount goes to support a health care sector, moreover, that is generally acknowledged to be unnecessarily expensive, full of holes, inequitable, and lacking in access for the poor and other demographic categories. In short, Americans pay more for less—vastly more for much less.

Medicare is, of course, a separate matter from aggregate health care costs. But Medicare, by itself, is still a huge program. In 1990, for instance, the number of enrollees was 34 million, a population that is still increasing and growing older. The total program expense for 1990 was 107.4 billion, a number that continues to increase at about twice the rate of inflation for the economy as a whole.[1] Except for Social Security, Medicare is the largest domestic program, dwarfing other entitlements. The Medicare budget by itself is over one-third the amount of the *entire* defense budget.

Medicare is not just a large program in aggregate dollar amounts, especially of Federal government outlays. Because of its rate of increase, it has been, along with national defense, a major factor driving the domestic budget deficit. Understandably, in an era of budget deficits and "no new taxes" (or very few of them), Medicare is a major target of deficit reduction strategies. For these strategies, hospital and physician payment reform are important. To the extent that they encourage efficiency, they hold out a hope of reducing expenditures or moderating their increase. And, to the extent that they establish a fair price or one that providers can live with, they can guide budget cuts that are both sensible and acceptable. Medicare payment reform could be, and has become in practice, a major tool for budget-balancing and long-term deficit reduction, matters of the highest domestic priority.

The concept of payment reform implies more than cost containment or ratcheting down the Federal payment to providers. Cost containment is important for those involved with the budget, especially Congress and the Administration. But providers, policy analysts, and Medicare beneficiaries have other objectives as well, among them encouraging efficiency, providing for a fair and equitable payment, and assuring access to care. Thus, a payment system aimed exclusively at cost containment would be unacceptable, especially for providers or Medicare beneficiaries. It could help win immediate skirmishes over cost containment and deficit reduction, but fail to achieve other important objectives such as changing the attitude and behavior of physicians and hospitals or redressing regional inequities in the provision of care.

Given the existing Medicare payment system, a reform that would meet these various constraints was a tall order. That payment system was largely taken over from the practices followed by private insurers such as Blue Cross and Blue Shield. It incorporated the existing regional and specialty differentials in charges and fees and the historic patterns of maldistribution of health care facilities and professionals. Over time, regulation piled on regulation, report on report. And the payment system was shot through with vested interest and protective arrangements, so that even incremental changes were difficult to make.

In 1980–1981, as a new decade began and the presidency changed from Jimmy Carter, a moderate Democrat, to Ronald Reagan, an avowed conservative Republican, few would have bet much on the prospects of a fundamental reform in the Medicare payment system. Many domestic programs were put "on hold" or slated for demolition in accord with the new administration's deregulative and "contractionist"[2] ideology. Anything resembling either the prospective payment system or the Medicare fee schedule that ultimately developed would probably have been vetoed. Yet necessity begets innovation, according to an old saying, and sweeping changes were made, particularly by devising new means and ends. In part, this entailed abandoning some objectives and shifting priorities. But Medicare payment reform was also made possible as a result of the almost revolutionary transformation in the separation of powers and relations between the executive and legislative branches of government. It is, itself, a part of institutional changes of constitutional significance.

Although the Reagan Administration was an unlikely time for change, the fact remains that, together, the Medicare hospital and physician payment reforms were the most drastic and far-reaching changes in Federal health policy since the passage of Medicare itself. They are remarkable for the comprehensiveness and sophistication of their design—indeed, the sheer technical achievement is astonishing. The changes in the payment system and its restructuring of rewards and incentives are fundamental and vast in their scope. Both the Prospective Payment System and the Medicare Fee Schedule represent consistent and rigorous applications of a coherent policy, grounded in the best design and methodology available. Moreover, these innovations were quickly developed and enacted into law, largely with the acquiescence and active support of the hospital industry and the physicians' associations. These are rare occurrences in the development of public policy, and it is even more astonishing that most of them took place under a right-wing, ideologically conservative regime.

Both of these ventures, the Prospective Payment System and the Medicare Fee Schedule, are instances of regulation, something that Americans are prone to do and an activity in which they have developed a formidable expertise. Yet regulation, as a method of controlling health care costs, had not fared well and was in particularly low esteem in both the Reagan and Bush administrations. So, it is worth noting that Medicare payment reform not only succeeded in this adverse environment, but that it also represents regulation with a difference. Both the Prospective Payment System and the Medicare Fee Schedule rely on technically developed estimates of resource use—not the physician's charges or the hospital's costs—as a basis for payment. In principle, hospitals are paid according to national DRG rates and physicians according to relative values that are national, uniform, and based on technical calculations of the amount of work or resources appropriate for a particular hospital admission or physician service. The "in principle" is important to note, for there are many regional and specialty variations and particular accommodations. But this emphasis on an objectively determined number was an important element, perhaps essential, for securing provider acceptance. It was intended, as well, to encourage continuing acquiescence in the regulatory system and its outcomes, even when they worked to the disadvantage of particular providers or the government. Regulation generally relies on some measure of mutual confidence and continuing good faith on the part of the regulated and the government, but Medicare payment reform involved this kind of mutual trust in dramatically larger measure than any previous regulative attempts.

Another objective of Medicare payment reform, other than cost containment, was to create new incentives for providers and to bring about some desirable changes in the health care industry itself. The Prospective Payment System not only aimed at a fair price for a hospital stay with a particular DRG designation, it set a *prospective* price of which the hospital could be assured, encouraging that hospital, through efficiencies it might realize, to earn a "margin" or profit and then keep it. Hospitals were, at once, relieved of the constraints of the Medicare Cost Report and invited to manage efficiently with increased dollars as their reward. OBRA 1989 (P.L. 101-239, December 19, 1989) provided, in addition to the Medicare Fee Schedule, for an extensive program of research into and the dissemination of information about appropriateness of care evaluations, practice guidelines, and medical technology assessments. The goal was to find out and to say what constitutes good medical practice. So, the Fee Schedule, in addition to offering physicians a "fair price," gave them an opportunity to do what they had always said they wanted most to do but were prevented by government regulations from doing, to practice "good medicine." In summary, each of these statutes combined regulation, incentives, and a large measure of hopeful expectation with respect to the behavior of providers. Over the long term, both involve a risky but exciting venture in "winning the hearts and minds" of the hospital industry and the physicians.

A large burden of positive expectations has been put on Medicare payment reform. It could prove to be too much. Americans have a penchant for regulation, and they often resort, in this endeavor, to gadgets and gimmicks. The Prospective Payment System and the Medicare Fee Schedule are, in a sense, two high-tech gimmicks expected to cut Medicare costs, pacify the hospitals and the medical profession, transform medical practice and industry behavior, and provide the leverage with which to redress gaps and inequities in beneficiary access to care. They must also survive as functioning and intact systems in the pathological conditions created by a perennially divided President and Congress and the vagaries and turbulence of deficit reduction politics. Whether these payment methodologies will last and whether they will prove to be effective tools for achieving these purposes depend on how well they have been designed and the will and purpose with which they are used. Therein lies some of the interest in following the implementation of the Prospective Payment System and the Medicare Fee Schedule. For now, both the providers and the government are acting as though they can and will work.

For the public enterprise in a wider sense, the stakes riding on the outcome of this venture in payment reform are large and probably growing larger. The United States may be able to put forth a better effort at Medicare cost containment and reform, but it seems doubtful. How these experiments turn out would seem to have important lessons with respect to the reform of Medicare itself, possibilities for a workable system of national health insurance, and prospects of regulating the health care industry generally. Much of this legislation was born out of deficit reduction strategies, so it is important for this reason, for the dollar amounts involved, even more for the prospects of deficit reduction and our capacity to shape the future.

Medicare payment reform is an instance in which great effort was brought to bear on a comparatively narrow issue, in which a small number of variables were controlled and many of the effects of intervention ignored or left unconstrained. Consequently, this study provides a good example of action and reaction in health policy, of the kind of unanticipated consequences that are sometimes important. For instance, we are now (1991) in the midst of another health care "crisis" or, at least, a period of great turbulence. A perennial factor behind this development has been the continuing rise in overall health care costs, exceeding $660 billion in 1990. But another influence has been the effectiveness of constraints on Medicare hospital payments and the increasingly stringent controls on physicians. As Medicare regulations have begun to bite, providers have sought to collect more from nongovernmental payers, i.e., from other insurers, corporations, and private patients. They have also made realistic assessments of what the future holds for them. So Medicare payment reform has made some contribution to this "crisis." As one response to this situation, and for the first time in American history, "Fortune 500" corporations, trade unions, the American Medical Association, the hospitals, health insurers, and advocates for the poor have begun actively to urge schemes for national health insurance. National Health Insurance (NHI) was a proposal that many thought dead and safely buried, especially with the coming of the Reagan Administration in 1980. That it has been revived so quickly owes much to the Reagan and Bush administrations and their policies toward Medicare reimbursement. It is a truism that reform often leads to revolution. Even more paradoxically, one of our most conservative presidents may prove to have been a major influence in leading, ultimately, to a comprehensive system of NHI. Meanwhile, these case studies may help point to what lies immediately ahead in Medicare policy.

I. THE POLICY ENVIRONMENT

The next chapters examine in detail two major policy initiatives: The Prospective Payment System and the Medicare Fee Schedule. These amendments to the Medicare program can be evaluated in their own terms, as sensibly calculated to solve particular problems or not and as entailing a variety of incidental costs. Yet these reforms also merit consideration in a larger context, for they reveal much about the limits of policy in the field of health care financing and what we have reason to hope for, or fear, in the future. A major theme developed in this book is that the making of health policy in the United States is severely, even perilously, constrained by the limits set by our own political institutions and the legacy of past decisions. The original Medicare program was seriously flawed, needing fixing from the day it began. Nevertheless, determined efforts by the Federal government to reform its health care financing provisions began late, moved slowly, and faltered until a state of increasing muddle and near crisis demanded action. Despite these circumstances, the Prospective Payment System and the Medicare Fee Schedule are remarkably well designed to achieve some limited objectives. But an adequate appraisal of these payment reforms—a measure of the achievements and their limitations—requires some introductory discussion of their historic background and the policy environment: specifically, the Medicare legislation that gave rise to the need for payment reform and the major institutions responsible for developing and implementing these changes in health care financing.

In his authoritative work on Medicare, Robert Myers[3] attributes the genesis of Medicare to groups such as the American Association for Labor Legislation, founded in 1906, and the Progressive Party, that included a national health insurance plank in its 1912 platform (Myers 1970, 3, 4). It is worth recalling origins, for they identify important sources of initial and continuing support for governmentally funded health insurance. But they also call attention to the long history of struggle and failed attempts that preceded the passage of Medicare in 1965 and to ways in which the American path diverged from that followed in other countries. With this background in mind, it may be well to acknowledge, at the outset, that the Prospective Payment System and the Medicare Fee Schedule may be seen from a future historic vantage point as little more than installments or short-term expedients in the continuing effort to control health care costs.

The Medicare–Medicaid legislation, or more technically Titles 18 and 19 of the Social Security Amendments of 1965,[4] was regarded as one of the most significant achievements of the Kennedy–Johnson administrations. It was passed after President Kennedy's assassination and the 1964 elections, by a heavily Democratic Congress that saw its mission, in part, as that of redeeming pledges to the American people and a dead president. In recognition of the occasion, President Johnson flew to Independence, Missouri, to sign the legislation in the presence of Harry S. Truman who, as president in 1950, had suffered a humiliating defeat in an earlier attempt to enact a program for national health insurance.

One reason for the congratulatory mood was that Medicare–Medicaid was, for then, a large achievement, substantially greater than even its principal supporters had expected. It was passed after a series of defeats in the Kennedy Administration and despite the formidable opposition of the American Medical Association. Moreover, it included not one major initiative, but three. The Medicare–Medicaid legislation began with an Administration-backed King–Anderson bill, that would extend the social security benefit to cover hospital and nursing home costs. Excluded was medical and surgical coverage or medical care for the poor, not entitled to social security benefits. But two alternative proposals were in competition with King–Anderson. One was the AMA-sponsored "Eldercare," an expanded version of the Kerr–Mills program, which was a grant-in-aid scheme that provided medical assistance for the aged poor. The other was the Byrnes[5] proposal, similar to the Federal employees program, for a contributory plan covering medical and surgical benefits.

Making the most of a historic opportunity, Congress combined all three into what Wilbur Mills, Chairman of the House Ways and Means Committee, called a "three-layer cake." With various modifications, the King–Anderson bill became Part A of Title 18, a hospital insurance benefit. The Byrnes bill became Part B of Title 18, a contributory medical–surgical benefit, without coverage for drugs. And the AMA version of Kerr–Mills became Title 19 or Medicaid.[6]

The analogy of a "layer cake" has some expository value. It suggests one truth: that the American people got a lot at one time in the Medicare–Medicaid legislation. But it also serves to illustrate another, lamentably common, characteristic of health policy-making, then and now. That is the tendency to deal with or avoid difficulty by combining partial, even potentially conflicting, policy elements into a package that is less than a synthetic whole. Such was the case with Medicare–Medicaid; and with that comment as a point of departure, several observations are in order, particularly about ways in which the original legislation has shaped the subsequent development of policy.

It is instructive, for a moment, to view Medicare–Medicaid as a system of national health insurance. From that perspective, it is a singularly limited and badly designed version. It dealt with two of the most important categories of need, the elderly and the indigent. But the two programs were very different. Medicare grew out of a tradition and philosophy of social insurance. Payroll taxes were contributed to Trust Funds, and there was a strong sense of entitlement to the same medical care that anyone else got. Medicaid, by contrast, built on a public assistance mode. People had to establish "eligibility" and they often got welfare medicine. From the beginning, then, the American version of "national health insurance" established as policy and law a two-tiered system of mainstream medicine and care for the poor. Aside from the issue of fairness or equity, this difference has divided energies devoted to reform between advocacy of a universal scheme of health insurance and pursuing Medicare or Medicaid only strategies. And because Medicaid was chronically underfunded and still covered a minority of the poor, many went without health care or the costs for uncompensated care were shifted to Medicare providers, insurance companies, or other payers.

Medicare itself was divided between Part A and Part B, establishing the hospital and physician benefits, respectively. This dualism helped gain provider support and eased the pinch for beneficiaries, especially by limiting the liability for expensive hospital stays. But it built in two different forms of payment: cost reimbursement for hospitals and payment of charges for physicians. As a result of this difference in payment method, Medicare created incentives to overutilize hospital care and underutilize less expensive physician's services. And it made difficult to achieve some measures, such as capitation, that might encourage efficient combination of resources or substitution of less costly modalities of care. Mostly, reforms directed at Part A or Part B have developed separately and at different times, almost never together or as part of a comprehensive strategy.

Another important feature of the original Medicare–Medicaid legislation was the way in which it approached cost containment—which was to put much of the burden on beneficiaries rather than providers. Medicare provided for reimbursement of the hospitals' "reasonable costs" and for the payment of physicians' "reasonable charges," language that would appear to contemplate stringent cost containment measures. But the statute also specified that claims processing would be handled by the traditional "carriers" and "fiscal intermediaries," i.e., pretty much the private insurance agencies that the providers had dealt with before Medicare. Moreover, many of the early administrative decisions implementing Medicare were permissive and conceded much in terms of accounting practices and allowances on claims (Feder 1977). At the same time, the legislation came down rather heavily on the beneficiary and the demand side. Medicaid, like the earlier Kerr–Mills program, continued to be a grant-in-aid program in which the states paid up to half of the total costs, sometimes severely taxing the resources of the poorer ones and leading them to raise eligibility standards and cut funds for care. Medicare had numerous exclusions, deductibles, and co-pays intended to limit utilization. Physicians (though not hospitals) could also bill for additional payments, over and above the amount allowed by Medicare. In summary, the cost containment features were weak, and much of the incentive for restraint in utilization was put on the beneficiary, not the provider.

Despite the victory celebration in Independence, Missouri, the advent of Medicare was viewed with ambivalence, not least within the Department of Health, Education, and Welfare, among those who helped create the program and those subsequently engaged in its implementation. There was, from the beginning, a sense of unfinished business and an awareness that the task would be harder because of decisions already made. Early on, officials within the Social Security Administration and members of HIBAC[7] puzzled over how much to indulge providers in order to get the program firmly established and over how many of the concessions already made to try to win back. As provider fees and aggregate program costs rose, forward-looking administrators and Congressional staff began thinking about authorizations and money for research and development and about how to devise cost containment strategies. These efforts came to fruition in the Social Security Amendments of 1972, which created the statutory authorizations for research and demonstrations and funded, initially, research that laid the conceptual foundations for the Prospective Payment System and the Medicare Fee Schedule. Viewed from this perspective, then, Medicare was not just a flawed and incomplete piece of work but also the beginning of a number of efforts at cost containment and payment reform that culminated in the Reagan–Bush administrations and the decade of the 1980s.

In this modern saga, a dominant theme has been that of payment reform, primarily to contain costs, but also to protect beneficiaries and to redress other inequities. The Medicare–Medicaid legislation and its initial implementation are important because some of the early decisions channeled subsequent reform attempts and continue to influence them both directly and indirectly. One strategic decision was the division between Medicare and Medicaid and with Medicare, that between Parts A and B. Almost as important was the balance established between the public and the private sectors, in the use of traditional payment methods, including the carriers and fiscal intermediaries, and in the heavy reliance on deductibles and co-pays, on beneficiary disincentives as cost containment expedients. Medicare began as a heavily mortgaged program and the American people continue to pay in many ways. That important Medicare payment reforms were successfully carried through, despite this liability inherited from the past, makes the achievement the more remarkable.

One useful way of regarding the course of policy development and implementation—for instance, Medicare payment reform—is by identifying obstacles to or constraints on good outcomes. For payment reform, the burden of past partial solutions was important. At this level of generality, two other major factors that created difficulty should be mentioned. One is the nature of health policy itself. And a second is the character of American political institutions, particularly as instruments of policy-making.

In essentials, good policy requires the development and evaluation of alternatives, choice of the best option, and effective advocacy to get it adopted. This could also be described as bringing knowledge and power together. In this respect, health policy and especially that part involving medical care presents some special difficulties of its own. To begin with, it tends to be arcane—scientifically difficult and employing little understood procedures—so that otherwise good proposals may fail to meet a burden of persuasion or be defeated by arguments that invoke the authority of science or technology. Medical care also requires organization in order to deliver services to patients. And organization is both power and interest. This is to state the obvious, that physicians and hospitals have a lot to defend and are alert in doing so. They also have some special advantages in fending off regulation, so that effective reform may require concessions acknowledging such advantages or aimed to win over the regulated without sacrificing at the same time the coherence and integrity of the reforms themselves. Both the Prospective Payment System and the Medicare Fee Schedule were self-consciously devised to meet these constraints. How successful they will be on this account or in maintaining program integrity for the longer term remains to be seen.

Like war, health policy and, increasingly, medical care are too important to be left to the professionals, which is another way of saying that they have become increasingly politicized. This holds as well for medical care financing. Once almost entirely private, it has become increasingly subject to public scrutiny and regulation. But as the origins of Medicare illustrate, delegation and a sharing of public and private control may be essential and are certainly characteristic: in the development of regulations, the processing of claims, the monitoring of quality, and so forth. This antagonistic–symbiotic relation of the public and the private in health care regulation compounds the problem of bringing knowledge, or adequate technical solutions, together with political power and the effective resolution of policy conflicts. With the complex system of private federalism sustained by health care financing, the technical problems are difficult, both conceptually and practically, in developing and applying workable regulations to providers. So, too, is the politics, engaging an array of governmental agencies and requiring, on occasion, a sensitive diplomacy and, at other times, the use of great aggregations of power strategically and ruthlessly. It is a protean kind of activity that leads provider groups to exploit their access and leverage and the public authorities to negotiate and bargain with whatever resources they have or can develop. As health policy, including health care finance, has become increasingly politicized, the scope of conflict has widened, both with respect to the issues and the parties involved. This tendency greatly increases the incentives to exploit some characteristic strengths and weaknesses of American government.

The most distinctive feature of the American polity is the combining of federalism and separation of powers as a double security against the accumulation of power. In this "compound Republic of America," as James Madison termed it,[8] power has not remained as dispersed and fragmented as he envisioned. But it is rare for it to be concentrated enough to resolve any large domestic policy issue, either as a coherent unity or within a short span of time. As for health policy, this feature of

American politics has meant that organized professional and political power on the provider side (Freidson 1970) is met, for the most part, with institutional weakness on the governmental side. Health policy has been much influenced by this institutional weakness, which, in terms, means that it tends to follow the ups and downs of the electoral cycle; the relations of Congress and the President as determined by party majorities and the constitutional separation of powers; the congressional committees, their jurisdiction and structure; and the particulars of administrative organization in the executive branch. These are all important factors in shaping policy and especially in affecting the way in which knowledge (i.e., technical and economic rationality) and power (interest and politics) get connected. Therefore, a brief characterization of some of these institutions may be useful as a prelude to the case studies that follow.

The Department of Health and Human Services (DHHS) is a good place to begin, since it has long been the administrative agency most important for Federal health policy (Figure 1). As the organizational chart indicates, in addition to the Social Security Administration and other programs for the aging, families, and children, the DHHS has a wide range of responsibilities in health and medicine including support for biomedical research and the training of health professionals, communicable disease and community health, the Food and Drug Administration, and the Health Care Financing Administration, which administers Medicare and the Federal part of Medicaid. Environmental health was transferred out when the Environmental Protection Agency was formed (1970); and the Veterans Administration and medical care for military dependents are separate.[9] But aside from these, the Department has administrative responsibility for all the major Federal health programs and policy changes often begin here, though less frequently since the beginning of the Reagan presidency.

The DHHS is the successor to the Department of Health, Education, and Welfare (DHEW), which was organized in 1953, by bringing together the Social Security Administration, the Public Health Service, the Office of Education, and the Childrens' Bureau. The Food and Drug Administration was later transferred in. The first Secretary was Oveta Culp Hobby, a millionaire sportswoman of no pronounced policy views, largely named to mollify the A.M.A. In October 1979, President Jimmy Carter established a separate Department of Education, so that the DHEW became the DHHS, with education removed.

Origins can provide important clues to present reality, and that is very much true for the DHHS. One important variable, from the beginning, has been the Secretary of DHHS: both the character of the individual appointee and the prominence accorded the office by the President. As

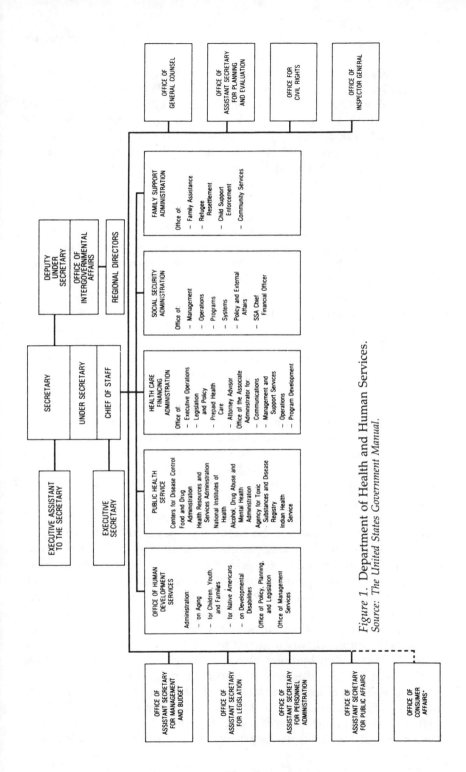

Figure 1. Department of Health and Human Services.
Source: The United States Government Manual.

13

the example of Mrs. Hobby suggests, secretaries have varied greatly. Some like Marion Folsom (1955–1957) or Caspar Weinberger (1973–1974) were capable. Others, like Joseph Califano (1977–1978) or Richard Schweiker (1981–1983) enjoyed, for a time at least, strong presidential support and an important role in the Administration. Just as often, the Secretaries have been relatively ineffective, accorded little status in the Cabinet or White House circles, and targeted by hostile provider or clientele groups. As the dates would indicate, few have stayed long in office, two years being the norm. In general, Secretaries have had to be personally and politically effective and have the support of the President if they were to accomplish much. And an initiative like Medicare payment reform, both technical and controversial, would not be likely to get much support at higher levels, either because the Secretary was unable to give it or because it was not high in priority for him or her.

As these origins might also suggest, the DHHS, even with the Office of Education removed, remains a large and diverse organization, resembling a holding company rather than a single firm or an integrated corporation. With 120,000 employees, down from a high of 147,000 under the Carter Administration, it is the largest Federal department except for Defense. Its responsibility is vast and its missions varied. Organizationally, this translates into a complex assemblage of scientists, technicians, professionals, and clientele advocates and an array of programs, regulatory activities, and funding streams that generate an enormous variety of political interest and loyalties. The Department also sprawls about, with much of its leadership in Washington but other parts in Maryland, Atlanta, Georgia, and the 10 regional offices. Created from diverse parts, the Department's centrifugal stresses are strong, and a sustained unity is rare.

Within this organizational structure, the Health Care Financing Administration (HCFA) should be mentioned separately because of the importance it has for Medicare payment reform. The HCFA was created in March 1977 under the Carter Administration, in order to bring Medicare and Medicaid together under one administrative agency. It was established as an "Administration," coordinate with the Public Health Service and the Social Security Administration and assigned important program development responsibilities of its own.[10] However, the HCFA's development was troubled by weak leadership, organizational difficulties, and then by the partisan onslaught of the first Reagan Administration. Despite this inauspicious beginning, it successfully undertook the design and implementation of the Prospective Payment System and the initial implementation of the Medicare Fee Schedule. Within the DHHS, it is the main source of expertise and program initiatives for Medicare and Medicaid. It also develops and implements the regulations for these programs. The HCFA enjoys the further distinction of carrying the responsibility for the second largest chunk of money within the DHHS ($156 billion) with the smallest staff (4000).

One consequence of pluralism and diversity is that many of the DHHS constituent agencies were, and continue to be, "in business" for themselves: that is, developing and cultivating their own clientele support, access to congressional committees and subcommittees, and support within the executive branch. A long-familiar notion in public administration is that of "triangles" or "iron triangles," the ententes of mutual interest that develop between an administrative subdivision, a Congressional subcommittee, and an interest group that lead to increased appropriations, regulatory concessions, or statutory change. They exist largely because of separation of powers and fragmentation of responsibility that allow cozy relations to persist and that maximize opportunities for shallow manipulations of power to achieve particularistic benefits. Right-thinking public servants have decried these "iron triangles" as putting special advantage above the public interest. At the same time, DHSS programs have often had particular advantages in an administrative politics of this sort because of program sponsorship by physicians, biomedical scientists, and various "helping" professions that bring a dynamism and persuasiveness to the activities of program innovation and support. Also going for these programs was the material interest and self-righteous advocacy of many of these same professions as well as the genuine need and pathos of elderly beneficiaries, children, the "homeless," and so forth. Though the program politics of the DHHS was sometimes crassly particularistic, it was also more than that, so that there was both a moral imperative and a political dynamic pressing for program enhancement.[11]

Some institutional features of Congress have important effects on the development and implementation of DHHS programs, including Medicare and Medicaid. These include traditional arrangements, such as the division of program jurisdiction between various committees and the separation of the authorization and appropriation process, as well as more recent developments, such as the increasing power of subcommittees as centers of program initiative and control and the growing "individualism" of Congressional members, particularly in seeking to provide constituency services and raise campaign "war chests" from individual and PAC contributions. Fragmentation in Congress complements pluralism within the DHHS, a pairing that gives opportunity for innovation but also prompts demands for legislative or budgetary concessions and particularistic interventions in the implementation of programs.

One institutional peculiarity of great significance for Medicare, as well as for health policy generally, is the sharing of jurisdiction between committees. Specifically, this means that Part A of Medicare, funded by a Social Security payroll tax, falls within the jurisdiction of the tax committees: Ways and Means in the House and Finance in the Senate. On the other hand, jurisdiction over Part B or physician services, and over Medicaid is shared with Energy and Commerce in the House and Labor and Human Resources in the Senate. For long-term care and for a variety of issues of general concern to the elderly, the two Committees on Aging have important roles. This shared jurisdiction complicates procedures. It also introduces some specific elements into the making of Medicare policy that are both peculiar and important. The leading role of the two powerful tax-writing committees—in the first instance, their health subcommittees—ensures that Medicare legislation can get decisive backing, though often their support is impressed with a narrow, "bottom-line" practicality that makes short work of professional sensitivities or procedural niceties. This is one way that dispersed power gets effectively concentrated in the present-day Congress, although at some cost. Another result of this divided jurisdiction is that policy-making for the different program elements of Medicare and Medicaid proceed independently of each other and sometimes in ways that may work at cross-purposes and have remote and unintended consequences. Of course, these committees and their staff consult and often agree, especially with Democratic majorities in both houses. The budget reconciliation process also provides a kind of planning and negotiating framework that helps establish a rough ordering of priorities. But committees have a well-earned reputation as power centers and their divided jurisdiction over programs marks that power and its limits. As legislated, the hospital benefit, physicians' services, and a separate provision for the "medically indigent" are dealt with separately, by committees with overlapping jurisdictions and, at times, divergent philosophy and purpose.

The budget process was just referred to and deserves a comment because of the special impact it has had on the Medicare program. Budget creep, the deficit, and other budgetary pathologies predated the Reagan era, and Congress itself enacted a major reform in the Budget and Impoundment Control Act of 1974 that established the outlines of its budget procedures. Most important, it sets overall target figures that help sort priorities and negotiate outlays down over the budget cycle. The procedure is complex, arduous, and time-consuming; but more of this later. One reason that it has been important for Medicare is because of the amount of money involved in the program and the need to reduce it. Another has been the widely shared conviction that hospitals and physicians were making out too well under the Medicare payment system. Further, the Gramm–Rudman legislation of 1985 made Medicare a special deficit-reduction target, not only giving sanction to this particular expedient, but encouraging specific cost-saving amendments to the Medicare program itself, many of which had little else to commend them except that they represented a short-term budget "fix" and gratified some Congressman or constituent. An important point, then, is that much of the policy with respect to Medicare payment reform has been made in a political environment that tended to push cost containment first and foremost and often encouraged a rather mindless incrementalism.[12]

This last statement might suggest that innovation in health programs, including Medicare and Medicaid, ought to be approached thoughtfully, even with a modicum of suspicion. These programs address the vital needs of a large part of the American people, including young people and the very old, least able to fend for themselves. Yet, as noted, they are quintessentially programs for clienteles, promoted as well with the persuasive cant of lobbies, health care providers, and other "helping" professions. For longer than the Department or Medicare has existed, advocates for these programs have bubbled with innovations of a sort, surfacing scores of new proposals for meeting a need or spending additional dollars. Not only is such activity productive of expense, it can often be carried on successfully, perhaps most successfully, when little attention is paid to how much lasting good it does. To this kind of politics must be added elements contributed by the congressional environment, such as divided jurisdiction, subcommittee dominance, and the constituency concerns of individual members. Urgent needs, powerful interests, and specific institutional mechanisms impel Federal health initiatives toward a follow-your-nose policy of something for everyone.[13] Indeed, an important question, sometimes puzzling and not easy to answer, is why Federal health policy turns out well, when it does.

Given the political environment in which the DHHS operates, managing this sprawling, pluralistic, ever changing enterprise as a corporate entity is hardly possible. It is more useful to think about how some of the centrifugal and particularistic tendencies get checked and how specific priorities are set and pursued. With this in mind, several features of departmental organization and the objectives giving rise to them are important in characterizing the Department's activities. One such development, pursued steadily since the Kennedy–Johnson era, has been the gradual strengthening of "staff" and oversight activities: adding an Inspector-General and a Chief of Staff, and enhancing the roles of the Department's own Office of Management and Budget and Office of the General Counsel. A second development testifies to the importance of external relations, with Congress and the White House as well as provider and clientele groups. This is the creation of a high-level policy apparatus, especially the Assistant Secretary for Planning and Evaluation and the Assistant Secretary for Legislation. Creating posts at the assistant secretary level was important for enhancing their status and especially for increasing staffs assigned to these functions. Other individuals and staff participate in policy planning and development, including a number from the Office of the Secretary. Their purpose is, in formal terms, to advise the Secretary. More descriptively, they have a large role in winnowing and helping to identify and develop promising policy initiatives and alternative proposals.

As for program developments such as the Prospective Payment System or the Medicare Fee Schedule, organizational tendencies such as those just described could cut differently, work advantageously in some ways and not in others. Centralization and integration could help concentrate energies and encourage a longer and more comprehensive view and did so, for instance, with several programs under the Carter Administration such as national health insurance, long-term care, and several other Medicaid initiatives. At the same time, any Secretary of DHHS must, perforce, either choose a few major priorities or have, practically speaking, none at all. At the secretarial level of program policy, moreover, there are certain DHHS hardy perennials, such as national health insurance, long-term care, and child health that get first place while initiatives such as hospital and physician payments that are technical and anger the providers tend to get ignored or crowded aside. Earlier mention was made of the difficulty of getting power and knowledge together, and from this perspective, such DHHS organizational changes could be a way, in effect if not in purpose, of creating an obstacle in such policy developments, "layering" them rather than facilitating their emergence. It happened that Secretary Schweiker favored the hospital prospective payment initiative and made it a top priority; but that was a particular situation. In this respect, the fate of physician payment reform within the DHHS provides an instructive comparison, for it languished without effective executive branch support until Congress acted and passed a version of its own.

Beyond the Department are the Cabinet, the presidential staff agencies, and the White House Office. With respect to this apparatus, an important development of recent years has been a tendency for the President and his close aides to relate differently to the major cabinet departments and presidential agencies, dealing with one group as an inner circle and a second as an outer and less significant one. Within the first are included the Departments of Treasury, State, Defense, and Justice, together with a few key agencies such as EOMB, the CIA, and the NSC. Outside are the departments that serve clients or manage resources, such as Agriculture, Education, and Interior. To apply a homely image to the President's agenda, these could be thought of in terms of "front burner" or "back burner" concerns, with the first group important because it represents the immediate and urgent, and the second getting priority only when it occasions political embarrassment or presents a major opportunity. Needless to say, DHHS has been in the second group, particularly with the Reagan and Bush Administrations.

A second development of major significance, especially since the Kennedy–Johnson Administrations, has been for the Presidency to be controlled by the Republican Party and the Congress by the Democrats. Since then, the only Democratic president has been Jimmy Carter. On the legislative side, the Republican Party has held a majority in the Senate for one period only, from 1980 to 1986; and has not held a majority in the House since 1946, almost half a century.

As for DHHS programs, these tendencies converge in an important way. On the one hand, they are programs that are important to providers and popular with beneficiaries. They lend themselves to Congressional initiatives and tinkering. And, with the Republican Party controlling the executive, these programs represent one way in which Democratic legislators can shape the domestic agenda. Yet from the perspective of a Republican president, this kind of agenda building and encroaching control could lead not just to a weakening of the executive chain of command and diminished control over departmental policy, but to a surrendering of the domestic agenda to a Democratic Congress.

These developments help to explain why people in the inner circle of the presidential advisers sometimes speak of their own departmental secretaries and the outer cabinet in "us–them" terms and treat them less as allies and more like unruly provinces to be pacified and kept in subjection. In the second Nixon term, a determined attempt was made to assert presidential control over the executive branch, an effort that contributed to the Watergate crisis and legislation aimed at curbing the "Imperial Presidency" (Nathan 1983). Important in the present context, though, is that the Reagan Administration picked up where President Nixon left off with a number of strategies and procedures designed not just to establish and follow through on President Reagan's domestic priorities, but to ensure that the congressional subcommittees with their various constituency demands and the departmental bureaucrats with their program ambitions would not be able to reverse this momentum. Again, there will be occasion to explain in detail ways in which these developments affected payment reform, but in comprehensive terms, these measures included identifying key posts and staffing them with political loyalists, closely monitoring any new program initiatives to ensure conformity with Reagan policies, and blocking attempts by Administration officials, high or low, to lobby Congress with their own proposals (Benda and Levine 1988).

The rigor and the effectiveness with which these measures were pursued varied over time. Much was made in the Reagan presidency of "windows of opportunity" and there was a consensus that the new Administration had to strike fast and hard at the entitlement programs then seek to hold the ground taken. There was some relaxation of controls, especially in the second Reagan Administration and the general executive branch reshuffling. But many of the same techniques and the philosophy animating them have persisted in the Bush Administration, so that they have both a historic and continuing relevance to Medicare policy.

Along with the budget deficit, this particular temporal phase in the constitutional separation of powers and the divided partisan control of the Presidency and the Congress were major supervening factors in determining the political environment in which Medicare payment reform was accomplished. At times, these powerful influences hindered reform efforts; at other times they provided a powerful impetus for change. In the largest sense, they limited options and shaped the alternatives themselves, so that both the Prospective Payment System and the Medicare Fee Schedule are responses to institutional circumstance as much as they are solutions to technical problems.

A part of the background to the account that follows is the Medicare legislation itself—a landmark achievement, but flawed in its fundamental design. Weakness in our political institutions and the power of organized medicine help account for these defects and continue to affect attempts at reform. Where we were and the constraints imposed by our own political institutions help reach an informed and fair assessment of the achievement represented by these two efforts at Medicare payment reform. They, too, fall short in important ways and leave much undone. Yet, in the immortal words of Yogi Berra,[14] "It ain't over until it's over." A major purpose of this study is to help understand the past in order to move foreward.

NOTES

1. Projected to reach $124 Billion in FY1992.
2. A term in vogue then, referring to strategies that would reduce the size of the Federal government.
3. Chief Actuary for the Social Security Administration 1947–1970.
4. P.L. 89–97 (July 20, 1965).

5. John W. Byrnes (R., Wisc.), House Minority Leader.

6. For a more extended account of these events, see Marmor (forthcoming).

7. The Health Insurance Benefits Advisory Council, a representative body created to help with the implementation of Medicare. Cf. Feder (1977 pp. 144 ff.).

8. *The Federalist;* No. 10.

9. The Veterans' Administration is an independent agency. CHAMPUS, or the Civilian Health and Medical Program, Uniformed Services, is administered by the Department of Defense. The Federal Employee Health Benefits Program, which provides a contributory system of health insurance for Federal employees, is under the Office of Personnel Management.

10. For instance, it had its own Office of Program Policy, its own Office of Research, Demonstrations and Statistics, and its own Actuary.

11. Heclo (1978) uses the term "issue networks," which may more nearly describe the politics of such programs than the older, and perjorative, "iron triangles."

12. OBRA1990 suspended Gramm-Rudman, replacing it with discretionary spending caps and a five-year schedule of deficit reductions. This arrangement may not endure, but will probably last until the 1992 elections so that, for the present, the budget reconciliation process is less significant. *Congressional Quarterly,* January 26, 1991, pp. 232–237.

13. A former OMB official recalls a saying in that agency: "There goes HEW again, 'Nation wide and an inch deep.' " In other words, responding to every one but with little cumulative result.

14. Catcher and later manager for the New York Yankees.

2

Prospective Payment System: Development

The prospective payment system (PPS) that was enacted into law as part of the Social Security Amendments of 1983 and initially implemented in October of that year is, arguably, the biggest single change in the American health care system since the passage of Medicare, almost 20 years before. The legislation changed the system of hospital reimbursement from one that was cost-driven by the individual decisions of physicians and health care professionals to one in which the Federal government would prescribe a set price for an entire episode.[1] It changed *what* was paid for as well as *who* determined the price, and *how* that price would be calculated.[2] In changing the method of hospital payment, PPS also transformed fundamentally the economic incentives that hospitals would face, the tools of calculation and control needed by them and by public officials, and the political relations of the hospital industry and the government. As change in the health care sector goes, PPS could be called "revolutionary," and much of the interest in this episode lies in trying to explain why change of this magnitude came about.

If PPS is a "revolution," it is also uniquely American. The diagnosis related groups (DRGs) that provide the basis for setting the price and are the conceptual foundation for the system resulted from the remarkable kind of public-private initiative in government, academia, and private industry that is especially characteristic of American policy development. The system is built on the data bases, computerized information systems, and expertise created over the years by the hospital industry, the fiscal intermediaries (FIs), and the government. It is peculiarly American in its combination of administrative pricing or regulation and its provision of incentives for management efficiency. It may prove to be, alas, peculiarly American also in its attempt to resolve fundamental difficulty with a "high-tech" gimmick, as some critics have argued. That remains to be seen but, in any event, such an outcome would certainly be much in the American style.[3]

Despite the magnitude of the change that PPS represented it was, somewhat paradoxically, a quiet revolution. It was enacted into law with little controversy and with the united support of the hospital lobby, that viewed it as less than ideal but clearly better than any of the alternatives being discussed. The American Medical Association largely ignored the entire episode. It passed Congress, not as a bill in its own right, but appended to the Social Security Amendments of 1983, virtually without committee hearings and with the briefest of floor debates in the House and Senate. Indeed, once PPS became law, the HCFA administrators and technicians spent many hours over the next few months explaining to Congress what had been done and reassuring them that nothing terrible had occurred.[4] The explanation for this quiet revolution lies in an unusual conjuncture of political circumstance and technical expertise, the subject of this chapter.

I. HOSPITAL COST CONTAINMENT

Unlike policy development, which tends to be continuous, national politics has a convenient periodicity about it, marked by the elections and the four-year terms of the presidents. Accordingly, the administration of President Jimmy Carter (1976–1980) served as a preparation for and a prelude to the far reaching changes in hospital payment policy that followed in the next administration.

The Carter administration, with Joseph Califano serving as the Secretary of the Department of Health, Education, and Welfare, had begun with an ambitious proposal for national health insurance. Hospital cost containment was an essential complement to that proposal, since a demonstrable ability to control hospital costs was deemed a prerequisite for national health insurance. After national health insurance was shelved, hospital cost containment remained as the major health initiative of the Carter administration. The bruising and embittered struggle over hospital cost containment lasted from early 1977 until the closing days of the administration. It was a fight of sizable proportions. The bills and proposals from the White House, the Congress, and the health care lobbies canvassed most of the alternatives and cost containment stratagems as they were then known. And while the hospital cost containment effort ended in an inglorious defeat for its proponents and seemed to leave little behind but the smoke of battle, it was important especially in helping to shape attitudes, both within industry and in government, in exploring a variety of possible methods for controlling hospital costs, and in revealing deficiencies in the "state of the art," especially inadequacies of concept, data, and technology.

During the Carter administration and partly because of the hospital cost containment effort, important shifts of attitude took place in government and within the industry. Both became increasingly disenchanted with the potential and the practice of the regulatory approach to health care, whether for purposes of health planning, quality assurance and utilization review, or cost control. Journal articles documented the failure of regulation; younger Congressmen, such as David Stockman (R., Mich.) and Richard Gephardt (D., Mo.) espoused "competition" approaches and hospital representatives complained of burgeoning cost-reimbursement manuals that kept them in regulatory leading strings. When the Carter cost containment initiative was ultimately defeated in November 1979, with the passage of the Gephardt Amendment, substituting a "voluntary effort" for the Administration bill, it was not so much because of any faith in another VE, which had failed once and dismally, but because of a growing disillusion with regulatory approaches including hospital cost containment. Whether one counts this as "the death of a paradigm" (Goldsmith 1984) or not, there was a strong sentiment that there ought to be a better approach.

One effect that the cost containment effort had was to unify many of the hospital trade associations and industry leaders in opposition to it, leading them not only to articulate their policy objections but to come forward with proposals of their own, such as the Voluntary Effort, and to recommend specific methods for reimbursement. Hospital industry representatives, in recalling that era, reported a strong and shared sentiment that they did not wish to repeat the experience, along with an awareness that the industry would have to take increased responsibility in the future for seeing that "something was done" about rising hospital costs, something more than another VE.

Although the hospital cost containment effort remained essentially regulatory in approach, it was important for introducing or raising to prominence a number of proposals or methods that would be important for the future. Among these were such notions as payment on a per case basis, incentive reimbursement, peer group classification of hospitals, hospital budgets, indexing of rates of increase, and total expenditure caps.[5] One bill in particular, S1470, the Talmadge–Dole–Long bill, incorporated many of these ideas in a way that anticipated subsequent legislation. This bill, the product of the Senate Finance Committee, and especially of its staff, would have classified hospitals by size, type, and other criteria. It provided for payment by average per diem routine operating costs applicable to each category of hospital with reductions for costs above average and a bonus for below average. Since it was "Medicare only" rather than "all payers" and also excluded "ancillaries,"[6] it would have controlled only a small part of total hospital costs; but it strikingly anticipated some of the later legislation, especially TEFRA,[7] and it broke the link between cost and automatic revenue increases, an important prerequisite for any prospective payment system.[8]

The hospital cost containment experience gave a number of ideas new prominence and a legitimacy in the policy debate that they had not previously enjoyed. Some of the proposals might have actually worked and been tolerable from the perspective of the hospital industry. Yet, as participants recalled that period, neither the political mood nor the policy proposals that had been developed were right for a successful outcome. As one observer put it, the "burden of proof" was too much on the government; and the "hospitals had too many answers."[9] Also, at the level of the policy analysts, there was an awareness that a better methodology was needed—better ways of controlling total costs, yet doing so fairly and rationally, whether through a better method of classifying hospitals or of putting a price on the services they provided.

A paradox of health policy—though not of health policy alone—is that sometimes more progress is made under Republican administrations than under Democratic ones. Many new programs were begun under the Nixon and Ford administrations, among them Health Maintenance Organizations (HMOs), the Professional Standards Review Organizations (PSROs), and the Health Systems Agencies (HSAs). And two of the biggest changes in Medicare since its original passage in 1965— the prospective payment system and the addition of coverage for catastrophic illness—were both enacted in the Reagan Administration. No doubt, a major reason is that Congress has continued under these administrations to be mostly controlled by the Democratic Party, that is insistent on protecting or enhancing the big entitlements, such as Social Security and Medicare, under such circumstances. But the fact that HMOs and PPS, two of the most successful and original policy innovations since 1965, came about not only under Republican administrations but were also expressions in some considerable measure of a "pro-competition" or, at least, of an anti-regulatory philosophy, is a comment not only on the need to seek wisdom from all quarters but also on the fact that "solutions" to the intractable problems of health care costs may well require imagination and non-obvious approaches.

The anti-regulatory philosophy that the new administration brought with it probably helped considerably in getting PPS enacted, most particularly by encouraging a "Medicare only" approach. Given the anti-spending, contractionist views of the Reagan administration, hospital cost containment was an agenda item of importance, But "all payer" approaches that would have sought to constrain all hospital costs, for private patients as well as for Medicare and Medicaid, were "off the table," not to be considered, most immediately because they would have entailed extensive regulation of the private sector. Not only would this be obnoxious to the hospital industry, but from the perspective of the Reagan Administration, it was unneeded since the point was to control government outlays, of which the main source was Medicare. Medicaid, as a policy area, came under the devolution strategy of the Administration: that is, to be left as much as possible to the states. Underlying policy preferences, or "ideology" as it was often termed, argued for a Medicare only approach and, as events unfolded, that approach proved to be strategically advantageous as well and, just possibly, the only alternative that could have succeeded.

Another favoring circumstance was the choice of former Senator Richard S. Schweiker as the new Secretary of the Department of Health and Human Services. Having been a Senator, Schweiker knew legislation and the ways of Congress. He had been the ranking minority member of the Health Subcommittee of the Finance Committee and regarded health affairs as his specialty. On taking office as Secretary, Schweiker announced four main priorities for the Department. Two of these came from President Reagan's White House: budget reduction and block grants. Two were Richard Schweiker's own priorities: the drug approval process and health care costs. According to Schweiker, the latter was his highest priority, and for him, it meant primarily some form of hospital prospective payment system.[10]

Throughout this period, the burden of proof as between government and the hospital industry was also shifting. As noted before, in the course of the hospital cost containment episode, the hospital lobby began to organize itself and to respond with greater unity as well as to recognize the need for putting forward policy proposals of its own. Late in 1980, for instance, and after all of the hospital cost containment alternatives had been legislatively defeated, the hospital representatives were negotiating with the HCFA over possible approaches to a prospective payment system.[11] These talks were suspended when Ronald Reagan won the election but they were an indication of this important and lasting shift in attitude.

Meanwhile, within Congress, hospital costs were an issue that would not go away. With national health insurance no longer an immediate possibility, Medicare hospital costs were a natural candidate for top priority, which is to say that congressional committees and their staffs find ways to employ their time. Also, as one AHA representative observed, "the numbers were going the wrong way."[12] Despite a second

Voluntary Effort, hospital costs kept escalating. Congress, for its part, having twice agreed to wait and see, was pretty much convinced that it had seen enough, that more decisive and drastic measures were needed.

Several converging trends produced a sense of urgency requisite for action. One was the mounting budget deficit, resulting from the tax cut of 1981 and the worst recession since the 1930s, both of which sharply reduced government revenues. Yet in a time of recession and budget slashing, hospital costs and revenues kept increasing as rapidly as before. And, more pertinent for the Federal government, these escalating hospital costs combined with declining payroll tax revenues threatened imminent exhaustion of the hospital Trust Fund. Congress responded swiftly, in August of 1982, with the hospital payment limits generally known as TEFRA.[13]

II. A DECISIVE TURNING POINT

Although there was an Administration version developed within DHSS, TEFRA was mainly the product of the House and Senate committee staffs, who drew largely on proposals that had first appeared during the hospital cost containment skirmishes. It was a makeshift piece of legislation, put together in great haste, but despite this, it was of great importance, both conceptually and practically. It was also a decisive turning point in the struggles over hospital costs and led quickly to the eventual prospective payment system.

TEFRA dealt only with Medicare hospitals. In essence, it provided for an average per case[14] reimbursement, the average being for a particular hospital class. The hospital class was determined by case-mix indexes. Per case reimbursement was limited by the amount of inflation in a hospital market-basket (plus 1%), and by a downward ratchet that, each year, reduced the "applicable percentage," which was the amount by which the average per case reimbursement for a particular hospital could exceed that of the other members of its class. If a hospital came in under the limit, it could keep some of the savings. For cost overruns, the hospital was penalized: the government would pay only a fraction of the difference. The legislation was hastily assembled and something of a patchwork; and yet some of its features were noteworthy and deserve some additional comment.

The singularly unattractive denomination, TEFRA, by which the hospital legislation is commonly known, is an acronym for "Tax Equity and Fiscal Responsibility Act of 1982." In addition to hospital costs, the legislation—P.L. 97–248—made major changes in the existing peer review program, Medicare HMOs, and other reimbursement methods, and dealt, as well, with a number of other titles of the Social Security Act. The bulk of P.L. 97–248 deals with provisions affecting taxes and other revenue provisions wholly unrelated to either Medicare–Medicaid or the Social Security Act—except, of course, for the fact that all of these provisions come within the jurisdiction of the Ways and Means Committee in the House and Finance Committee in the Senate. As a piece of legislation, it illustrates two legislative practices important for health legislation. One is the tactic, illustrated here, of combining health measures with other legislation in order to expedite passage. The other is the increasing tendency to bundle many bits of relevant legislation into an omnibus bill, a practice that Congress had begun prior to 1981, but became increasingly accustomed to, or inured to, in the early years of the Reagan Administration.

TEFRA provided for "per case" or "per discharge" reimbursement. This was a significant step and directly anticipated the approach taken, ultimately, in the PPS legislation. Under TEFRA, hospitals would still be reimbursed for their costs, but for their average costs per case as indexed annually and within limits prescribed for a particular peer group of hospitals. There was an additional provision of percentage incentives. Hospitals stood to gain or lose depending on how they managed. Per case reimbursement also removed at least some of the cost-reimbursement incentives then existing for hospitals to load more and more into "ancillaries" or to shift their billings from the "per diem" or routine bed charges to the ancillary RCCs—i.e., the more lucrative nursing, laboratory, and specialized services.[15]

By combining or "bundling" all of these bills into one, annually determined, average payment per discharge TEFRA introduced an element of prospectivity into hospital reimbursement. It also greatly increased the potential for Federal administrative control, since the government would set annual limits on various hospital specific cost factors and would, as well, determine a national hospital "marketbasket" figure and annual allowable increase or "caps."

The notion of setting "caps" or annual rates of increase had figured prominently in the hospital cost containment controversy, especially in the Administration proposal and in the Talmadge bill. TEFRA established two kinds of caps. One was the annual update factor, set at "marketbasket + 1%" applied, after a one-year transition, to the preceding year's rate. This established a "target amount" for per case reimbursement and, thereby, an incentive for hospitals to manage efficiently through a provision for sharing in cost savings or cost overruns. A second cap was more innovative and also much more objectionable to the hospital industry. This cap was termed, in a piece of governmen-

talise worthy of the IRS, the "applicable percentage." It was designed to
ratchet down the annual rate of inflation in hospital costs, eventually to
no more than 10%—a grim prospect for the hospitals considering their
past and recent history of relatively unconstrained cost increases.

An especially innovative feature of the second cap was its use of a
case-mix index, a state-of-the-art concept that figured prominently in the
eventual PPS. Since the unit of reimbursement was to be an average
"case" or "discharge," and the cap on inflation applied ultimately to the
individual hospital, a method for weighting the hospital averages was
needed. Hospital cases differ greatly in the use of resources as between,
say, a simple leg fracture and a heart transplant. Also, some hospitals
treat much sicker patients, for instance, the medical school hospitals and
major medical centers with their staffs highly trained in the "super-
specialties" and their sophisticated equipment that attracts these patients because of such resources. It would be inefficient, unfair, and
potentially a threat to patients to pay a community general hospital the
same average per case as a medical school center. Such a flat payment
would be a windfall to the community hospital and would either bank-
rupt the medical center or lead it to "game" the system, for instance, by
turning away patients, transferring or "dumping" them, or resorting to
a variety of other stratagems designed to reduce the hospital's cost per
case. TEFRA met this problem by directing the Secretary, practically
speaking the HCFA, to develop "case-mix indexes" for each hospital and
then assign hospitals to appropriate peer groups, based on these indexes. The case averages would then apply to groups that made sense in
terms of likely resource use: for instance, rural hospitals, community
general hospitals, or major teaching centers. Though this approach was
still crude and would have delegated an enormous amount of discretion
to "the Secretary," the underlying methodology was, in conception,
quite sophisticated and dealt with some major sticking points unsuc-
cessfully confronted in earlier cost control efforts, especially how to
devise controls that were fair as between large and small hospitals, and
that did not, at the same time, put Medicare beneficiaries at risk, either
with respect to quality of care or access to it. These constraints were as
important politically as they were ethically, and bed rock for the hospital
and Medicare constituencies as well as for Congress.

The TEFRA hospital provisions are an interesting example of legislation that was not intended to last.[16] It was hastily done over the Spring
of 1982, mostly from leftover parts of earlier legislation, to be used as
another weapon in the ongoing skirmishes over hospital cost containment. Although some of the concepts, such as case-mix indexes and per
case reimbursement, were sophisticated methodological innovations,
the legislation itself was crude and covered many issues of great com-

plexity. Not surprisingly, it left the hospital industry unhappy. Under TEFRA, hospitals would still have a continuing paperwork burden of cost reporting. Yet they would share very little of any savings realized. Moreover, simulations known both to Congress and to the hospital industry revealed that the TEFRA caps would have generated large regional differences in hospital income. The third year under the "applicable percentage" or overall cost limits would have brought acute financial distress, if not outright ruin, to a number of hospitals in specific states.

Some of the more cynical or disgruntled observers believe that TEFRA was intentionally designed to be so obnoxious and threatening that the hospital industry would welcome any reasonable alternative. Congress clearly had an alternative in mind, for it wrote into the TEFRA legislation a mandate for "the Secretary": to report back to them on a PPS proposal. At the same time, the need for quick action on hospital costs was manifest. Those in Congress closest to the legislation say that TEFRA *was* needed as a cost containment measure and especially if no alternative system of prospective reimbursement could be developed. But they add that TEFRA was also intended as a signal to the hospital industry that Congress meant business and that they would not be unhappy if TEFRA encouraged the hospital industry representatives to come in and "deal." A somewhat more positive perspective is that TEFRA gave an entree and legitimacy to proposals that they might advance. In any event, the consensus is that TEFRA was perhaps *the* decisive step—that there would be a system of hospital cost containment, preferably one based on prospective payment.

As a final observation, the mandate to the Secretary was an interesting one. The Secretary was directed to develop a proposal for prospective reimbursement "in consultation with the Senate Committee on Finance and the Ways and Means Committee of the House of Representatives," a novel provision that indicated bipartisan commitment[17] to the enterprise and expectations of an unusual amount of ongoing collaboration between Congress and the DHSS in developing such a system. In addition, Congress called for the Secretary to come back with his report by December 31, 1982, less than five months away, an absurdly short period of time for such a complicated and difficult endeavor. Obviously, there was more here than meets the eye. In fact, the design for a prospective payment system was already well under way in the DHSS and there were assurances from Secretary Schweiker that the Department could have a report to Congress by December 1982 and a system in place by October 1983. For that matter, it was Richard Schweiker who had prevailed on his former colleague, Senator David Durenberger (R., Minn.) to propose inclusion of this mandate in the TEFRA legislation. Therein lies another part of the tale: how the DHSS and especially the

HCFA had been working on the vehicle or the payment methodology at the same time that the Congress had been developing the political resolve to make a drastic and radically different change in the system of hospital reimbursement.

III. A DECADE OF DEVELOPMENT

There is no necessary reason why the prospective payment system that was eventually developed used the DRG methodology. The important elements of a prospective system are (1) that hospitals know in advance what they will be paid; (2) that the system be effective in controlling costs; (3) that it compensate fairly; and (4) that it not harm the beneficiaries or patients. Additional important objectives are that it not be administratively burdensome and that it provide desirable incentives for the hospitals to manage efficiently without deteriorating the quality of care or violating the constraints of the system. At the time that PPS was developed, there were probably a dozen or so methodologies that might—or might not—have been ultimately developed to meet these objectives;[18] but no one knew, and the DRG methodology was available. That it was available owed something to lucky accident, but much more to planning, vision, and ultimate faith in rationally devised solutions on the part of individuals and organizations within government and outside, in academia and the hospital industry.

In the field of public policy, as elsewhere, a rapidly moving object attracts the eye. Certainly, that was true of hospital costs, which began increasingly after 1965 to invite the attention of legislators and administrators as well as health policy researchers and consultants. Hospital costs also helped inspire an important part of that landmark legislation known as the Social Security Amendments of 1972 (P.L. 92–603), with two sections especially important for the development of PPS. Section 223 authorized the setting of "reasonable cost limits" for hospital reimbursement and Section 222 provided for researches and demonstrations into methods for the prospective reimbursement of hospitals as well as authorizing waivers enabling states to participate in rate-setting programs.[19]

An important result of regulation, as of any major governmental initiative, is that it begets a response, sometimes unreasonable, but often both reasonable and reasoned. One part of the hospital industry's response, especially among larger urban and teaching hospitals, was to argue that fundamental changes in cost reimbursement, to be fair, had to take appropriate account of case-mix differences.[20] Initially, much of the stimulus for this interest on the part of the hospitals came from the Economic Stabilization Program of the Nixon Administration. Under Phase IV of this program, hospital rates of increase would be limited on a per case basis, but hospitals that could demonstrate a case-mix increase could get more.[21] Although Phase IV was never implemented, it stimulated interest in case-mix measures within the hospital industry. Then, as the Medicare administrators began to implement the Sec. 223 limitations and states experimented with rate limits of their own, the notion of case-mix differentials began to acquire greater currency, especially as a way to argue for increases or exceptions. Of course, the notion of case-mix differentials can be used to get prices down as well as to raise them; and the government began funding studies of its own and developing expertise in a variety of alternative case-mix measures (Bentley and Butler 1980, 5).

The DRG methodology was, initially, one among several varieties of case-mix indexes and was only incidentally related to its eventual use as a technique of cost control.[22] Indeed, therein lies a commentary on the value of nurturing promising ideas, even when their eventual payoff is unknown. The initial research proposal, developed in the Yale School of Organization and Management by Robert Fetter, John Thompson, and Richard Averill, was awarded one of the first grants made under the authority of the Social Security Amendments of 1972. At that time, there was no HCFA. The research was funded by the Health Services Bureau of the Public Health Service, not with any special interest in cost containment as such, but in the hope that it would lead to clinically coherent categories that could serve as a basis for monitoring quality and appropriateness of care. Much of the later work, funded primarily by the National Center for Health Services Research and by the HCFA, was for the refinement of DRGs as an internal management tool for hospitals, helping them to identify wasteful uses of resources in costly cases. But their research also included a small, secondary proposal to investigate the applicability of DRGs for interhospital comparisons and for cost reimbursement. On the strength of this work, the HCFA put out a "request for proposals" (RFP) for demonstrations testing the feasibility of this methodology to which New Jersey quickly responded, providing an important working example of DRGs in action during the period that Federal legislation was being contemplated.

During this period, the HCFA was also working on routine cost limits and funding research and demonstrations under its Sections 223 and 222 authorities. This work revealed the limitations of some of the relatively crude methods of getting at resource use variations, such as classification or peer grouping of hospitals; but it also showed that there were serious problems with DRGs as they then existed. If DRGs were to serve as a basis for payment, they must be sufficiently precise and "coherent" to identify the specific clinical diagnosis or procedure[23] that is paid for. They would also have to be rich enough to predict the resource use, i.e., the average amount of resources needed for a patient in that particular DRG. The original DRG research, though, was based on ICD A-8,[24] an earlier classification of diseases. It had only 383 DRGs, and lacked clinical adaptations and the richness needed to explain enough of the observed variation in resource use.[25] Some of the extramural projects funded by the HCFA were making these limitations clear. One of these was a project with Blue Cross–Blue Shield of Western Pennsylvania, directed by Wanda Young, that showed the importance of clinical content for Medicare patients and that a number of the existing DRGs were "split" or lacked clinical coherence.[26] Another study, directed by Susan Horn of Johns Hopkins University, dealt with severity of illness and showed that the initial system failed adequately to predict resource use, especially for sicker patients or those with complications. Interest in case-mix indexes and in DRGs remained strong among researchers, the hospital and insurance industries, and a small number of technicians within the HCFA. But at this early stage, in 1978, they did not seem especially promising. DRGs apparently lacked the predictive power to serve either as a management tool or for price setting. Worse, they might be one of those attractive nonsolutions that look as though they work, but do not.

At this juncture, the World Health Organization published a ninth edition of the *International Classification of Diseases*, adding clinical modifications in 1979. This publication was both an action-forcing event and an important opportunity. ICD-9-CM called for an updating of the existing system of DRGs, and it also afforded an opportunity to refine them, especially by employing the clinical modifications. The HCFA quickly let another contract to the Yale group, this time for a revision of the DRGs based on ICD-9-CM. Mindful of the promise of DRGs for a prospective payment system, the HCFA staff took steps to learn about this system for themselves, by establishing and participating directly in an elaborate project advisory committee. For two years, HCFA technicians, outside academics, and representatives of the fiscal intermediaries (FIs) sat with the Yale group in all-day sessions, at least once a month, to monitor progress and to learn. In 1982, the revision was completed, proving to be a significant improvement.

Meanwhile, a study by Julian Pettengill and James Vertrees—technicians within the Office of Research in the HCFA—was being conducted to determine how well this new system would perform as a basis for hospital payment and whether it was the best alternative available. The study was encouraging. It also moved some of the way toward an ultimate design for a system of payment, taking into account various possible difficulties with the DRG methodology as well as some politically sensitive variables, such as local hospital wage variations, urban–rural differentials, and allowances for teaching hospitals.

The Pettingill-Vertrees report was not published until December 1982, even though the work was completed by March 1981 (Pettingill and Vertrees 1982, 101). It is an elegant, though understated report, written in the cool prose of the technician. Yet it cannot be read without emotion and a strong sense that it celebrates the work of many. It marked the culmination of more than a decade of effort and was, most likely, a historic turning point.

By this time, in 1981, the DRG methodology had been only partially evaluated. It was, in fact, never really field tested, for the New Jersey experiment was quite different from the prospective payment system that was eventually adopted. For that matter, PPS was enacted before the New Jersey demonstration was evaluated. Nevertheless, the course of events that led up to maturing of the DRG methodology provides a good example of successful research and development and repays consideration from that perspective. Sections 222 and 223 of the Social Security Amendments of 1972 provided the necessary statutory authority and the resources. The private sector, especially academia, came forward with ideas and research proposals; and the civil servants had the imagination to spot good prospects and nurture them. They also had the in-house capabilities to evaluate and assimilate the result. By 1981, there was at least one—and perhaps only one—methodology that might provide a viable alternative to more cumbersome and less attractive alternatives, such as TEFRA. Among a small number of people in the health services research community, in the hospital and insurance industry, and within the HCFA, there was also a rationally grounded assurance that it would work.

IV. DEVELOPING A PROPOSAL

The prospective payment system that emerged as the Secretary's proposal in December 1982 was a remarkable piece of work for a number of reasons. One was the swiftness with which it was developed. Another was the originality and the technical sophistication of the proposal. But even more astonishing than either of these was that such a proposal should have emerged during the Reagan Administration at all.

One of the top priorities of the new administration was deregulation or, as President Reagan was fond of saying, "getting government off the backs of the people." Accordingly, deregulation task forces were an early order of the day, and the Executive Office of Management and Budget (EOMB) was charged, under Executive Order 12291, with review of all new regulations to ensure that they were not unduly burdensome and that they would pass a benefit–cost test. A prospective payment system based on a DRG methodology, whatever else one might call it, was a system of administered pricing, not a welcome policy option in the new administration. DRGs were viewed in this unflattering light by the new leadership of the HCFA—so much so that a former deputy chief of the Bureau of Program Policy recalls that they were "like the worst of four-letter words" and not to be mentioned.[27]

The new administration was unusually political, even ideological in character. Much of this attitude was deliberately encouraged, since this was an administration that intended to make a difference, especially in its impact on many of the programs administered by the DHHS and the priorities attached to these programs. As part of the transition planning for the new administration, many posts within departments were designated as politically important. Candidates for these posts had to be cleared for political acceptability and for ideological commitment to the President's objectives. In addition, the number of posts designated "Schedule C" was substantially greater than in any previous administration, including that of President Carter, notorious in this respect. During the transition, the Heritage Foundation went so far as to sponsor seminars on the importance of keeping the conservative faith and on ways to avoid being "coopted" by the career civil servants.

The HCFA, that ultimately would carry the main responsibility for designing the prospective payment system, was designated as one of the sensitive agencies. Instead of one political layer, there were three. Particularly with respect to program development, this meant that above the career civil servants and technicians, most of them in Baltimore, there were three layers of political appointees within the HCFA alone, again divided between Baltimore and Washington. Under the new Administrator, Carolyne K. Davis, there was a layer of Associate Administrators, one of whom, Patrice Feinstein as Associate Administrator for Policy, was a central figure in the development of PPS. At a tier below her were two deputies, one in charge of research and demonstrations,[28] and the other the Bureau of Program Policy.[29] Within the Department, above the HCFA, were two more political levels important for program development, the Assistant Secretary for Planning and Evaluation, and the Chief of Staff (a Schweiker innovation that has lasted). Each of these political appointees had their own "staff," some of whom were technical experts. Yet this administration took a strong line that political people developed policy and the civil servants carried it out. The political appointees were more than usually wary of the civil servants and of being "coopted" by them. Most were Reaganites and in varying degrees "ideologues," that is, strongly committed to the President's pro-competition, deregulation, and private sector priorities. Almost none had any previous experience in government,[30] and none had ever administered a government program or worked as a civil servant. Certainly, if the Reagan Administration wished to make a difference, this was one way to go about it. The situation was mitigated by the fact that all of the key political appointees had some background in health affairs, variously in research, teaching or academic administration, and the private sector. Possibly, a fresh perspective not closed in by the civil service view that everything has been tried before was important to ultimate success. This group brought with it energy and a willingness, indeed a determination, to try something new. Yet, these were not auspicious circumstances under which to begin a sustained course of program development.

Richard Schweiker, the newly designated Secretary of Health and Human Services, was by all accounts the single most important figure in the development of PPS. Having served for 20 years in Congress, 10 of them in the Senate, where he was the ranking minority member of the Senate Finance Health Subcommittee, he was knowledgeable about health affairs and many of the substantive programs administered by the Department. Knowing Washington politics and being a person of considerable stature in his own right, he was able in large measure to bypass the clearance process and bring most of his Senate staff with him, some of whom had worked with him for nearly 20 years. With an experienced staff and with a developed sense of his own priorities, Schweiker was able to move quickly and effectively in the new administration.

According to Schweiker, some form of prospective payment was high on his list of priorities. As he reported,[31] a strong element in his own thinking was the failed Voluntary Effort on the part of the hospitals, which Rostenkowski (D., Ill.) as Chairman of Ways and Means had sponsored in the House and which Schweiker had supported in the Senate. Apart from the interest that any Secretary of Health and Human Services would have in rising hospital costs, Schweiker regarded this area as one in which he had a personal involvement and some responsibility for "cleaning up the mess." One of his first acts as Secretary was to direct his Assistant Secretary for Planning and Evaluation, Robert J. Rubin, to lay out several options for him, with hospital reimbursement as a top item on his health agenda.[32]

Throughout the entire Reagan Administration, however, substantive domestic programs—health care included—had to take second place to larger presidential objectives. This was especially true during 1981, the

first year of the new administration, when tax and budget cuts and
attacks on entitlements were of highest priority. For the Department,
1981 was the year of the Stockman "budget revolution" and also of a
crisis over the Social Security Trust Fund, both of which figured prominently in the future of health policy. From the Trust Fund crisis came a
series of administrative proposals for taxing benefits and cutting back on
Social Security entitlements that failed so disastrously in Congress (and
in the country at large) that to this day no one in the Reagan or Bush
administrations has seen fit to try again. Indirectly, this event had an
important effect on health care financing, since any sizable dollar savings in Social Security outlays, which is the biggest single item of domestic expenditure, would have to come, perforce, from some source other
than taxing benefits or reducing entitlements. And when looking for big
savings, no target was more attractive than hospitals, both because of
the enormous amounts of money they sopped up[33] and because they
were generally viewed as grossly overpaid. Also of great strategic importance was the role of EOMB and the approach to budget policy initiated
by David Stockman. Called then a "top-down" approach, it has been
described by a former PAD[34] as "budget reduction and optimization
within those constraints." What this meant in practical terms was that
getting the dollar outlays down was primary while the means to do so or
the impact on substantive programs were secondary, so long as other
presidential objectives, such as deregulation, were met.[35] Although
1981 was, so far as the DHHS was concerned, mostly the year of the
budget and the Social Security debacle, these developments helped
make proposals for the reform of hospital reimbursement more acceptable in 1982.

In addition to the work done early in 1981 within ASPE at the behest
of Secretary Schweiker, various approaches toward hospital cost containment had been previously discussed within the Department and
partially developed, with varying degrees of sponsorship for each of
these approaches. These ranged from capitation and competitive bidding to individual hospital budgets. Of more than passing interest, one
of these approaches strongly resembled the later TEFRA legislation, and
included in it a prospective payment methodology based on a case-mix
index utilizing DRGs. Intensive work had begun on this specific option,
leading to a detailed proposal in August of 1980.[36] Because of the impending election that November, the Administrator of the HCFA—at
that time Howard Newman—decided not to press forward with this
approach. However, it surfaced again as one of the proposals submitted
to Secretary Schweiker by the departmental "Competition Task Force,"
an initiative of the new Administration, the purpose of which was to
develop "pro-competition" proposals. Oddly, this TEFRA-like option

was regarded as "pro-competition" and put forward in good faith as such. Although it was not immediately pursued, the proposal was notable especially for its inclusion of a case-mix index and for basing it on DRGs.

Meanwhile, Secretary Schweiker had decided that he wished to have a prospective payment proposal ready for the legislative session of 1982. Accordingly, he directed ASPE late in the Spring of 1982 to begin reviewing the alternatives.[37] He also directed Carolyne K. Davis, the new Administrator of the HCFA, to begin the staff work necessary to bring forward a fully developed proposal for introduction in Congress a year from then. From the Fall of 1981 until December 1982, when the Secretary's Report on "Hospital Prospective Payment for Medicare" was forwarded to Congress, work on this task was continuous and a top priority for the Secretary, the Department, and especially the HCFA (Oday unpublished, 6).

An initial step was to lay out the major alternatives. Accordingly, an Options Paper was developed within the Bureau of Program Policy (later BERC), and used by HCFA policy-makers as a basis to evaluate seven major alternatives in terms of their cost control potential, feasibility, administrative advantages, data requirements, etc. This original Options Paper was used as the basis for the deliberations of an HCFA task force, chaired by Thomas R. Burke.[38] The task force drew on the expertise of technicians within the HCFA. It was later expanded, in January 1982, to include representatives from the hospital industry and the health affairs constituency (Oday unpublished, 17). Aside from canvassing the issues, one purpose of this activity was to put the hospital industry on notice that significant changes were impending; and these stirrings within the Department were immediately noted in the trade journals. At the same time, the task force was instructed *not* to come forward with any specific recommendations, in order to forestall an early mobilization of opposition by the industry. Aside from the tactical astuteness of this decision, the memories of the bruising battles during the Carter hospital cost containment struggle were fresh in the minds of the HCFA administrators.

In addition to exploring alternatives, the Burke Task Force was useful because it reduced the number of options, some on grounds of practicality, others because of unacceptable policy implications. Capitation was an attractive methodology, for instance, but not viewed as technically feasible at that time. Expenditure caps with rate of increase limits might well have worked, but they were too similar to rejected Carter Administration proposals. Negotiated rates, that might have been the most effective cost containment device, were seen as interfering too directly with hospital management. Four of the seven options were rejected by the Burke committee, leaving three for further and more intensive consideration. These were competitive bidding, a TEFRA-like option, and "individual case rates," an approach similar to the eventual PPS. With a final recommendation that a number of fundamental issues required resolution, the Task Force was disbanded and further work referred to the Bureau of Program Policy (Oday unpublished, 6–20).

A notable historic fact is how little attention DRGs or "individual case rates" received at this stage of policy development. Thomas Burke, who chaired the Task Force, reports that he was aware of the work and advocacy of a group in ORDS. For his part, though, he favored a variant of competitive bidding and opposed DRGs as an "administered price system." Policy-makers within the HCFA, from Carolyne Davis on down, were also much of that mind, and either slow to appreciate the DRG conceptualism[39] or opposed to it as "too much like New Jersey."[40] In any event, DRGs were not viewed as a desirable alternative. Those who persisted in advocating them were derisively termed "DRG Weenies" one of whom recalls that DRGs did, in fact, barely survive as an option reported to the Secretary by the Burke Task Force.[41]

After the Task Force completed its work, emphasis shifted to a next phase, the development of a proposal for PPS. Patrice Feinstein, as Associate Administrator for Policy, was put in charge of the development group within the HCFA. She recalls a request from Secretary Schweiker, at this juncture, for a meeting with the senior staff of the HCFA in Baltimore.[42] For Schweiker, PPS had a high priority because health initiatives were faring badly at the moment and he had just suffered a symbolically important budget defeat on the childhood immunization program.[43] In a dramatic and effective gesture, he came alone to Baltimore and spent several hours with the HCFA staff and policy people, urging them to "get the job done for me."[44]

At the request of Secretary Schweiker, this phase was to be "closely held," kept confidential so as to prevent extensive interest group involvement at an early stage, a stratagem that, in his view, was essential if they were to move quickly and effectively toward an ultimate design. In Feinstein's opinion, this stricture also made sense, because at that juncture, "we didn't know what we were doing."

In the working pattern that developed, a very small group of people met together on a daily basis. Aside from Feinstein, the most important were Larry Oday, her deputy and the director of the Bureau of Program Policy; Michael Maher, the director of Provider Reimbursement; and, more occasionally, Carolyne Davis, the HCFA Administrator. This working group developed issue papers and decision memoranda that were sent up on a weekly basis to a committee chaired by Richard Schweiker and staffed by the Assistant Secretary for Planning and Evaluation,

Robert Rubin. Consultations with and briefings by technical people were frequently required, but confidentiality was maintained by using Maher as a liaison with the technicians and charging them not to report elsewhere the substance of their discussions.[45]

One of the first important steps of the working group was to develop a decision memo for Secretary Schweiker with respect to four major issues left for resolution by the Burke Task Force. On March 19, 1982, these options were discussed with the Secretary and on each of these he made clear his preference:

1. There should be no additional beneficiary liability under PPS.
2. PPS should provide incentives for outpatient modes of treatment.
3. Regional hospital costs, especially labor costs, would be recognized.
4. PPS should make an explicit adjustment for case-mix (Oday unpublished, 23–24).

This meeting was important for setting parameters. The last decision, opting for a case-mix adjustment, deserves a specific comment, for it drastically narrowed the number of choices and the range between them. Deciding to recognize a case-mix differential raises directly the question of what to use for a case-mix adjuster and how to use it. Peer group classification, for instance, by size, type, and location of hospital, would be one method. This kind of classification scheme had been used as part of the Sec. 223 methodology for setting routine cost limits for hospitals. It had also figured in some of the legislative proposals during the Carter hospital cost containment episode. Yet, lacking a precise case-mix adjustment, the peer group approach failed to get beyond the most basic routine costs, and especially were inadequate to capture the increasingly expensive "ancillaries." Here the DRGs could be used as a refinement, as contemplated in TEFRA and in an earlier HCFA option. They could also serve, directly, as a measure of payment for the individual discharge. However, the issue of a specific method of payment was not to be resolved for several months, at the very end of this initial phase of development.

Meanwhile, this small group worked away—daily, over weekends, at lunch—on the many issues entailed in a prospective payment system: some technical, others conceptually difficult; still others plumbing issues of fundamental principle. Items for decision included such matters as whether there should be urban–rural differentials, what provision to make for capital expenditures, adjustments for teaching hospitals and "disproportionate share" hospitals treating large numbers of indigent patients, what wage indexes to use, the role of the Medicare cost reports, whether there should be a transition or phase-in, and so forth.

Patrice Feinstein, with a gift for metaphor, said "it was like a mother telling her ten-year-old daughter to bake a cake": in other words, a messy learn-as-you-go process of devising means to ends and shaping ends to means, entailing uncertain steps, false starts, and uneven, uncertain progress.

During the early months of 1982, the trade journals were picking up on administration activities and the hospital industry was coming forward with some of its own proposals. In March of that year, several variants of prospective payment were endorsed by sectors of the industry, with especially strong support from the Federation of American Health Systems, the trade association of the for-profit hospitals.[46] With TEFRA and other administrative proposals known to be under consideration, it was a time for "coming to the table," i.e., for seeking agreement.

Then, early in May, occurred one of those decisive events in which one person seeking a solution met another person offering one. The American Hospital Association was holding its annual convention in Washington. In attendance was the newly appointed Washington representative, Jack W. Owen. Owen had been president of the New Jersey Hospital Association for some 17 years, during which time he had seen seven different systems of reimbursement. But among them was the current system of prospective reimbursement based on DRGs, and about this system, Owen was enthusiastic. Richard Schweiker, for his part, was interested in the New Jersey system as "something different," and also as a working model of prospective reimbursement. So, on Schweiker's invitation, the president of the American Hospital Association, Alexander MacMahon, paid a courtesy call accompanied by Jack Owen, during which they discussed, *inter alia*, the New Jersey approach with its DRG methodology.[47]

According to Schweiker, the experience was for him a remarkable one, bringing the recognition that the DRG methodology was the approach he "had been looking for." He liked especially the idea of setting a case-mix adjusted price. For such a price would leave the hospital free to manage within these limits and provide, as well, incentives for efficiency and for shifting treatment to outpatient sites. At the same time, with a case-mix adjuster, the price could be set at a "fair" level so that the hospital would have neither the incentive to nor justification for skimming off the most profitable patients or "dumping" the money losers. Later investigation on Schweiker's part revealed to him that the "Yale studies" and the HCFA data base were both "farther along," i.e., more fully developed, than he had expected. So, to his mind, a PPS based on DRGs was both an attractive and a feasible alternative. At the time of this historic meeting, Schweiker recalls, the fact that this approach would apparently be acceptable to the largest hospital association, the biggest of the big three, was not lost to him.[48]

Schweiker shared some of his enthusiasm with the PPS working groups and with a few acquaintances in Congress. Carolyne Davis recalls that he showed her a book about the New Jersey system with suggestions that this alternative be given weighty consideration, and that he asked so many questions that she and Patrice Feinstein made several trips to New Jersey to learn about the system.[49] At this time, he refrained from more specific directions, wishing to see what the HCFA would develop.[50]

For the HCFA working group, price-setting by DRGs had never been the preferred alternative. One reason was that this method was viewed as too regulative, especially if it were to be closely modeled on the New Jersey system. An addition concern was that the industry would see the approach as too revolutionary. And some were frank to confess that they did not fully understand the methodology and had doubts about the capacity of the HCFA to implement it.[51]

The preferred option within the HCFA—at least among those privy to the decision process—was to set a flat rate per discharge, using DRGs only to establish total cost limits for individual hospitals. The flat rate per discharge would be based on the individual hospital's historic cost experience trended forward in a way that accounted for inflation. But upper and lower limits on total payments per hospital would be set using a case-mix adjuster employing DRGs. This approach resembled TEFRA as then being developed in Congress. It also shared some features with a proposal advanced by the American Hospital Association. For its proponents, it had a particular advantage of being highly "prospective," i.e., letting hospitals know in advance what reimbursement they could expect to receive. Also, it was minimally "regulative." It did not entail medical audits and would reduce reporting requirements. This was an approach, furthermore, that would be easy to develop. In fact, the HCFA had already prepared a draft regulation.

Events were now moving rapidly, and by early Summer of 1982, a version of TEFRA had reached the Secretary's desk. On July 21, 1982, the HCFA working group met with Schweiker to discuss the all-important issue of the payment mechanism to be used for the proposed system. By then, the choice had narrowed to two options: one, the flat payment approach mentioned; and a second that would employ DRGs as the price setting device for individual discharges. At the meeting, there was much discussion of the two, airing the pros and cons of each. Toward the end of the meeting, a consensus seemed to be converging on the flat payment alternative preferred by the HCFA. At this juncture, Schweiker canvassed the opinions of those present, all of whom expressed a preference for this alternative, including Schweiker's own Assistant Secretary for Planning and Evaluation, Robert Rubin.[52] This outcome would have settled the matter, except that Schweiker said that he preferred the DRG approach and would like the members of the group to go back to work and see what they could do to develop a PPS methodology based on DRGs. And his was the vote that counted.

In recalling the meeting, Richard Schweiker said that this was the only time in his political career that he made such a "Lincoln decision." He had not been more directive, earlier, because he wanted to see "what they could come up with." But he was "flabbergasted" at their final recommendation. People knew about his meeting with Jack Owen, and he had certainly imparted the message that he was "intrigued with DRGs." He was surprised that they had not taken these indications or messages to heart. For him, the flat rate approach was clearly unacceptable, for at least two major reasons. The first was that it would encourage hospitals to "skim off" the healthier patients and avoid the sicker ones. The second was that it offered hospitals little incentive to change their technology or manage more efficiently. These were matters of prime concern to him, and a large part of the reason he wanted a prospective payment system.[53]

There remained a number of important, even pivotal, decisions to be made by these two working groups. But once having decided to employ the newly developed DRGs as the pricing mechanism, the important issue was *how* to make them the vehicle for achieving or expressing policy objectives such as deregulation or management efficiency on the one hand without sacrificing equity or cost control on the other. In this respect, the HCFA group took a strong line, urging that the prospective features of the system be enhanced. Especially they argued, and successfully, that the old cost–reimbursement philosophy should be reduced to a minimum: that DRG rates be treated as a price and hospitals allowed to keep any margins; that "outlier" payments, which would reimburse hospitals for especially severe or long-term cases, be reduced to a minimum; that rates be national, with no urban–rural or regional differentials; and that the system be implemented immediately, without a transition period.

This was strong medicine for the hospital industry, accustomed to pass-throughs, bail-outs, and hold-harmless clauses. It implied capitalism and Social Darwinism, large profits for some hospitals and bankruptcy for others. This was a prescription that some within the industry approved and others abhorred. It proved, ultimately, too rigorously consistent and draconian for the Congress. But it certainly had the merit of proposing something new and radically different. In retrospect, and given the legislation that emerged from Congress and the way in which it was subsequently implemented, PPS may have survived as well as it did because of the rigorous line taken at this point.

After the July meeting, Schweiker moved quickly to commit the Department and to commit it to a tightly constrained time limit. Through the Senate Finance Committee's Health Subcommittee, he and Thomas Donnelly, then the Assistant Secretary for Legislation, got included in the impending TEFRA legislation a section mandating the development "in consultation with the Senate Committee on Finance and the Committee on Ways and Means of the House of Representatives" of proposals for the "prospective reimbursement of hospitals, skilled nursing facilities, and, to the extent feasible, other providers."[54] Significantly, the Secretary was directed to submit his report not later than December 31, 1982, a clear indication that key figures within Congress were aware of developments within the DHHS. In August, Schweiker also held a press conference announcing progress in this area and saying that PPS could be implemented, that is, fully developed and paying bills by September 1, 1983.

Since the date announced by Secretary Schweiker was less than 13 months away, he was setting an ambitious agenda. He acknowledged as much, but said that he hoped that the challenge of the task would elicit exceptional effort. Also decisive for Schweiker in this venture was his own favorable view of the "Yale study" and the data base already developed within the HCFA.[55] Nevertheless, it was a vast and daunting undertaking. Here, in bare outline, is a list of the major tasks to be accomplished over the ensuing year:

1. Writing and approving the Secretary's Report to Congress.
2. Drafting the Department's legislative proposal to Congress.
3. Negotiating with the White House, EOMB, and the Congress over passage of the legislation.
4. Evaluating and accommodating to the legislative changes.
5. Assembling the actuarial and other data necessary for PPS calculations. Auditing the hospital cost reports; cleaning up data files.
6. Developing a strategy for and writing the regulations to implement PPS; also regulations for the exempt hospitals; for certain inpatient physician services, etc.
7. Developing operational procedures, data, and computer capabilities to pay hospitals using the PPS methodology.

8. Developing strategy and procedures for monitoring hospital response to PPS (ways to monitor both utilization and quality of care).
9. Holding meetings with the FIs, PROs, hospitals, and provider representatives to explain the new system.
10. Publication of rules for notice and comment; clearing the final rules with amendments.

This list outlines, in barest terms, something of the scope of the task. What it fails to impart is the issues of policy yet to be resolved, the amount of task coordination, the intricacy of detail, and the sheer enormity of putting in place an entirely new payment system. What it also does not convey is the working reality of a busy agency that, in this case, had to create, in addition to PPS, a whole alternate system of payments for the TEFRA hospitals, involving 17 sets of regulations with all their operational implications. It was, furthermore, an agency that had never been unified or enjoyed a stable, continuous leadership, that was smarting from reductions in force (RIFs) and personnel freezes, and riven by mutual suspicions between career civil servants and Reaganite political appointees. Moreover, it had never undertaken a task of this scope.

In October 1982, Carolyne Davis announced to the HCFA staff the plans, until then still highly confidential, for developing and implementing PPS by October 1983. Understandably, reactions varied. Some welcomed the challenge and the new policy initiative. Others felt differently: for instance, reimbursement specialists accustomed to one system and routine, and program policy people who saw the enormity of the task involved. A common response was "that's impossible—we can't do that."[56] It was a bold venture, and the outcome was by no means assured, even late in the process of development.

The most immediate task was to draft the Secretary's Report to Congress. Since the Report was due for delivery in December of that year, and one month had to be allowed for clearances, that meant that it had to be written by the end of November. Development of the Report was assigned to ORD, and particularly to the new head of research, Allen Dobson. It was, at the same time a group effort, incorporating policy decisions up to that point and the review and comment by the HCFA working group and the Schweiker committee, especially Robert Rubin and his staff. Containing over 100 pages of closely reasoned text, the Report is remarkable for its technical sophistication and clarity as well as for its careful explanation of theoretical difficulties and data limitations. A reading of it evokes speculation about how so much could have been brought together so quickly. About this point, the Report is appropriately silent. There is only the brief acknowledgment:

This report is the direct result of several months work and analysis but draws heavily from nearly a decade of research and demonstrations by the Health Care Financing Administration (HCFA) as well as other components of the Department of Health and Human Services. The Department has also benefitted by discussions with health care industry representatives as well as Congressional staff involved in health care. (U.S. Department of Health and Human Services 1982, 1)

True enough. But how much would need to be read between these lines to explain why and how the process had been brought successfully to this point!

Drafting of the legislative language for a bill to be introduced in January had already begun, in October 1982, within the Legislative Division of the Office of General Counsel at the departmental level. This proposed legislation, only a few pages in length, closely followed the policy recommendations already reached. Its introduction into Congress was to be Richard Schweiker's last major act as Secretary.

V. LEGISLATING THE PROSPECTIVE PAYMENT SYSTEM

The legislative progression for this proposal was extraordinarily rapid for a topic as controversial as PPS, taking less than six weeks from the first Ways and Means subcommittee hearings on February 14 to the final conference report on March 23. At the same time, the resulting legislation was complex, including a number of arcane formulas, special provisos, and exceptions. It is important not to lose sight of the major theme in these developments. Simply put, almost everyone in Congress wanted a prospective payment system, but each wanted one that would not impact too severely on their state, district, or favorite hospital. Consequently, the DHSS proposal was extensively and minutely amended, so much so that some believe that a substantially different system of reimbursement was created: *ad hoc* price regulation by Congress and Commission rather than a prospective system. Whether this assessment is correct or may prove to be increasingly true to reality as PPS unfolds over time, the legislative process did reveal a systematic and persistent difference of priorities between the Administration, especially as represented by the HCFA, that wished to emphasize prospectivity and incentives for management efficiency and the Congress, more concerned with equity, fairness, and hospital margins. The difference is hardly a surprising one; but it is important both for making sense of the legislative process and for understanding many subsequent developments in the implementation of PPS.

Some of the developments most important for ultimate legislative success took place either in advance of or outside the legislative process itself. One such development was the close relationship established between Congress and the DHSS. For an item, TEFRA not only blessed this good work in advance, it directed "the Secretary," i.e., Schweiker and the Department, to work closely with Congress in developing the proposal. Schweiker, for his part, took great personal interest in PPS and spent much of his remaining time as Secretary in breakfasts and on the Hill, lobbying old acquaintances. One good feature of PPS, he recalled, was its dual aspect: it could be defended as hospital regulation among Democrats and as pro-competition when talking to Republicans.[57] In addition to the Secretary himself, Rubin and his staff, Davis and Feinstein, and a number of HCFA technicians including Maher, Dobson, and Pettingill worked actively and closely with the Congress and its committee staffs.

After the Department went public with its plan for PPS in August 1982, the HCFA and other Department officials began increasingly to include industry representatives, holding meetings with hospital delegations, fiscal intermediaries, and trade associations to explain PPS and solicit views. This advance work was valuable. As one consequence, influential association representatives such as Michael Bromberg of the Federation of American Hospitals[58] and Jack Owen of the American Hospital Association could reassure their constituencies, thus diminishing some of the alarm and potential controversy over the proposed legislation. Also, the industry groups, accepting the reality that some form of prospective payment system was inevitable and even desirable, could argue knowledgeably for the technically best solution, which greatly facilitated the discovery of common ground as between legislators, the administration, and the industry.

One of the most important features of PPS had a curious, extra-legislative history. This is the constraint of "budget neutrality," with its additional implied proviso of a limit on the size of the dollar pool from which incremental adjustments in hospital reimbursement are made. Within the HCFA, there was strong support for the idea that PPS should be budget neutral with respect to TEFRA: entail, at least initially, no more total outlays than TEFRA. Equally important, especially with their concern about prospectivity, was the other side of the proviso: hospitals should get *no less* than the budget-neutral figure, i.e., they should be allowed to keep their profits (Oday unpublished, 58ff). There was also recognition of the idea—indeed, strong support for it—that the payment methodology would then be "zero-sum," that is, additional compensation for one hospital, say, in the form of an adjustment for case-mix or technology advances would at the same time reduce the standardized amount for all.

What one hospital got was still an "add-on" for it; but it also subtracted from the common pool. No longer could there be an easy assumption of more for all, as in the past. Each hospital was potentially a competitor with its neighbor for a share of the aggregate amount. Therefore, each had a strong interest in a fair decision-rule. These were potent ideas, even revolutionary, as the HCFA working group realized. For this reason, this part of the Secretary's Report was deliberately left obscure.

"Budget neutrality" was not a term in currency within Congress at that time and, strictly speaking, PPS is not "budget neutral" even though it has come to be very much governed by deficit reduction constraints since 1986. But PPS was made "budget neutral" with respect to the first two years of TEFRA: that is, outlays should be *no more* than they would have been under TEFRA. This provision came about through a "deal" concluded by Stockman, Schweiker, Pepper, Foley, and others while bargaining over budget reconciliation. Deficit reduction was serious business in 1982, and the bargaining was intense. Toward the end, 5% reduction in hospital outlays was still needed to reach a target amount; but the venerable and doughty Claude Pepper (D., Fla.) balked at taking any more Medicare savings from Part A. So, the group concluded, specifically with respect to the upcoming legislation, that the 5% could be gotten by assuming the enactment of PPS and making it "budget neutral" with respect to TEFRA, at least for two years.[59] PPS did not remain budget neutral, to be sure, but this language became part of the legislation, and budget neutrality is often thought to be an ideal, to be sought as far as possible, within constraints of reason and equity. Moreover, the "zero-sum" aspect of PPS *is* both a fact and an ideal, with enormous practical consequence, both in constraining ProPAC and in dividing the hospital community as a political constituency.

A major obstacle faced by PPS was EOMB clearance, not only because DRGs were viewed as regulative, but because of fears that they might well prove inflationary. David Stockman knew rather little about this specific area, but he and others shared a view that more dollars could probably be saved with TEFRA.[60] The provision for budget neutrality with respect to TEFRA helped the case, but doubts remained within EOMB because the DRG methodology was relatively new and unproven.[61] Here, Schweiker along with Rubin and his staff were able to intervene at a high level, going to the White House to argue for PPS. They were also able to prevail on Martin Feldstein, then Chairman of the Council of Economic Advisors and a highly respected economist, expert in hospital finance, to adopt a stance of "benevolent neglect"[62] and even of indulgence. Feldstein's acquiescence helped, in turn, to gain acceptance by Stockman.

The most important pre-legislative development was the decision within the House Ways and Means Committee to incorporate PPS into the Social Security Amendments of 1983. Including Medicare amendments with other Social Security legislation was not new, but "fast-tracking" legislation in this fashion was not an ordinary occurrence in 1982. It was important for the fate of this bill, though, since there were many technical and controversial provisions in the proposal and PPS might well have gotten stalled in committee, on the floor, or in conference. Making it part of the Social Security Amendments did much to ensure its passage, since millions of social security beneficiary checks depended on this bill. According to Schweiker, he was called by Daniel Rostenkowski, Chairman of the House Ways and Means Committee and an old friend, to ask if he objected to including PPS as a title in the Social Security Amendments. Schweiker was quite pleased and assented with alacrity. But he left office within a matter of days, so that subsequent negotiations had to be conducted through Tom Donnelly, then the Acting Secretary, and Robert Rubin, the Assistant Secretary for Planning and Evaluation. According to John Salmon, Counsel for Ways and Means, he asked Rubin how quickly the Administration could move on the bill:

> Rubin responded, "In six weeks." At this point, Salmon said, "How about eleven days?" and then explained to him the merits of "one of the greatest legislative engines we'll ever see—the Social Security bill." (Iglehart 1983, p. 1430)

And so, PPS was added to the Social Security Amendments. Nevertheless, it was put in as Title VI, the last major part of the bill, so that it could be quickly jettisoned should its contentious features endanger the passage of the rest of the bill. The Senate, with its more flexible and generally speedier procedures, had no need of such a provision, and the Majority Leader, Senator Robert Dole (R., Kans.), initially opposed this inclusion, but others saw its advantageous features and prevailed.[63]

Early in February 1983, brief introductory hearings were held in both the House and Senate, partly as a courtesy to the departing Secretary Schweiker who appeared to explain and discuss the proposal. These were followed on February 24 by a first mark-up session in the Health Subcommittee of Ways and Means in which several important amendments were adopted, an interesting exercise in itself, illustrative of the speed with which Congress intended to move, since the Administration proposal was not formally sent to Congress until several days later. Rather like the fabled Cheshire cat of *Alice in Wonderland*, that disappeared leaving a grin behind, here were amendments that came into being without a bill present on which to act (Oday unpublished, 63).

When the Administration bill did appear, it produced some consternation in both the House and Senate. It was but a few pages in length, and without any provisions for a transition, for regional and other variations, exemptions, and provisos, all dear to the hearts of legislators. Among the milder appraisals was "wholly unacceptable" in its present form.[64] Others were more forthright, denouncing it as a "technician's dream" and saying that the HCFA bureaucrats must be "nuts."[65] HCFA officials said, later, that the Administration version was spare and rigorous by design. Part of the strategy was to keep it simple and clean with the hope that after Congress had added the "bells and whistles," i.e., amended it, the essential features and underlying structure of incentives would survive. However that may be, Congress set about with a will to make a series of major amendments.

One of the first changes in the Administration draft was to provide for two separate DRG rates, one for urban and the other for rural hospitals. There was little controversy about this change, either in the House or the Senate, since preliminary impact studies made clear the huge differences in actual payments that would result from one national system of DRG rates and how dollars would move from region to region.[66] This change was adopted initially in the first House mark-up session. It was also adopted, independently, by the Senate Finance Committee on March 10, one day after passage of the House version of PPS. There was no serious controversy about this provision, since the impact studies, even scanty as they were at that point,[67] largely concluded the issue. But it was an important step, especially for the future of PPS, since it institutionalized a bicameral division of interest with respect to future legislation, as between the House as sponsor of urban, core-city hospitals and the Senate as the champion of rural ones. Indeed, within the Senate, among the "bells and whistles" soon added, largely at the behest of Senator Baucus (D., Mont.), were amendments dealing with sole community hospitals and regional referral centers.[68]

A next step was to regionalize the DRGs, a move that resulted from complicated negotiations prior to the mark-up by the full Ways and Means Committee. The Administration draft provided for a wage adjustment, using the SMSA[69] as a base for calculation—this in recognition of the fact that hospital wages varied considerably and were largely beyond the control of hospital administrators. Congress added an urban–rural differential. But an early CBO study of DRG impact showed that within the nine census divisions of the United States, many individual hospitals would still gain or lose substantially, even with the urban–rural differential. Catholic hospitals, especially, appeared to fare badly and their representatives[70] lobbied hard on this issue, using the CBO figures and one-page impact study. It was equally clear that a number of teaching and disproportionate share hospitals would suffer under the national rates. Consequently, in the Ways and Means mark-up session, the Committee adopted a provision for nine different regional rates, in addition to the urban–rural differential, so that now the legislation would establish 18 regional rates, an urban and rural one for each of nine census regions. A later Senate version had only four regions, but the Conference Committee accepted the House proposal for nine regions.

At this stage, the House also made provision for the transition from hospital specific to national rates. The Administration version made no provision for a transition and some hospitals, especially the for-profit ones, actually preferred this alternative.[71] But transitions are customary with such legislation and definitely the normal expectation for the Congress. Indeed, this feature of the Administration draft was received with disbelief and comments such as "surely, they're joking!"[72] The only real issue for Congress was what kind of transition to create. One of the earliest moves within the House, accordingly, was to establish a transition from the historic, cost-based rates for each hospital to national ones: at first, allowing a one year phase-in, later, adopting three years. The transition feature was added to regions so that rates for an individual hospital would be a changing blend of hospital specific, regional, and national, with the national rates expected to be fully in force at the end of three years.

One matter dealt with by the House in a curious fashion was the "indirect" medical education (IME) allowance. Teaching hospitals, because of their use of residents and academic physicians, have a number of additional expenses that enhance patient care, but are difficult to track or assign appropriately for billing purposes. Over the years, an elegant formula had been developed, essentially a ratio of residents to hospital beds. This formula was agreeable to the teaching hospitals and had been accepted by the HCFA as a basis for reimbursement. It was also incorporated into the TEFRA legislation. But it had now to be factored into PPS with its own specific per-discharge payment. The existing indirect teaching adjustment produced a number, but both CBO and HCFA impact studies showed that with it, the teaching hospitals would fare badly. So, there was general agreement that the teaching allowance had to be increased by some ratio, but no consensus on what that ratio should be. HCFA studies suggested a figure of "1 and ½," but Ways and Means thought "1 and ½" risky because it was more difficult to argue persuasively, and so proposed a flat doubling, i.e., rounding to "2." CBO numbers seemed to support this conclusion.[73] And the HCFA went along, believing that this ratio would at least give the teaching hospitals the kind of benefit of the doubt that others were receiving. So, the teaching adjustment was doubled, the Senate concurring, thereby conferring on the teaching hospitals what proved to be a substantial windfall, built into the system, that continues to vex policy debates to this day.

Particularly sharp differences between the administration and the Ways and Means Committee developed over the issue of the "outlier" pool, i.e., how much of the total amount of dollars should be set aside for "outliers"—cases that entailed especially lengthy hospital stays or much higher costs than the norm. This issue brought to the fore some philosophical differences between the HCFA and Congress, with the former arguing for a bare minimum of 1 or 2% outlier payments and Congress just as insistently demanding 5 or 6%. The theoretical nub of this issue for the HCFA was that hospitals ought to learn to manage efficiently and, if they did not, they ought to absorb the losses. For Congress, what was at stake was equity and access. Hospitals ought not to be punished for treating "outliers," by definition cases beyond the statistical norm. Nor should they have compelling incentives to select against such outliers or to "dump" them on neighboring hospital steps. Accordingly, possessed of this philosophy, Ways and Means wrote into the law a proviso that not less than 4% of the pool should be allotted to outliers. This figure was later raised to 5% by the Senate.

By and large, the administration was opposed to exempting hospitals or making special allowances for specific categories. Here, too, Congress thought differently. Ways and Means agreed to the HCFA's minimal list of exempt categories: cancer, psychiatric, pediatric, and rehabilitation. But, contrary to the HCFA's desires, Congress both extended and liberalized the authority for granting "waivers" to states such as New York, New Jersey, Massachusetts, and Maryland, engaged in hospital reimbursement experiments. The Committee also continued provisions, long built into Medicare reimbursement, that provided specific consideration for "sole community" hospitals, and for those serving a "disproportionate share" of low income and Medicare beneficiaries.

There were a number of additional amendments adopted by the House, but these were the major ones. Aside from transforming the administration proposal quickly and effectively into a bill that was tolerable and even generous, the House amendments are interesting because of the way in which they tended to be shaped and justified. PPS was, to say the least, a novel approach and one imperfectly understood, especially within Congress. A natural way to approach such a relatively unknown proposal was to ask how it would play out, that is, to see where and to whom the payments would go and who would be advantaged or disadvantaged. But that approach tended to shift attention from the system as a whole—either its putative merits such as cost containment or incentives for efficency, or its procedural requisites such as consistency—to the voiced complaints and statistical evidences of regional inequities and hurts suffered by individual hospitals. This was precisely what the HCFA administrators had wished to avoid. Such an approach could well produce a system of hospital payment that *neither* encouraged efficiency *nor* ensured cost control.

Although the Senate began committee hearings on PPS as early as February 2, 1983, the Finance Committee did not hold a markup session until March 10. As a consequence, the Senate made fewer important substantive changes than the House. The Senate did, however, contribute several amendments dealing with procedural aspects of PPS that were of theoretical import and practical effect.

One topic of concern, both within the House and Senate, was data on impact, especially by region and type of hospital. The HCFA was slow to respond and chary of providing the data—so much so that both House and Senate had to rely for much of their discussion on sparse and hastily assembled tables supplied by CBO. This lack of responsiveness on the part of the HCFA resulted, in part, from genuine doubts about the reliability of some of their data, given that much of it was based on the comparatively new 20% MEDPAR sample.[74] But another reason was, quite simply, a reluctance to give Congress information that, from the HCFA's perspective, could be used to the detriment of the grand design. Carolyne Davis, for instance, was asked by the House Ways and Means Committee for hospital specific data by Congressional district. "I asked myself," said she, "why do they want that?" Accordingly, she instructed her already busy staff *not* to give that one high priority. The insistency on the part of Congress increased. At one point, Andy Jacobs (D., Ind.) of Ways and Means threatened to take PPS off the "fast track" if more data were not forthcoming. Robert Hoyer, then of the Senate Finance staff, recalls requesting data from HCFA representatives at any and every occasion on which they appeared before the Committee, though largely to no avail. They finally got data on outliers, but little else.

A general concern about responsiveness of the HCFA, especially as exemplified in the tug-of-war over impact data, was one important element in leading the Senate Finance Committee to add to the bill a provision creating an independent body, the Prospective Payment Assessment Commission, to advise the Secretary and the Congress on how to "update" PPS. One feature of PPS that the HCFA had not dealt with in detail was the issue of how the payment system would be amended, year by year, to add new DRGs, change the rates, take account of annual hospital cost inflation, and make recommendations on a number of unresolved or newly developing issues. The administration bill provided for an advisory panel, appointed by the Secretary. The Secretary could then do as he or she saw fit about these recommendations. This arrangement satisfied neither the House nor the Senate. Another worry, occasioned by the spareness and procrustean spirit of the administration bill, was the vast discretion it would give to the Secretary, with the prospect that PPS might be administered in that same procrustean spirit. This fear was strengthened and given substance by the HCFA's lack of response to requests for data, especially impact data. It happened that Bob Hoyer of the Senate Finance staff had developed a 24-page proposal for just such a commission, a pet project of his for some time.[75] This was adopted as one of the Senate amendments, fortunately in a shortened version, establishing a 15-member commission to advise the Secretary and the Congress.

A question that had until now received little attention was how PPS would affect quality of care. This was a remarkable omission since PPS was intended to change hospital incentives drastically. Practices such as selecting against sicker patients and transferring or dumping especially costly ones would seem to be expected behavior. But within the HCFA, the policy emphasis was on cost saving and, necessarily, much attention was absorbed in details. Quality of care tended to be pushed back in the agenda, with the thought that the PROs could take care of it, but without specific provisions being made for quality assurance. Some advocacy groups, such as the American Association of Retired Persons (AARP), and some committees, such as those on Aging in both House and Senate, expressed concern about the issue. Ways and Means considered the issue and provided an amendment of its own. But peer review and the PROs had long been a concern of the Senate. As part of TEFRA, Senator Durenberger (R., Minn.) had gotten included the Peer Review Improvement Act, extensively revising and extending peer review. This legislation was given further effect by requiring all PPS hospitals to contract with PROs for review of utilization and quality of care and providing in some detail for monitoring of their activities by the PROs.

Finally, there were several "pass-throughs" to deal with: i.e., items that would be reimbursed on a cost basis rather than factored into the DRGs. So-called "direct medical education" costs was one of these: costs for classrooms and teaching. Others were capital expenditures, return on equity (RoE),[76] and Medicare bad debt (Oday unpublished, 36ff). By and large, the HCFA knew a quagmire when it saw one, and had opted to pass these costs through for the time being, since they lacked an adequate methodology to include them in the DRG rates. The House tinkered with the capital issue and also adopted a provision on RoE. The Senate, perhaps wisely, chose an approach to capital that has since become common: a pass-through with a mandate to the Secretary to report back to Congress in 18 months with a proposal. A number of other mandated studies were also in the bill as passed: the impact of DRGs, the feasibility of physician DRGs, outliers and severity-of-illness indexes, the urban–rural differential, sole community and disproportionate share hospitals, rural teaching hospitals, and more. Without fully realizing the implication of all these mandated studies, Congress was moving incrementally toward a new form of policy-making, involving a new relationship between the executive and legislative branches.

A brief, but dramatic episode occurred near the end of the Senate mark-up when Senator Russell Long began to express reservations about the legislation and a desire for "further study." According to one account, he had been reached by John B. Connolly on behalf of Methodist Hospital in Houston.[77] However that may be, Long was both popular with members of the Finance Committee and much respected for his knowledge of health affairs, even though no longer chairman and now in the minority. Realizing that time was of the essence, since PPS could easily be severed from the Social Security Amendments, an AHA lobbyist passed an urgent note to Senator Durenberger, the Committee sponsor of the bill. Durenberger asked Russell Long how much time was needed. According to one observer, "You could have heard a pin drop. If he said 'two days', this thing was going South. But then he said 'two months' and that blew it."[78] The Committee voted for immediate passage and PPS cleared. Had it come off the "fast track," many believe there would have been no PPS, at least not for that session.

The Senate Finance Committee began and concluded its mark-up on March 10. PPS was briefly debated on four different occasions on the floor, eventually passing the Senate on March 23. The Conference Report made only minor amendments. As a final illustration of the speed with which this legislation moved, the House–Senate Conference was assembled and completed its work within 12 hours after Senate action. On March 24, PPS was passed in both houses. It was signed into law by President Reagan on April 20. Not only was this close to a record for speed, but one of the most important single laws dealing with health care since the passage of Medicare in 1965, with the possible exception of the Social Security Amendments of 1972, passed both houses of Congress with the most perfunctory of hearings and virtually *no* debate. Perhaps it could have only been passed in this way. But the implications of these statements for democratic government are not reassuring.

VI. INITIAL IMPLEMENTATION

A few weeks after the President signed PPS into law, Carolyne Davis held a party in her office to celebrate their success. At the party, she and

Patrice Feinstein were presented with a plaque memorializing their completion of this

> adjusted, averaged, standardized, regionalized, budget-neutralized, blended, recalibrated, back-it-out-the-base, unbundled, hold the Mayo, hula-hoop, dog-sled, and pass-through capital during transition and study everything else prospective payment act of 1983 (a simplified version). (Oday unpublished, 80–81)

Laurels were in order, for the passage of PPS was a great achievement. But there was no respite, for within five months after passage of this legislation final regulations had to be written and ready for comment and within six months the fiscal intermediaries must start paying bills. That was a logistical and technical feat similar in proportion to the task already completed.

Those who lived through that five months of maximum effort say that they were hectic but thrilling. Specifications of the new system existed, but could it be built? and would it perform? Even more, could the HCFA, shaken by the Reagan Administration and considerably reduced in staff, that had never as an organization done anything of this scope, accomplish this monumental task and do it in five months? Richard Schweiker had considered it a calculated risk. So did the HCFA leadership. Patrice Feinstein recalls that until very late they doubted they could pull it off. People had to believe that it could be done, to go forward, and trust colleagues to provide the necessary support. For the first and perhaps the only time in its history, the HCFA confronted a huge and possibly overwhelming challenge. But its members were well led, they pulled together, and they did their best, and that proved to be enough.

Central for translating the new statute into operative language were the hundreds of pages of regulations that would prescribe and explain how PPS would work and what changes it would entail for particular hospitals. This job entailed not just one set of regulations, but rules for the various categories of exempt hospitals and a number of subsidiary regulations on aspects of Medicare reimbursement affected by PPS. Important, of course, was that there was to be a prospective payment *system*, such that definitions, resource use, payment methodology, and overall monetary amounts all related with precision. This meant, in practice, an enormously complex job of relating numbers and devising precise language to implement a coordinated set of policy objectives. Policy analysts, regulations writers, and data specialists had, for their part, to get their work done on time and coordinate it with that of others. They had to understand how the system as a whole would articulate and be able to explain to their chiefs the significance of choosing one alternative over another. Busy policy people had to be able to delegate many decisions to the regulatory technicians within BERC with confidence that their priorities and policy choices would be faithfully expressed in the regulations. Here, both Oday and Maher, who had participated in developing the original proposal, were enormously important in seeing to it that the underlying policy of PPS was not lost in the vagaries and myriad incremental decisions involved in the crafting of regulations.[79] Yet as Patrice Feinstein recalled, often policy people simply did not know and trusted the technicians to decide.[80] The scope of the work was so enormous that it could only be done with a maximum of cooperation, trust, and good faith.

Regulations could not be written without data. This was an interdependent system in which the parts related and summed and in which wage and case-mix indexes, urban–rural differentials and regional rates, and outlier thresholds all had to be computed with data extracted from various files. As this was being done the Bureau of Program Operations (BPO) audited the individual hospital reports so that the pass-throughs and the hospital specific portion of the rates could be computed. Perforce, these processes went on simultaneously: as BERC wrote the regulations, the Bureau of Data Management and Strategy cleaned data files and spun the computer tapes to supply the numbers, while the BPO began the huge and laborious task of auditing thousands of individual hospital cost reports to establish individual base year figures. One observer invoked the image of an inverted pyramid because at times the whole operation seemed to depend on the files and the canny knack of a few data experts. But it was more like a team assault on an objective, in which success depends on the common understanding of the objective and skilled improvisation as to means.

Before any regulations or numbers could be made final, there was the intellectual headache of determining what set of assumptions would make PPS "budget neutral" with respect to a hypothetical first two years of TEFRA: a bit like calculating the path needed to hit a spot on the far side of the moon two years from date. These calculations waited on the Chief Actuary Roland (Guy) King and his medicare actuaries, statisticians, and economists who had, for their part, not only to make a number of accurate assumptions about mortality and morbidity, the state of the economy, technical developments in the health industry, and behavioral changes induced by PPS and TEFRA, but to compute the cost implications of operating under both. Moreover, the Actuary could not proceed until policy decisions had been locked up, while decisions about implementation depended in turn on the Actuary's figures. It was an operation requiring coordination and precision and yet haste and adaptiveness: almost a contradiction in terms, like improvising a minuet.

As early as April 1983, the Bureau of Program Operations began notifying the fiscal intermediaries and contractors and explaining the new system to them. Fortunately, some of their work could proceed in stages. Audits began in May, along with instructions for the hospitals on determining base year costs that would provide a foundation for calculating the per discharge payments (Oday unpublished, 104). But much of their work could not be completed until late. BPO writes the instructions and manuals for the fiscal intermediaries who, in turn, pay the hospitals. These instructions must be precise. Therefore, to put them in final form, the BPO technicians had to wait on the results of audits, final data determinations, and the outcome of decisions still being made by Congress, EOMB, and BERC. Then, BPO had to develop its own final instructions and manuals and communicate and explain the contents to the fiscal intermediaries. In the words of one participant, "Somehow it all got accomplished" (Oday unpublished, 105).

During the Spring and Summer of 1983, two systems of computer software were put in final form for use by the intermediaries in paying the hospitals: Grouper and Pricer. This development illustrates both a problem with the implementation of PPS and a solution to the problem. To be credible, PPS had to pay hospitals accurately according to formula. PPS was both novel and mysterious, and inexplicable variations or high rates of error in payment could prevent its acceptance. Yet the payment system depended on sorting by diagnosis with many opportunities for subjective and varying interpretations by physicians, record clerks, fiscal intermediaries, and so forth. The elegant solution to the problem was to develop an elaborate and sophisticated system of computer software to assign DRG classifications to the discharge abstracts submitted as a basis for payment. The Grouper system had to be put into final form quickly, but work on it had begun as early as 1979, led by some DRG enthusiasts within the HCFA, especially Julian Pettingill, James Vertrees, Rose Connerton, and John Nice. The HCFA administration had also let a contract to support work by Health Systems International and the Yale group on such a system.[81] When the legislation passed, the HCFA "went live" with the system and put the software in final form. Having this sophisticated system in place made the development of an additional Pricer program comparatively simple. This was completed over the Summer of 1983 and offered as an additional module to the FIs, who accepted it with enthusiasm. A final point is that the development of these two computer systems makes clear both the importance of time and sequence constraints in implementing PPS as well as the need for clarity and precision in the underlying concepts.[82]

Carolyne Davis and the policy leadership of the HCFA had, throughout, an important job, or array of tasks. Many difficult policy decisions had to be made along the way, difficult because their implications were hard to discern without other system components in place. There was a further task of explaining and defending their decisions, and the impact they would have on providers and beneficiaries, to other groups within the Department, especially ASPE, to EOMB, and to the Congress, all of whom sought to take a hand in shaping the final product. Davis, Feinstein, and others within the HCFA, spent many hours and days explaining PPS and how it would work, scotching rumors, and reassuring the Congress, FIs, and hospital representatives that the system would work as predicted and would work equitably.[83]

Those closely involved in the implementation of PPS give much credit to Carolyne Davis for her determination, singleness of purpose, and inspiriting role. In the mangled metaphor of one observer, "That time, Carolyne was really captain of the ship and everyone marched to her tune."[84] Many spoke of how the various offices and bureaus had worked together and struggled toward the common objective. They said that it was the Administration's "finest hour" and they had accomplished more than they believed possible. Probably, that appreciation speaks both to a quality of leadership and, as well, to a latent potential within the organization never fully exploited before.

There were surprisingly few big mistakes or omissions, especially considering the size of the task and the haste with which it had to be accomplished. In retrospect, HCFA officials recognized that they concentrated so intensely on possibilities for "gaming" the system through increased admissions and abuses of coding that they largely ignored the danger of premature discharges—the so-called "sicker and quicker" issue. Here, two observations. One is that "sicker and quicker" failed to become much of a problem. There were some true horror stories, but not a large number of instances. Second, as for "gaming," the Actuary told the HCFA that it was unlikely to occur on a large scale, at least initially, since hospitals would not be able to predict accurately in advance what their experience with particular DRGs would be and therefore could not effectively game the system. In other words, the HCFA officials had the right actuarial prediction in hand, but thought it too optimistic to be acted upon safely.

A second problem, that of overpayment, proved to be more troublesome, of which more anon. The overpayment, which amounted to a large sum, came about because of circumstances not entirely of HCFA's making and because of events difficult to anticipate. One source of overpayment was the double allowance for indirect teaching costs, a responsibility that the Congress shared along with the HCFA, and other similar allowances such as that for "disproportionate share" for which Congress deserves more exclusively the praise or blame, depending on how one appraises these matters. A substantial overpayment also resulted from trending forward 1981 figures to get a 1983 baseline. Although this method made sense, given that 1981 was the last year for which complete data existed, the trended figure turned out to be too high. Hospital costs rose less than anticipated, in part because of the unexpected severity of the recession. And hospital occupancy declined more than anticipated, a phenomenon still not adequately explained. Another overpayment resulted from a failure to audit current hospital costs, which affected especially the cost-based portion of hospital payments and update factors.[85] Explainable though the overpayments were, they were an imperfection built into the system that gave rise to a continuing and important issue of hospital "margins" that had important consequences for the implementation of PPS.

These mistakes did not detract from the moment and a lasting satisfaction for the HCFA people of doing better than ever before and more than supposed possible. One participant compared their performance with earlier years of the Social Security Administration, "that fabled agency that could do it right." Another contrasted the PPS experience with the HCFA's own recent past in which cost reports lagged and final payments ran years behind: "We took a $40 billion system and we got it in place between April and October 1, and the claims were right and they were on time."[86] After their success, there was a new pride in the agency and enhanced morale. Reports began to come in on time. New initiatives were suggested. In acknowledgment of the achievement even some personnel lines and research appropriations were restored.

CHRONOLOGY: PROSPECTIVE PAYMENT SYSTEM

1. Social Security Amendments of 1965 (Medicare/Medicaid—P.L. 89–97, July 30, 1965).
2. Social Security Amendments of 1972 (P.L. 92–603, October 33, 1972).
3. Carter Hospital Cost Containment bill (HR 6575; S1391) introduced, April, 1977; last initiative defeated, November 1979.
4. ICD-9-CM, January, 1979; Pettengill–Vertrees evaluation of DRG methodology completed, March 1981.
5. Carolyne Davis task force (Burke Committee) meets to consider hospital payment options, Fall 1981.
6. Patrice Feinstein Committee begins developing specific alternatives, March 1982.

7. Richard Schweiker meets Jack Owen of American Hospital Association, May 6, 1982.
8. Schweiker opts for DRG-based PPS, July 1982.
9. TEFRA passes Congress, August, 1982 (P.L. 97–248, September 3, 1982).
10. Secretary's Report to Congress on PPS, December 1982.
11. Initial Hearings, Health Subcommittee, House Ways and Means, February 3, 1983.
12. Social Security Amendments of 1983 pass Congress, March 23, 1983 (P.L. 98–21, April 20, 1983).
13. Publication of "Interim Final Rule" containing PPS regulations, indexes, DRG weights, September 1, 1983.
14. PPS officially begins, October 1, 1983.

NOTES

1. Not only was there a set, "prospective" price, but the payment "bundled" all the hospital costs into one global payment.
2. For this perspective, the author is particularly indebted to Lynn Etheredge.
3. The author was in Great Britain when PPS was enacted. There, PPS was regarded with a mixture of awe, indulgence, and curiosity—rather like a domestic version of "Star Wars"—a piece of Yankee ingenuity that was, no doubt, wrong-headed in its aims and methods but probably had better be studied. Since then, serious foreign interest has grown enormously as countries from Great Britain to Italy and Australia see in PPS a method for creating a different mix of incentives in their own health care systems.
4. Carolyne K. Davis, who was the Administrator of the HCFA at the time PPS was enacted and a principal figure in its development, reports a continuing series of requests from the United States and abroad for explanations and "briefings" on the system.
5. Interviews with David Abernethy (Staff, Health Subcommittee, House Ways and Means Committee, January 21, 1988); Jay Constantine (formerly Staff, Senate Finance Committee, February 2, 1988); Michael Bromberg, Federation of American Health Systems, November 24, 1987.1.
6. "Routine" hospital costs are, essentially, room and board. "Ancillaries" are the various medical services provided by hospitals, such as staff medical and nursing care, use of operating and recovery rooms, drugs, and some tests.
7. TEFRA (P.L. 97–248, 1982) is the "Tax Equity and Fiscal Responsibility Act of 1982." Among its provisions, it contained a sweeping and draconian revision of hospital reimbursement, generally credited with paving the way for PPS.
8. Interview with David Abernethy, January 21, 1988.
9. Ibid.
10. Interview with Richard S. Schweiker, former Secretary of the Department of Health and Human Services, June 3, 1988.

11.   Interview with Peter Bouxsein, majority staff, Health and Environment Subcommittee, House Energy and Commerce Committee, January 29, 1988.

12.   Interview with Mike Hash, Health Policy Alternatives, formerly AHA staff, March 2, 1988.

13.   The part that dealt with hospitals was actually only 5 or 6 pages in a huge, omnibus statute, but "TEFRA" still means to most people, especially those in the field of health policy, the hospital payment limits established in 1982.

14.   Technically, "per admission" or "per discharge," since the hospital stay was the basis for payment.

15.   An explanatory note. Historically, Medicare hospital reimbursement was subject to the limitation that costs be "necessary for the efficient delivery of needed health services." Some thought that meant "reasonable" cost limitation and others did not. In any event, few controls on cost reimbursement were applied in the early years except to ascertain that incurred costs were legitimately for health care (and not for parking lots or vacations in the Caribbean isles). In the Social Security Amendments of 1972, Congress established (Sec. 223) limits, providing a mandate to tighten cost controls and emphasizing disallowances when costs were not "reasonable," a constraint with considerable accounting and legal potential. Using this "223" authority, the Social Security Administration and later the HCFA were fairly successful in enforcing routine per diem limits (essentially room and board) but much less effective in dealing with the "ancillary" services and supplies. One reason was that the first was a flat fee, even though hospital specific. Ancillaries were paid on a variable ratio of allowed costs to charges (hence RCCs). The latter, therefore, carried with it both the management incentives and the auditing difficulties that could be expected to arise from a system of á la carte pricing. In addition, ancillaries were numerous, rapidly changing in technology, and varied greatly from hospital to hospital. Not surprisingly, as Medicare technicians reported, they never succeeded in "getting a handle" on the ancillaries. But with the increasing sophistication of the hospital product and a continuing incentive to shift all legally assignable costs from per diem to ancillaries, reasonable cost limitations were proving less and less effective in controlling total hospital costs. Consequently, a system that would "bundle" the whole package was even more desirable.

16.   At least the major part of it. There were several categories of hospitals put under the TEFRA system, mostly because of the difficulty of devising DRGs applicable to them. The categories were (1) psychiatric, (2) childrens, (3) rehabilitation, and (4) long-term (and later, cancer). Periodically, Congress and agencies such as the Prospective Payment Assessment Commission (ProPAC) worry about how to bring them under PPS. Meanwhile, as Stuart Altman, the chairman of ProPAC, has observed, the two systems exist side by side as one of the more interesting "natural experiments" waiting for some enterprising researcher to subject them to comparative analysis.

17.   At this time, the House was controlled by the Democratic party and the Senate by the Republican party.

18.   Cf. Bentley and Butler (1980, 5ff) and *Technical Appendices to the Report and Recommendations to the Secretary, U.S. Department of Health and Human Services* (Washington, D.C., Prospective Payment Assessment Commission, 1985), pp. 14 ff.

19.   This brief reference may give a misleading impression of the Social Security Amendments of 1972, almost as important as the original Medicare legis-

lation and certainly the major basis for subsequent regulation. Title II, "Provisions Relating to Medicare, Medicaid, and Maternal and Child Health," resulted in large measure from a remarkable staff study done for the Senate Finance Committee in 1970, surveying the major problem areas. The legislation built on this study and on methods and concepts that represented some of the most advanced regulatory thinking of the day: within industry, academia, Congress, and the administration. Cf. *"Medicare and Medicaid—Problems, Issues, and Alternatives,"* Report of the Staff to the Committee on Finance, United States Senate (Washington, D.C., Government Printing office, 1970).

20.   There was some early work using the notion of case-mix differences, especially on the part of economists such as Martin Feldstein (1967) and Judith and Lester Lave (1971), primarily with the aim of explaining variation in hospital cost patterns rather than devising a method of payment (Bentley and Butler 1980, 2).

21.   Under the Economic Stabilization Program, industry could use a product mix index to argue for increases. A similar method was to be used for hospitals under Phase IV (Bentley and Butler 1980, 2). Also, interview with Stuart H. Altman, chairman of ProPAC, June 10, 1988. See, generally, Zubkoff (1976).

22.   Interview with Edward L. Kelly, National Association of Private Psychiatric Hospitals, January 4, 1988. An explanatory note: Not surprisingly, given the enormous amounts of money at stake, the 1970s were a period of pioneering research into hospital management, including various techniques of monitoring quality of care and the utilization of hospital resources. The DRG methodology was one technique for measuring case-mix, or, from a different perspective, the resource use that should normally be expected for patients with a particular diagnosis. The diagnostic categories had to make sense to practitioners and be "coherent" clinically as well as predict with sufficient accuracy the actual resource use. Depending on how well they performed, DRGs could be used, in principle, to identify outliers for purposes of utilization review or quality assurance, compare the management of different cases within a hospital so as to eliminate inappropriate use of resources, or pay hospitals on a per case basis.

23.   The version of DRGs on which PPS is based uses medical *diagnoses* but surgical *procedures*, the reason being that for surgery, procedures did a better job of explaining resource use. The ultimate version had 468 rather than 383 DRGs, a change that gave the DRGs much greater predictive power.

24.   ICD A-8 is International Classification of Diseases, American Modification, 8th Edition. This system was designed primarily for mortality and morbidity reports and lacked the clinical refinement needed.

25.   Interview with Julian Pettengill, Congressional Research Service, Library of Congress, September 28, 1987.

26.   Ibid.

27.   Peter Bouxsein, later on the staff of the Health and Environment Subcommittee of the House Energy and Commerce Committee.

28.   Brian R. Luce, Office of Research and Demonstrations.

29.   Later renamed BERC (or Bureau of Eligibility, Reimbursement, and Coverage) because the current administration disliked the "policy" emphasis. Larry Oday, who became the head of BERC in 1982, was, along with Carolyne Davis and Patrice Feinstein, one of the political appointees most important in the development of PPS. He has written an account of this development on which the author has relied heavily, and with gratitude.

30.   Brian Luce had worked in the Office of Technology Assessment and

David Newhall and Robert Rubin had been members of Richard Schweiker's congressional staff.

31.   Interview with Richard Schweiker, June 3, 1988.

32.   Ibid. Also interview with Robert J. Rubin, M.D., Lewin-ICF, December 12, 1987.

33.   Several former and present EOMB officials referred to the "Willie Sutton" principle, a reference to the famous bank robber who, when asked why he robbed banks, replied "Because that's where the money is."

34.   Program Associate Director.

35.   Interview with Don Moran, Lewin-ICF. As the same former PAD said, "we would have taken anything, including atomic warfare, to wipe out every other hospital."

36.   Since 1977, the HCFA had been working in a major way on a prospective payment methodology, especially within the Office of Research, Demonstrations, and Statistics (ORDS). The particular emphasis on case-mix began late in 1978. Julian Pettingill, a case-mix and DRG proponent was given lead responsibility in developing the report within ORDS. One difficulty with the proposal, however, was that it was based on the earlier form of DRGs—less suitable as a payment mechanism because of its failure to predict accurately enough the hospital's cost experience within specific DRGs. Interview with Julian Pettingill, February 23, 1988; also Oday (unpublished, 4–6).

37.   Interview with Robert J. Rubin, December 12, 1987.

38.   Later to become Chief of Staff for the Department under Secretary Otis R. Bowen.

39.   Carolyne Davis reports as much, and so does Patrice Feinstein, then Associate Administrator for Policy. Peter Bouxsein recalls that, despite briefings and a visit from the Yale research group, Carolyne Davis showed little interest in DRGs, and then only when their "competitive" aspect was stressed. According to Julian Pettingill, he and others began to lobby for the DRG approach as early as the Fall of 1981, pressing the argument that they were the "only ballgame in town," i.e., the best workable technology. According to him, they were viewed as "horrible," with policy people "losing their lunch" over the mere thought of them. James Scott, who was at that time the Deputy Assistant Secretary for Legislative Affairs, recalls that DRGs were "not the preferred option" and that he was, himself, insistent that they be retained as one of the alternatives presented to Secretary Schweiker. Some of these accounts may have gained vividness over time and deserve to be seasoned with a judicious skepticism; but they all affirm the essential point that the DRG approach was, at this point, the favored option of a few "technicians," i.e., permanent civil servants, mainly in ORDS.

40.   Interview with Patrice Feinstein, June 9, 1988.

41.   Interview with James Scott, American Healthcare Institute, November 5, 1987.

42.   And also their all-day rehearsal for the meeting.

43.   Interview with Richard Schweiker, June 3, 1988.

44.   Interview with Patrice Feinstein, June 9, 1988.

45.   Interview with Michael Maher, Coopers and Lybrand, September 27, 1988.

46.   *Drug Research Reports—The Blue Sheet*, March 10, 1982, p. 6

47.   Interview with Richard S. Schweiker, June 3, 1988; Oday (unpublished, 26). The New Jersey system was, in fact, quite different from the PPS eventually

adopted, particularly in applying to all payers and in allowing a very large per
centage of cases (as much as 33%) to be treated as outliers. Cf. Hsiao et al. (1986).
   48. Interview with Richard Schweiker, June 3, 1988.
   49. Interview with Carolyne K. Davis, Ernst and Whinney, March 10, 1988.
   50. Interview with Richard Schweiker, June 3, 1988.
   51. Davis, Feinstein, and Oday all shared this view.
   52. Interviews with Richard Schweiker, Patrice Feinstein, and Larry Oday.
   53. Interview with Richard Schweiker, June 3, 1988.
   54. P.L. 97–248, Sept. 3, 1982, Sec. 101.
   55. Interview with Richard Schweiker, June 3, 1988.
   56. Interview with Patrice Feinstein, June 9, 1988. According to Feinstein,
some of the reimbursement staff acted as though they were "being told their
mother had just died."
   57. Interview with Richard Schweiker, June 3, 1988.
   58. Now Federation of American Health Systems.
   59. Interview with Don Moran, Lewin-ICF, January 5, 1988.
   60. Ibid.
   61. Interview with David Kleinberg, April 11, 1988.
   62. As Richard Schweiker put it.
   63. Interview with Sheila Burke, Senate Minority Leader Staff, March 8,
1988.
   64. Interview with Robert Hoyer, National Association for Home Care,
November 7, 1988.
   65. Interview with Sheila Burke, Senate Minority Leader Staff, March 8,
1988. Some other descriptions of the Administration proposal were scatological.
   66. Ibid.
   67. The HCFA had not made their impact data available to Congress and
Congress was relying on hastily performed impact studies from the Congressional Budget Office.
   68. Interview with Robert Hoyer.
   69. Standard Metropolitan Statistical Area, a Census Bureau concept, often
used for governmental programs involving various indexes. Since changed to
"Metropolitan Statistical Area."
   70. Especially Tom Gilligan of the Catholic Health Association. Interview,
October 30, 1987.
   71. Carolyne Davis believed that a transition would be needed, but preferred
to let the Congress write in its own version. Interview with Carolyne Davis,
March 10, 1988.
   72. Interview with Edward Grossman, Office of the House Legislative Counsel, February 4, 1988.
   73. Interview with Lisa Potetz, Office of Legislation and Policy, the HCFA,
October 20, 1987.
   74. HCFA personnel were only beginning to work with some of the statistical problems involved. Also, given the size of some of the samples and the
number of hospitals, inferences about particular data cells were of questionable
validity.
   75. There was limited precedent for this kind of commission, though there
was the Postal Rate Commission created in 1970 to advise the Postal Corporation. The House had a proposal, at that time lying dormant, for a similar commission to deal with physician reimbursement. In dealing with the administration bill, the House had already dealt with the update provisions, calling for an

independent advisory group. The Senate provided the particulars that were ultimately enacted into law. Since the passage of PPS, this particular type of commission has been adopted for physician payment and resorted to again, as part of the Medicare Catastrophic Coverage Act (P.L. 100–360, July 1, 1988) to advise on drug payments.

76.   Return on equity was an allowance for stockholder dividends, of great importance to for-profit hospitals. The legislation also provided a pass-through for certified registered nurse anesthesiologists for years 1985–1987.

77.   Interview with Tom Gilligan, Catholic Hospital Association, October 30, 1987. Robert Hoyer, a staff director when Long was Chairman of the Finance Committee, doubts this version. Long, in his view, had a number of reservations and doubts about the bill.

78.   Ibid.

79.   Interview with Allen Dobson, Consolidated Consulting Group, May 20, 1988.

80.   Interview with Patrice Feinstein, June 9, 1988.

81.   Interview with John Nice, Bureau of Data Management and Strategy, May 18, 1988

82.   Interview with Robert Streimer, Associate Administrator for Management and Support Services, the HCFA, June 7, 1988.

83.   Not the least of their public relations activities was explaining to members of Congress what they had just passed.

84.   Interview with Allen Dobson, May 20, 1988.

85.   Since everyone was moving at breakneck speed to get PPS in place, auditing current accounts would have been difficult. Another minor source of overpayment were some past excessive allowances for capital costs.

86.   Interview with James Scott, American Healthcare Institute, November 5, 1987.

3

Prospective Payment System: Implementation

The prospective payment system was especially remarkable for the political unity that accompanied its initial implementation. Secretary Schweiker had a coherent vision of what he wanted the legislation to achieve and gave prospective payment the highest priority. The Congress knew that it wanted *something* to contain Medicare hospital expenditures and accepted PPS as a welcome substitute for the doomsday device it had constructed with TEFRA. The hospital industry—particularly its association leadership—accepted PPS, some with alacrity and others with the awareness that the medicine could have been even more distasteful. And the HCFA administrators and technicians were able to put in place implementing regulations for a statue that they had initially designed and that had largely withstood both the political assaults and vagaries of the legislative process.

If there was political unity, there was also a coherent and precisely articulated design. Both Congress and the DHHS agreed that there should be a comprehensive and systematic solution, and PPS was that. In its development, all the plausible alternatives were evaluated. The DRG methodology was selected in the light of explicit criteria. Despite the add-ons and exceptions, that methodology survived intact. Indeed, the HCFA technicians incorporated it so integrally into the payment system that computer programs could be used to assign cases to their DRG classifications and calculate the dollar amounts to be paid.[1]

PPS was designed to work as a *system*. Within the HCFA, the original intention was that PPS be "budget neutral" and "zero-sum" so that whatever one hospital gained, another would lose. HCFA technicians sought to calculate the actual dollar allowances as closely as they could so as to prevent undue "slack" in the system. In addition to changing the "more for everyone" incentives of cost-reimbursement, these constraints would make the consequences of tinkering with payment formulas more evident and the system as a whole relatively "tamper proof."[2] This "logic" or rationale was not missed by observers, who referred to PPS as HCFA's "eighteenth-century machine," a contraption intended to work mechanistically and largely without human (i.e., political) intervention. That comparison is a metaphor carried too far, but there was a hope and some well-founded expectation that the system could be designed so as to insulate PPS and its implementation in a considerable measure from the political process and its attendant "fixes" for specific categories of provider need and greed.

Viewing PPS from this perspective could support an expectation that implementation would be relatively non-political and largely determined by technical considerations. Therefore, it is well to recall some of the ambivalence that attended the DRG methodology from the beginning. For an item, DRGs were not initially developed as a pricing mechanism and there persists to this day doubts about their suitability for this purpose. Moreover, when first considered as a policy option under the Reagan Administration, both the HCFA and EOMB viewed DRGs as an unacceptably regulatory form of administrative pricing. Within Congress Secretary Schweiker sold DRGs in part by taking advantage of their two sides: stressing to Democrats the regulatory potential of DRGs and to Republicans their merits as a prospective price. Congress amended the administration's proposal extensively, in the view of some[3] writing a statute that was more a substitute than an amendment. In other words, there was considerable room for disagreement about just what PPS was, suggesting that rather than a technical elaboration of the statute, implementation was more likely to entail a continuing controversy over which of various interpretations would prevail.

Some of those within the HCFA who participated in the development and initial implementation of PPS saw it in large measure as getting *away* from the evils of cost-reimbursement, a non-system that was becoming increasingly prolix, cumbersome, and unfair. What they liked about DRGs—if they liked them at all—was that they could set a fair and prospective rate for a hospital stay, dispense with the nit-picking regulations and the Medicare cost reports, and encourage hospital managers to manage more efficiently. What was important for these people within the HCFA was the uniformity, prospectiveness, and integrity of the system. They supported a speedy transition to national rates, going by the numbers, and as few special exceptions as possible.

Congress began with cost control as a prime concern. In the background was the hospital cost containment history of the Carter Administration and the Hospital Insurance Trust Fund crisis of the first years of the Reagan Administration. PPS was not their creation, but from the congressional perspective a substitute for TEFRA—which was very much a cost-containment bill, and derivative from the cost control initiatives of the recent past. Even the more knowledgeable members and committee staff knew or understood little about PPS at the time of enactment. They were, therefore, not remarkably impressed with its theoretical niceties or enamored of its rigor and systematic unity. One of their first and most urgent demands was for impact data showing how PPS would affect census regions, states, and congressional districts. Both the House and the Senate moved quickly to provide for urban and rural differentials and to establish a transition period. Consistently, the thrust of congressional efforts has been to adapt PPS so as to make it tolerable, that is, acceptable for individual constituencies.

There is, then, a continuing conflict between a technological imperative of consistent and rigorous implementation and an incentive to intervene for particular benefit or budget savings. Some administrators and even a few in Congress would let hospitals go broke or keep their "profits,"[4] no matter how large. Others see PPS as a wondrous machine for saving money or achieving deficit reduction. Still others, especially in Congress, want "equitable" exceptions for types of hospitals or individual hospitals and are mostly concerned with what PPS does for or to their own districts.

In principle, the tension between the particular and the general would be contained by the "anti-tampering" features of PPS, by the large discretion given to the Secretary (or to the HCFA) to implement the statute, and by the role of the Prospective Payment Assessment Commission (ProPAC), which would buffer PPS from interest group politics and mediate between the congressional committees and the HCFA. Yet aside from the unresolved issues in the statute itself, such as whether hospitals should be allowed to go broke, there have continued to be two other big and confounding influences. One of these is the continuing budget deficit, which makes hospital expenditures and especially excessive hospital margins an attractive target for budget and deficit reduction. A second confounding factor is the strained relations between Congress and the executive branch throughout the Reagan and Bush Administrations. These together have led the executive branch, and especially EOMB, to push hard for Reagan–Bush political priorities and for budget savings. They have also given Congress both incentive and excuse to respond in kind, especially with extensive and minute interventions into the implementation of PPS.

Diderot, the French Encyclopedist and philosopher, is credited with the slogan, "Despotism and statistics cannot coexist." This slogan rested on the kind of optimistic belief shared by many who helped design and implement PPS: that a fair and technically sound system of hospital payments could be designed, would win assent and be enacted into law, and could be administered without being destroyed by "politics." It remains to be seen whether that faith was in some measure warranted or whether PPS has been or will be subverted, either by being "exceptioned to death" or by being converted into a handy instrument for meeting budget reduction targets. In either event, the experience of implementing PPS has a wider significance, exposing the difficulties of regulating the vast, varied, and dynamic health care industry in the political context created by the semi-permanent partisan divisions between Congress and the Executive.

I. IMPLEMENTATION ACTIVITIES

An important background element with respect to the implementation of PPS was the early concern within Congress about the particular topic of legislative–executive relations. Not only was Congress made uneasy by the less than forthcoming attitude of the HCFA with respect to impact data, but the brevity and rigor of the Administration proposal made many in Congress sharply aware of the vast amount of delegation that this legislation would entail. The response within Congress was to write a highly prescriptive statute and provide in some detail for the manner in which it would be implemented. The statute is replete with formulas for calculating the payments, with "shall" mandates for the Secretary and specific deadlines, and with numerous provisions for the disposal of unfinished business. Notable also was the establishment of ProPAC, a novel commission created to advise both the Secretary and the Congress on the implementation of the statute.

This concern within Congress about implementation makes good sense, if one takes into account the way in which programs such as PPS are administered. With PPS, as with the vast majority of Federal programs, for that matter, implementation is not so much directed immediately to physical activities like planting trees or sorting the mail as it is toward developing and promulgating regulations. Specifically, for PPS, this means producing many reporting forms, "rules," and detailed instructions that will ultimately regulate the hospitals but that are directed initially to the fiscal intermediaries who, in turn, will pay the submitted claims, audit the records, collect data, and deal on a day-to-day basis with the hospitals. Such "rules" are sometimes mind-boggling in their scope and complexity.[5] For HCFA, especially, they are often supplemented or even displaced by less formal and less public manuals, letters of transmittal, and memoranda, which are more quickly implemented and less constrained either by clearance procedures, public comment, or potential law suits. Inevitably, a vast amount of discretion remains with "the Secretary," which is to say with the bureau directors, program analysts and regulations writers, and the technical advisory committees and consultants who help determine the content of the implementation regulations. The statute shows a cognizance on the part of Congress of this need for extensive delegation: for instance, leaving the annual "update" of the overall DRG rate of increase to the Secretary. At the same time, the legislation showed the ambivalence in the collective mind of Congress: a hope that the Secretary would administer PPS in a spirit acceptable to the Congress, and a substantial fear that he or she would not.

Both in the statute as written and in the subsequent administration of it, the major implementation activities fall under four major categories of concern. These are (1) setting the annual update, (2) DRG amendment and recalibration, (3) monitoring the system and proposing amendments to improve it, and (4) unresolved issues, including old and new mandates from Congress. Each of these can profit from some brief explanation before describing how the year-by-year implementation of the statute has been carried out.

The "update" factor, which is language deriving from the statute, refers to the percentage by which the "standardized" amount will be changed each year to account for price inflation and for a number of other changes in the hospital's production function. The basis for computing per case payments to hospitals is the "standardized amount," which is the payment for a DRG with a relative weight of one.[6] Separate standardized amounts are computed for urban and rural areas and multiplied by area wage indexes. During the transition period, each DRG hospital had also a hospital-specific and a regional portion that would be applied in determining the per case payments, but since November 1987 the basic standardized amounts are national, except that rates still differ for urban and rural areas.[7] The update factor or percentage is by law made up of two parts. The first of these is the "hospital market basket," a figure computed from a number of indexes that takes account of price inflation in the goods and services that hospitals must purchase.[8] The second is a production function, that makes allowance for changes in case mix and service delivery.[9] From a political perspective, the update factor is especially important because it is the multiplier for a number of other variables: DRG weights, the wage index, the allowances for medical education, and a percentage adjustment for disproportionate share hospitals. Since PPS is zero-sum and a national system, small percentage changes can have a large regional impact as well as life-or-death consequences for individual hospitals. At the same time, the annual update is one of the few ways in which the hospital industry can get

Table 1. Example of Calculation of PPS Payment

Hypothetical hospital located in Chicago, Illinois
  Beds = 300
  Interns and residents = 30
  Wage index = 1.2240
  Case-mix index = 1.08
  Hospital-specific cost/case in base year = $3,200
    (Fiscal year starts July 1; base year: July 1, 1982 to June 30, 1983)
Hypothetical case
  DRG 235 (fracture of femur)
  Discharged on January 15, 1985
  Weight = 1.7403
  1. Calculation of hospital specific portion
    Update cost/case to FY 84
      $3,200/1.08 × (1.12701) = $3,339.29
    Update cost/case to FY 85:
      $3,339.29 × (1.06300) = $3,549.66
    Multiply times DRG weight:
      $3,549.66 × $1.7403 = $6,177.48
  2. Calculation of Federal portion (which is 75% regional 25% national)
  Regional urban standardized amount =
    $2,452.00 labor related; $712.68 nonlabor related
  National urban standardized amount =
    $2,320.61 labor related; $664.44 nonlabor related
      Regional: ($2,452.00 × 1.2240) + $712.68 = $3,713.93
      National: ($2,320.61 × 1.2240) + $664.44 = $3,504.87
        (0.75 × $3,713.93) + (0.25 × $3,504.87) = $3,557.13
      Multiply times DRG weight:
        $3,557.13 × 1.7403 = $6,057.79
  Indirect teaching allowance[a]
    Scaling factor = 0.1
    Teaching adjustment factor = 0.1159
      (interns and residents)/beds/0.1 × 0.1159 × $6,057.79 =
        30/300/0.1 − 0.1159 × $6,057.79 = $702.10
  Total Federal portion = $6,057.79 + 702.10 = $6,759.89
  3. Since January 15, 1985 occurs during the hospital's first year under PPS,
    the formula is:
      (0.75 × hospital-specific + 0.25 Federal)
      (0.75 × $6,177.48) + (0.25 + $6,759.89) = $6,323.08

[a] Attributable to this case but paid at a later date in a lump sum payment (although the hospital receives interim payments every two weeks).

Table 2. Hospital Prospective Reimbursement Input Price Index (The "Market Basket")

Category of Costs[1]	Relative Importance 1981[2]	Price Variable Used
1. Wages And Salaries	56.53	Percentage change in average hourly earnings of hospital industry workers (SIC 806)
2. Employee Benefits	8.16	Percentage change in supplements to wages and salaries per worker in nonagricultural establishments.
3. Professional Fees, Other (Legal, Auditing, Consulting, Etc.)	0.56	Percentage change in hourly earnings index for production or nonsupervisory workers on private, nonagricultural payrolls, total private.
4. Malpractice Insurance	2.12	Percentage change in hospital malpractice insurance premiums.
5. Food..................	3.32	(a) Percentage change in food and beverages component for Consumer Price Index, All Urban (relative importance, 1.71). (b) Percentage change in processed foods and feeds component of Producer Price Index (relative importance, 1.61).
6. Fuel And Other Utilities	3.52	(a) a percentage change in implicit price deflator—consumption of fuel oil and coal (derived from fuel oil component of Consumer Price Index) (relative importance, 1.73) (b) Percentage change in implicit price deflator—consumption of electricity (derived from electricity component of Consumer Price Index) (relative importance, 0.80) (c) Percentage change in implicit price deflator for natural gas, derived from utility (piped) gas component of Consumer Price Index (relative importance, 0.67). (d) Percentage in water and sewerage maintenance component of Consumer Price Index (relative importance, 0.32).

(continued)

Table 2. (Continued)

Category of Costs[1]	Relative Importance 1981[2]	Price Variable Used
7. Drugs	2.61	Percentage change in pharmaceutical preparations, ethical component of Producer Price Index.
8. Chemicals And Cleaning Products	2.17	Percentage change in chemicals and allied products components of Producer Price Index.
9. Surgical And Medical Instruments And Supplies	2.09	Percentage change in special industry machinery and equipment components of Producer Price Index.
10. Rubber And Miscellaneous Plastics	1.73	Percentage change in rubber and plastic products component of Producer Price Index.
11. Business Travel And Freight	1.84	Percentage change in motor transportation component of Consumer Price Index. All Urban.
12. Apparel And Textiles............	1.45	Percentage change in textile products and apparel component of Producer Price Index.
13. Business Services	5.00	Percentage change in services component of Consumer Price Index. All Urban.
14. All Other Miscellaneous Expenses[3]	8.90	Percentage change of Consumer Price Index for all items. All Urban.
Total............	100.00	

[a]Costs not within the scope of the limits (i.e., capital, medical education and medical professional fees) were excluded in deriving the input price index.

[b]A Lasperyres price index was constructed using 1977 base value weights and the price variables indicated in the table. Base value weights (cost shares) were derived from special studies by the Health Care Financing Administration using primarily data from the American Hospital Association and the Interindustry Economics Division of the Bureau of Economic Analysis, U.S. Department of Commerce. In 1977 each price variable has an index value of 100.00. The "relative importance" changes over time in accordance with price changes for each variable. Cost categories with relatively higher price increases get relative importance values and vice versa. For an explanation of the basic methodology used, see Freeland, Mark S., Anderson, Gerard and Schandler, Carol Ellen, "National Hospital Input Price Index," *Health Care Financing Review,* Summer 1979, pp. 37–81.

[c]This is a residual category of costs not included in the 13 specific categories above. It consists primarily of miscellaneous and unallocated items.

Source: Technical Appendixes to the Report and Recommendations to the Secretary, U.S. Department of Health and Human Services, April 1, 1985, p. 28.

more for all. The significance of these properties has not been lost on the hospital industry, the Congress, or the EOMB, and the update factor has become *the* most contentious single issue respecting implementation.

A second major implementation activity is DRG recalibration and amendment.[10] Of the two, recalibration is technically the simpler one, referring to periodic changes in DRG weights to reflect more accurately the costs or resource inputs associated with a particular DRG. Initially, this recalibration was to take place every four years, but since 1987 it occurs annually. In essence, recalibration amounts to "repricing" the DRG to reflect changes in resource use for that particular DRG. DRG amendment including changes in classification or assignment, is a modification of the DRG itself, either to accommodate new technology or in recognition that a particular DRG is "broken," i.e., does not predict resource use accurately enough. A separate provision for multiple joint procedures or for magnetic resonance imaging would be examples of DRG amendment; assigning a higher DRG weight to reflect increased nursing care or use of drugs associated with heart attacks would be an illustration of recalibration. Amendment and recalibration seem, then, to be much the same kind of procedure, but economically and politically, there is a big and important difference. With recalibration, changes take place only *after* the cost experience for the industry as a whole shows the need for a change. Therefore, individual hospitals laying on new and expensive modalities of treatment or pioneering in new, high-tech equipment are at risk and dependent on eventual recalibration for adequate payment. DRG amendment, on the other hand, is money "up front," so to speak, available *before* the cost and charge reports are assembled and audited and *before* the new modalities and technologies are adopted industry-wide. DRG recalibration and amendment, therefore, affect vitally the adoption and spreading[11] of life-saving technology and treatment methods, making the HCFA and ProPAC the monitors and regulators of technological change in hospital care. Just as obviously, the establishment of these procedures greatly affects the politics of health care, by interesting hospitals, physicians, drug companies, and the manufacturers of medical equipment in the particulars of DRG recalibration and amendment.

PPS was both sweeping in scope and novel in method. Therefore, both the HCFA and Congress were concerned with monitoring the system and with providing modifications where and when needed. The annual update and DRG recalibration and amendment are, in themselves, important monitoring activities. They require, for instance, assessments of case-mix increases, of technological change and practice patterns within the industry, and of trends in hospital margins, or surplus income realized from hospitalizing Medicare patients. The HCFA was, from the beginning, especially attentive to possibilities for "gaming" the system and early on established techniques to spot trends toward excessive admissions or unjustified "upcoding."[12] Congress was, and continues to be, especially concerned about the impact of PPS on beneficiaries and on hospitals. For this reason, it gave PROs a large role in monitoring hospital admissions as well as appropriateness of care, and subsequently enacted legislation dealing with premature discharges and denials of payment for substandard care. Congress also charged the Secretary and ProPAC with periodic assessments or impact studies dealing with a wide range of topics: effects of PPS on hospitals and beneficiaries, area wages and wage-related costs, census region impact, special needs of sole community hospitals and regional referral centers, the urban–rural differential, and costs of uncompensated care. For an era of "deregulation," PPS is a continuously and closely monitored program. From the HCFA, ProPAC, and provider and beneficiary associations, moreover, have come continuing streams of proposals for amendments, which because of the budget reconciliation process are relatively easy to enact. There is a piece of folk wisdom that says, "If it ain't broke, don't fix it." Somewhat differently, the fear with respect to PPS is that it will be fixed so often that it will eventually be broken.

A last category of issues that crops up in the process of implementation is that of unfinished business, left over as problems unresolved in the initial design of PPS, addressed in the course of legislation, or widely perceived among health care experts or lobbyists as significant ways in which to improve the working of the system. Mostly, these are proposals to make PPS payments either more accurate or "fairer" by some other criterion. For instance, an issue left over from the legislative process is that of designing a "volume adjustment" that would make an appropriate allowance for economies of scale that can be realized by large-volume hospitals and reduce their per discharge payments accordingly.[13] Attempts to develop a "severity of illness" or "intensity of care" index that would increase the accuracy of payments within resource intensive DRGs was also mentioned by Congress and, for that matter, was being sought at the time PPS was being designed. At the time, no satisfactory method for folding capital into individual DRGs existed and so capital was left as a "pass-through," paid on a cost-reimbursement basis. But the statute contained a mandate to the Secretary to report back within 18 months on "the methods and proposals" by which capital and return on equity could be included in PPS. Similarly with disproportionate share and sole community hospitals: they were "grandfathered" into PPS, with directions to the Secretary to devise or report back to Congress on methods of payment that would take into account their "special needs" or "unique vulnerability." There have been many other mandated reports and directions to the Secretary for ways of improving PPS from studies of outliers to fees set for certified registered nurse anesthesiologists (CRNAs), but the examples cited are among the most important. One point that should be made is that such business is largely unfinished either because of political disagreements or because of a lack of technically feasible solutions. Consequently, how such difficulties eventually get resolved, whether by finding a technical solution or by some rougher and more political resolution, is significant in assessing the future prospects for PPS.

One received view is that implementation is "politics by another name" (cf. Bardach 1977; Pressman and Wildavsky 1973). With respect to PPS, one would hope not. It was designed to discourage political tampering. Even ProPAC, that represents the industry and advises Congress, was created in large measure to buffer decisions from direct political pressures and to provide an independent and expert perspective. So, the implementation of PPS is significant because it is more than "politics by another name," a process in which the best numbers often win. Why and how they do are important questions. At the same time, the previous description of implementation activities should make abundantly clear the fact that the implementation process *is* intensely political. Furthermore, it is marked by critical junctures, points at which the basic integrity of PPS is much at stake: whether it is to be primarily a technical, rational system or a politically driven, particularistic succession of fixes.

In broad and formalistic terms, the annual implementation process for PPS follows the model of administrative rule-making,[14] but with the special procedures added by the PPS legislation. Each year in May—before June 1, as mandated by law—the Secretary must publish a recommendation for the annual update. What actually comes forth at this time is one or more "proposed rules" giving the Secretary's recommendations not only on the annual update but also responding to scores of legislatively mandated changes, making recommendations on recalibration and amendment of DRGs, revising wage and other indexes, and addressing a large number of specific regulatory issues. In fact, the proposed rule or rules will run to several hundred pages of new wage indexes, DRG weights, modified formulas and definitions, technical regulations, explanations, and justifications, pretty much reviewing the entire range of activities covered by the PPS legislation.[15] It summarizes a year of monitoring activities, of data gathering and number-crunching, of policy analysis and decision-making, and regulation-writing and clearance.

The May proposed rule or rules is primarily the work of the HCFA, and much of the annual cycle of work, especially within the Bureau of Eligibility, Reimbursement, and Coverage (BERC) and the Bureau of

Data Management and Strategy (BDMS) is aimed at its completion. There are other activities within the HCFA important for PPS. The Bureau of Program Operations, for instance, translates PPS policy into operational instructions for the fiscal intermediaries, updates and checks the DRG Grouper and Pricer programs, and oversees the payment process. The Health Standards and Quality Bureau supervises the PROs that monitor utilization and quality of care under PPS. Moreover, hundreds of less comprehensive rules and notices dealing with specific coverage and reimbursement issues and the regulations of the providers and the payment process are published week by week throughout the year. But the May publication, often referred to as the Secretary's recommendations, like the budget process, relates many issues to a whole and brings into sharp focus most of the strategic choices.

Viewed as a collective intellectual process, preparing the annual proposed rule is a big and demanding task of developing and coordinating data, forecasts, and policy decisions. The central objective, one to which most other activities are subordinate or ancillary, is to set next year's DRG prices. To do so involves numerous assumptions and forecasts about the future hospital market basket, technical advances and case-mix changes within hospitals, projections of mortality and morbidity, hospital lengths of stay, and many other significant variables. It also requires cost projections for legislative mandates, for the DRG recalibrations and amendments, for all the add-ons and exceptions, and for any changes made with respect to payment procedures.[16] Supporting these projections are data and analyses, some developed in-house and some gotten through contracts with consultants, to make possible the determination of vital numbers such as area wage indexes, resource use for specific DRGs, outlier experience, hospital per case operating margins, and so forth. Inasmuch as PPS is zero-sum, i.e., limited by the annual update, these figures are vital not just for setting an annual update and recalibrating the DRGs, but also for assessing the impact of *all* the policy decisions made during the year: for a change in the definition of a regional referral center, for instance, or a decision to amend a DRG to pay for an expensive thrombolytic drug. Getting the "Secretary's Proposals" together, then, is not only a technical and intricate process, it involves coordination and logistics: data people, actuaries, policy analysts and regulation writers knowing each other's work, being able to rely on it, and collaborating effectively.

Viewing the development of the annual May proposed rule as a coordinated intellectual process makes an important point about the HCFA's role in the implementation of PPS. This implementation is dependent on knowledge of specialized data files and projecting and relating these to an ongoing system: which is to say, on a particular administrative *expertise*, not readily available to others and not easy to duplicate in another setting. Also, because the HCFA technicians can and must deal with the systemic consequences of individual decisions they have a strong motivation to fend off outside intervention, especially of a particularistic sort, and to insist on playing by the rules and the numbers. These are considerations that bear significantly on both the actual and the appropriate roles of ProPAC and the Congress in overseeing the implementation of PPS.

The preceding description deals primarily with the central part of the proposed rule, especially the update factor. The rule or rules will also cover such narrow but important items as modification of data files or the specifics of claims requirements, particular kinds of treatment such as kidney or liver transplants, and the definition of specialized facilities such as rehabilitation units or burn centers. In addition, an update and modification in cost-reimbursement methods will be promulgated for PPS-exempt hospitals, CHAMPUS hospitals, and other hospitals in Puerto Rico, Guam, Alaska, etc. This recital illustrates the enormous work-load carried by the HCFA, for this May publication is but one proposed regulation of many that will be published during the year, although it is the most important and comprehensive one.[17]

The practice with a rule of this scope is for it to go through a number of drafts with extensive comment from various bureaus within the HCFA and an extensive clearance process within the Department that will involve such staff divisions as the Office of General Counsel, the Office of Management and Budget within DHSS, and the Office of the Secretary. A critical step is referring the proposed rule to the Executive Office of Management and Budget (EOMB) that in recent years has regularly returned such rules with a "pass back" demand that more budget saving be taken from PPS or a proposed regulation or definition changed, a process that has had much to do with politicizing the PPS update factor.

Also important for the development of the proposed rule is the activity of ProPAC. In the original legislation, the Commission was required to submit its recommendations for PPS changes to the Secretary prior to April 1 (later March 1) to allow the HCFA and the Department an opportunity to evaluate and respond to ProPAC's recommendations. This report dealt with the major implementation topics outlined before: update factor, DRG recalibration and amendment, and other policy changes. Under this last heading, "other policy changes," the Commission would, each year, send forward a number of major recommendations, 19 in one year and over 30 in another, that were published in the June 1 proposed rule with the Secretary's comments. The process did not end there. ProPAC would then comment on the Secretary's comments in a November report to Congress. Given contemporary political realities, though, the initial submission to the Secretary seemed increasingly irksome and ritualistic, so that Congress discontinued it in 1991. The initial report goes to Congress, not the Secretary. The Secretary is directed only to explain differences between the Department's recommendations and those of ProPAC's.[18] But ProPAC still comments on the proposed rule and its position is known in time for budget reconciliation legislation that may be pending for that year and that will include most of the major changes affecting Medicare.

Since the Commission is important in the implementation of PPS and has also served as a model for various other Medicare commissions, it deserves more than passing comment, especially about its prescribed role and activities. As noted earlier, it was largely the conception of Robert Hoyer, then a chief professional staff person for the Senate Finance Committee. Aside from providing independent, expert advice and a "second opinion," both he and the Congress saw it as meeting other needs. One was to give Congress its own source of timely data and analysis, rendering it less dependent on HCFA and "the Secretary." A second was to buffer Congress somewhat from pressure group politics, thereby not only relieving the committees and their members from the importuning of lobbyists and constituents, but also increasing the legitimacy of the ultimate decisions.

The Commission, as such, is a body of 17 members, one of whom is the Chairman.[19] These members are primarily representatives of the provider community, which is to say, hospitals and medical schools, physicians and nurses, and health care association representatives. There is one designated "public" or "consumer" representative. This recital would make it appear that the Commission mainly represents the industry. Yet its background and expertise is broad and deep including, for instance, representation from HMOs, industry benefits and health insurance, health economics and planning, and former HCFA administration and congressional staff. This expertise and rich background not only add credibility to the advice that the Commission gives to Congress, but also promote unity among the commissioners, moderating their own particularistic concerns. The Chairman of the Commission since its inception has been Stuart Altman, dean of the Florence Heller School at Brandeis University and a former deputy assistant secretary for planning and evaluation in DHSS. An astute and dedicated health policy activist, he is also a remarkably skillful commission chairman and is widely credited with fostering consensus and public spirit within the Commission.

The main business of the Commission is to develop and approve three reports. Two of these have already been mentioned: the April (now

March) report submitting the Commission's recommendations to Congress and the November report evaluating the Secretary's final adjustments to PPS. In June, the Commission submits to Congress another, large report complete with technical appendices, reviewing salient trends in the hospital and health care industry, the working of PPS and its impact on hospitals and Medicare beneficiaries, and dealing broadly and in depth with a number of continuing and developing issues such as outlier policies and reimbursement for capital expenditures.[20]

In developing these reports, the Commission does much of its work through subcommittees. As its name would indicate, the Subcommittee on Hospital Productivity and Cost Effectiveness deals broadly with issues relating to the hospital industry as a whole and particularly with the PPS annual update: the hospital market basket and the components of the discretionary adjustment factor. The Subcommittee on Diagnostic and Therapeutic Procedures is charged with a broad oversight of changing technology and treatment patterns and, more specifically, concerns itself with new DRGs and DRG reassignment and amendment. A third Subcommittee on Data Development and Research is responsible for planning the annual research cycle and for developing the RFPs[21] and contracts for that research. With the exception of this last subcommittee, their meetings are open to the public and are well attended by hospital industry representatives and by other interested parties from various consulting firms, DHSS or the HCFA.

The Commission meets at roughly two month intervals, for six or more two-day meetings a year. At the meetings, the commissioners hear committee reports and expert witnesses and discuss major policy items such as the recommended update figure, what to do about a particularly troublesome DRG, or what approach to take in revising the teaching allowance or the reimbursement for capital. Many of the tougher decisions are made in the evening or during meal-time executive sessions. But the public meetings are well-attended and lively and set a high standard for pertinence and intellectual quality of the discussion. The meetings preceding the March and November reports are, of course, especially important ones since they give a preview of the recommendations to the Secretary and to Congress.

One reason that the Commission's recommendations are both timely and well received, especially by Congress, is the quality of its staff. The Commission staff is a small one of about 30 professionals, but in that number are included many advanced degrees and people with past experience in agencies such as the HCFA and the CBO who came to ProPAC with a policy expertise and an easy familiarity with the PPS world of statistics, computers, and megabyte data sets. While largely dependent on others[22] for their data and basic research, the staff is good at quickly assessing trends, interpreting the implications of data and research in readable prose, and meeting short deadlines, all capabilities that are important for the Commission and that have gained support for it in Congress.[23]

From the perspective of Congress, ProPAC has proved to be a successful innovation. Aside from the timeliness of its recommendations, there are two other major reasons for this acclaim. One is the Commission's "credibility," as the Chairman, Stuart Altman, often reminds its members. "Credibility" is a quality that is difficult to explain,[24] but as applied to the Commission would seem to derive especially from their capacity to develop recommendations that transcend group interest and are based on argument from the best, or at least good, technical and policy considerations. Although not generally formulated this way, part of the Commission's success would appear to be that it supplies some of the "neutral competence" that executive agencies such as the Office of Management and Budget once did. A second, and more expedient reason, is that ProPAC's recommendations fit so nicely, both temporally and by virtue of their scope and substance, with the budget reconciliation process. They give the Congress many of the proposals and alternatives that it needs at a time and in the form that it needs them.

The budget reconciliation process derives from the Budget and Impoundment Control Act of 1974, which was part of the post-Watergate reforms that also included the Federal Elections Campaign Act of 1974 and the "democratization" of both House and Senate procedures. "Reconciliation" was intended as a procedure that would enable Congress to curb its own spending proclivities by bringing the decisions of the authorizing committees into conformity with overall targets set by the House and Senate Budget Committees. Initially, budget reconciliation was largely piety and pretense on the part of Congress, but it became serious business after 1980, partly as a result of the Stockman "budget revolution" that showed what *could* be done, and partly as a result of the mounting budget deficits of the Reagan administration that showed that something *had* to be done. 1984 produced DEFRA,[25] a major effort. Then, in 1985, as deficits continued to mount, Congress laid on itself an additional self-denying ordinance, the Balanced Budget and Emergency Deficit Control Act of 1985,[26] popularly known as "Gramm–Rudman–Hollings" or simply "Gramm–Rudman." This act, among other things, identified special areas for mandatory percentage reductions (sequestration) if the total appropriations were more than $10 billion over the budget reconciliation targets. Not surprisingly, deficits have continued to this day, so that Gramm–Rudman has been a factor.[27] A number of programs, such as the national debt, Social Security, and Food Stamps, were exempt. But Medicare, specifically, was not. Moreover, about this time, it became increasingly apparent that PPS was producing large margins or profits for some hospitals. Both justice and expediency argued that hospitals should be targeted, and they were.

A growing practice has been to make budget reconciliation a vehicle for substantive legislation amending the ongoing programs, especially those involving entitlements, such as Medicare. The Deficit Reduction Act of 1984 (DEFRA) was the first time this expedient was used extensively, but since then, most substantive amendments to Medicare have been made in this fashion.[28]

In practice, the authorizing committees that write the substantive legislation have their budget or deficit-reduction targets, developed through a complex process of negotiation and budget resolutions. To meet these targets, the committee members—usually their staff aides—prepare lists of options. In the actual reconciliation, like ordering from a Chinese menu, so many are taken from list A, B, or C until the target is met. These recommendations go to the Conference Committees and are then sent to the House and Senate floors as huge "omnibus" bills. For Congress, the issue is to pass or not, largely without significant amendment. Furthermore, since the President lacks an "item-veto," such bills are almost veto-proof, though the OBRA of 1987 did lead to a threat of veto by President Reagan and a so called "summit" that produced an eventual agreement, including a relaxation of Gramm–Rudman. President Bush also threatened repeatedly to veto the OBRA of 1989. But the central point is that a number of spending programs such as Medicare get amended in detail and sometimes extensively modified at the subcommittee level or at the behest of individual members by a process that is largely exempt from effective review or from amendment by the House or Senate as collective bodies or by the executive branch of the Federal government.

With respect to Medicare, there are some particular features of budget reconciliation that merit special comment. Medicare falls within the jurisdiction of the House Ways and Means and the Senate Finance committees.[29] These committees are both powerful and expert. Almost anything within their purview affects the budget. Furthermore, unlike other authorizing committees, Ways and Means and Finance raise revenue through taxes, so that they can "offset" a proposal that increases expenditures against others that reduce outlays or raise revenue. For most Medicare or Medicaid[30] programs, and specifically for PPS, the budget reconciliation process provides a full-service apparatus for amending the statute in detail or for delivering marching orders to the HCFA and the Secretary.[31]

If the budget-reconciliation process opened up possibilities for micromanagement and for amending legislation in detail, PPS itself offered tempting opportunities. Aside from the dollars involved, the statute itself almost invited tinkering: with its transition dates, regions and categories of hospitals, and DRG rates, add-ons, and exceptions. As Patrice Feinstein, a former HCFA associate administrator said, "Under cost-reimbursement, there was no way for Congress to send money to Providence, Rhode Island; but under PPS, that's precisely what they can do." She went on to say that PPS had proven surprisingly subject to manipulation.[32] Her observation directs attention to the many temptations that bedevil the members of Congress. It also suggests both the importance of ProPAC and some ambivalence about its role: essential to prevent crude favoritism and corruption of PPS and yet, perforce, an accomplice in showing Congress how to "fix" it so as to benefit constituents.

II. SUBSTANTIVE POLICY

PPS has been described as an "eighteenth-century machine," a metaphor that conveys the implicit proposition that it would function in an automatic and timeless fashion whatever the historic circumstance or political milieu in which it had to work. Like all metaphors, this one both reveals an essential property and obscures another. PPS does have important features, like the update factor and the zero-sum constraint, that enhance its systemic qualities. But PPS is also an administrative device, a political institution, which is to say a system of norms that is more or less effective in mediating the forces of economic interest and parochial concern.

This observation is especially pertinent for PPS, since Congress, the Administration, and the hospital industry had and have different conceptions of what PPS is supposed to achieve, and even more, they differ about first priorities. From the perspective of DHHS and the hospital industry, PPS was not primarily a cost-saving device, but a method of payment that was less regulative and that would provide better management incentives. Congress wanted cost control, but also protectiveness and local advantage. Only the Office of Management and Budget, after initial misgivings, regarded PPS primarily as a way of reducing Federal government outlays. So, there is a continuing disagreement about the ends and means of PPS, which has made particular modifications of PPS at the expense of system imperatives both easier and more legitimate.

Domestic budget politics since the passage of PPS has been unsettled, encouraging political intervention and attempts to tamper with the system on the part both of Congress and the executive agencies, especially

EOMB. PPS began under bad auspices: distrust between the Administration and the Congress. From 1983 on, the deficit reduction tactics of EOMB and DHSS have nourished this discord and led to open struggles with the Congress over the budget that made PPS a prime and strategic target. During the tenure of Secretary Margaret Heckler, from early 1983 until 1986, the level of trust and cooperation between the Congress and the Department was at a historic low. In brief, PPS was a disputed prize in one of the perennial separation of powers struggles between the executive branch of government and the Congress: in this instance, a more than usually intense and protracted one that continues to this day.

Another source of trouble was that of "overpayments" to the hospitals: the consequences of miscalculations and excessive allowances that generated large hospital margins and big regional variations, especially in 1984 and 1985, the first full years of operation under PPS. The reasons for and the extent of these payments are a vexed issue, of which more will be said. But in the present context, these overpayments radically undercut arguments that Congress or EOMB should exercise forbearance. Far from being "tight," PPS needed drastic tightening. Moreover, these payments became especially apparent late in 1985, just as deficit reduction enthusiasm was highest, creating a mood that only the most sacred of cows could be spared, among which hospitals were not included.

For PPS, as this discussion would suggest, there has been a routine kind of implementation: applying the system according to its underlying "logic" and purposes, coping with the usual difficulties presented by technical problems, statutory omissions or inconsistencies, and responding to the complaints or solicitations of providers and other interested groups. This process has been somewhat confounded by the issue of hospital "margins." At the same time, there has been an ongoing, "higher" (or lower) politics of the budget and separation of powers. Although the HCFA and ProPAC and the congressional committees have gained experience and sureness in working with the routine, contemporary politics is a bigger, exogenous kind of influence that periodically or ultimately threatens to overwhelm the system, despite its slowly increasing legitimacy and efficacy. Which will win out is a question much at issue. Many say that PPS is already nothing more than an "administered price system," with Congress and EOMB largely doing the administering. Some take bets on how long PPS will last before being "exceptioned" to death, with the most common estimate being about five years (from 1989). Still others say that is the best system available, and that the chief participants—Congress, DHHS, and the hospital associations—know this and will ultimately do what is necessary to preserve it. While the eventual issue remains much in doubt, an examination of the way in which some of the representative and more important implementation issues have been handled will at least give a better sense of the prospects for the future.

During most of the first two years under PPS, until late in 1985, a large part of the activity on the part of the HCFA was devoted to monitoring the early experience and assuring themselves and others that PPS was actually going to work. To that end, much effort went into meetings with FIs and hospitals to explain and sell the system. As part of implementation, a high level committee within the Bureau of Program Operations, chaired by its director, John Berry, met weekly to review reports coming in from the FIs and HCFA regional offices monitoring such key data as numbers of admissions, outlier payments, and experience with high volume DRGs.[33] PROs were given special instructions on admissions. A study was begun to measure real case-mix increase and to develop estimates of legitimate as opposed to inappropriate upcoding. On these accounts, the evidence was reassuring. Admissions were not increasing: they were, in fact, continuing a historic decline. And case-mix increases, though somewhat higher than the expected legitimate upcoding, were not alarmingly so.

Program officials within the HCFA during the early stages of PPS implementation agree that they were worried about excessive admissions, so much so that they largely neglected the so-called "sicker and quicker" issue, the danger that sick, elderly patients would be discharged too early in order to cut length of stay (LOS) and increase revenues. This was an issue seized on by the American Association of Retired Persons (A.A.R.P.) and by Senator John Heinz (R., Pa.) then the chairman of the Senate Special Committee on Aging. The Senator paraded a number of PPS victims before the Committee who recounted their histories, blaming PPS and the PROs—seldom their physicians or the hospitals—for their maltreatment. Eventually the "sicker and quicker" issue produced some protective legislation, but little else of significance. There were a few horror stories and anecdotes, but no widespread pattern of events to back the allegations. When the Republican Party lost control of the Senate after the 1986 elections and Senator Heinz relinquished the chair, the issue subsided.

Another trend that was difficult to audit and potentially of great importance was the shifting of treatment from inpatient to outpatient sites and of claims from Part A to Part B of Medicare. Insofar as this shifting of patients entailed moving from expensive inpatient hospital care to outpatient departments and physicians' offices, it was a desirable trend and an intended effect of PPS. But this development also involved a substantial amount of cost-shifting, double billing, and unbundling, some of it legitimate and some of it illegitimate but difficult to track or estimate accurately. To this day, there persists a serious question of whether PPS has saved money or merely shifted costs to Part B and to the benefici-aries.[34] Moreover, as the rate of increase for Part A expenditures de-clined, that for Part B, for physician expenditures, began to rise rapidly leading to a politically explosive increase in Part B premiums and co-pays. This is not to say that PPS was, by itself, inducing this cost shifting from Part A to Part B, since the reality was more complex, involving changes in physician behavior and long-term trends in the hospital in-dustry that were independent of PPS.[35] Moreover, the HCFA bureau-crats were alert to such problems. As part of the original legislation, they had insisted on a strong unbundling prohibition. They were actively at work on a data system that would facilitate tracking such cost-shifting as well as monitoring episodes of care.[36] But this was a case of a trend moving faster and more powerfully than could be adequately anticipated.

During the first two years of PPS, ProPAC was primarily getting orga-nized and establishing its routines. The first 15 (later 17) Commissioners were appointed by the congressional Office of Technology Assessment late in 1983. They began recruiting a staff shortly thereafter. In some-thing like record time, the Commission and staff were able to begin the cycle of annual reports with its first "Report and Recommendations to the Secretary . . ." on April 1, 1985. This first cycle of reports, with their Technical Appendixes, established ProPAC as an important factor. It also revealed some of the characteristic features that have distinguished its work. Notable among these is the priority given to congressional man-dates or expressed desires. ProPAC has also tended to come down on the side of easing the shoe where it pinches: supporting a lengthened transition, allowances for inner city and rural hospitals, increased outlier payments, etc. From the beginning, though, their reports have been notable for their technical competence, their punctuality, and their use of timely data. Whatever the ultimate judgment may be with respect to the role assigned ProPAC by the Congress, the Commission and its staff have filled that role effectively.

Winning Some and Losing Some

Aside from the process, there is the product, or the general topic of the quality of decisions made in the course of implementing PPS, es-pecially after the first two years. Here, a useful organizing concept is that of a creative tension (sometimes destructive) between technical ra-tionality and local or provider interests. For the different issues that arise—such as urban–rural differentials the various add-ons and exceptions, recalibration, the inclusion of capital or DRG modifiers, and the annual update—this tension gets resolved in different ways, with the rational and system-like properties sometimes winning out and parochial or provider interest prevailing at other times. "What's the trend?" is one important question to be asked: whether the system-like qualities are being preserved or strengthened, or whether PPS is evolving toward an administered price "non-system." Also important, as part of the implementation process, are the ways in which Congress, ProPAC, and the HCFA or DHHS are able to adapt means and ends so that the tension is a creative one, sometimes leading to devised solutions that serve a larger or different conception of rationality, or that adapt effectively to intractable technical or political constraints. There is not one simple account of implementation to be given. For urban and rural issues politics seems to prevail. In other areas, such as DRG recalibration and amendment, technical considerations are more important. Items like "capital" are ambiguous; and the update is in a class by itself.

Urban–Rural Differentials. One of the earliest and most persistent subjects of contention has been that of urban and rural differentials. This issue was one of the first confronted by Congress in the consideration of PPS and the statute itself ended with a number of mandates or delegations to the Secretary to take various additional measures in respect to this subject: such as reviewing the impact of PPS on census divisions, adjusting the wage index, and assessing the feasibility of eliminating the separate urban and rural rates of payment. For the most part, the HCFA chose not to respond or not to pursue these congressional mandates or delegations vigorously. But as early as DEFRA of 1984 (July), Congress began adjusting the wage index by legislation, independently of the Secretary's actions. And one of ProPAC's recommendations in its first "Report and Recommendations to the Secretary . . ." (No. 13, April, 1985) was to establish a differential wage index for the inner cities, arguing that suburban hospitals benefitted disproportionately and inner-city ones suffered with the existing wage index. Since action on this account was within the discretion of the Secretary, the HCFA made no change, responding that it lacked an appropriate methodology and the data to make such an adjustment and that the line-drawing would be likely to create as many problems as it solved. The HCFA also disagreed with ProPAC, arguing that such a differential would further overpay some of the already well-paid urban hospitals, nicely illustrating the difference in approach between the two agencies. Needing little, if any, prompting on this issue, Congress in 1986 mandated a study, directing the Secretary to report by May 1987. The report was finally released by the Secretary on Christmas Eve, 1987, several days after Congress had already legislated a differential for "large urban areas" in the OBRA of 1987.

An issue that was both difficult and disturbing in its implications was that of the disproportionate share hospitals. This category of hospitals had existed prior to PPS and had been "grandfathered" in along with sole community hospitals. But there remained the issue of how to define such hospitals and how to calculate the special allowance under PPS. The statute directs the Secretary to make such "exceptions and allowances" as he or she "deems appropriate" to take into account the "special needs of public or other hospitals" treating a significantly disproportionate number of patients who are low income or who are Medicare beneficiaries. The premise was that such hospitals incurred higher costs because their patients were sicker and because of other factors beyond the control of such hospitals, such as higher labor and security costs, a lack of full paying patients, uncompensated care, and other expenses.

The difficulty with the disproportionate share allowance was that, from the perspective of the HCFA, it seemed either illegal, improper, or incalculable. To the extent that it was a proxy for Medicaid patients or uncompensated care, that was not legally chargeable to Medicare and if Congress intended differently, it should say so in terms by amending the Medicare statute. Moreover, the data did not clearly indicate that low income patients or Medicare patients were measurably more expensive or, if so, by how much. In any event, the case-mix index and the outlier payments make allowance for sicker patients and the urban wage index and the indirect medical education (IME) allowance are proxies for additional expenses encountered by inner city or large teaching hospitals. So, from the perspective of the HCFA, the case had not been made and, in any event, looked like double payment.

The quarrel over the disproportionate share allowance seemed to be a genuine disagreement between the HCFA, that saw no proper way to make such an allowance, and ProPAC and the Congress, who wanted it made. The issue was sharpened in 1984 when a group of hospitals sued the secretary over DSA payments and won.[37] In DEFRA (1984),[38] Congress directed the Secretary to define a disproportionate share hospital and provide a list of qualifying institutions. Eventually, the Secretary did so, and submitted a list of some 50 hospitals, a response that was far from what the Congress had in mind. In some exasperation, Congress wrote its own version of the disproportionate share allowance in COBRA of 1985 and directed CBO to study the issue.[39] Recognizing that the indirect teaching allowance was a proxy for some of the same variables, the disproportionate share allowance was subtracted from that pool so as not to increase the total outlays or pay twice for the same costs. The outcome has seemed generally acceptable. Yet the disproportionate share episode was a significant precedent: for it added a payment justified primarily by the needs of the hospitals and not because of any proven resource use occasioned by treating Medicare patients. It went by hospital need and not by PPS numbers.

The benefits being created for urban hospitals, largely at the insistence of the House, were being matched by an array of special provisions for rural hospitals, almost entirely the work of the Senate. In COBRA, Congress prescribed in detail special payments for sole community hospitals, just as it had written its own formula for the disproportionate share allowance. Soon to follow the latter, moreover, was a rural disproportionate share allowance and a shift to discharge weighting,[40] favoring the smaller hospitals. Also, in 1986, Congress provided for separate rates of outlier payments for urban and rural hospitals, and, in 1987, for differential update factors for urban, big city, and rural areas.

The treatment of regional referral centers was like that of the disproportionate share issue. These referral centers were typically rural or suburban hospitals that had additional expenses because of their need to maintain a range of specialized services and outpatient facilities. They were recognized in the original PPS legislation with a particular reference to "hospitals of 500 beds or more located in rural areas." Under HCFA policy, those hospitals designated as RRCs were paid at higher urban rates. Such a schedule, much higher than the one for rural hospitals, made designation as a referral center important to a number of larger rural hospitals and led them to seek more inclusive policies on the part of the HCFA. From 1984 through 1987, both Congress and the HCFA tinkered with the conditions of eligibility, using such indexes as case-mix, number of discharges, and staff and referral patterns. Although one might query the underlying policy of incrementally adjusting the number of eligibles upward, the criteria employed were consistent with the underlying philosophy of PPS, since they got at the underlying policy question of whether the activities and the economic circumstances of the RRCs were sufficiently like an urban hospital to justify the higher rate. But it was a slow, incremental process and, in truth, often did not reach the hospitals that Senators wanted included. Therefore, in 1987, at the behest of the Senate, Congress passed the "Quayle Amendment," lowering the number of beds requisite for eligibility to 275. Why the specific number, 275? Well might you ask. According to Senate Finance Committee staff, the method and its rationale were simple. When a list of desired hospitals was plotted against number of beds, 275 was the highest figure that would still include the desired hospitals.[41] If anything, this instance of special pleading was even more egregious than that of the disproportionate share allowance, since there was not even the pretense of an appropriate policy—just a desire to benefit the hospitals in the home state.[42]

The urban–rural exceptions and add-ons may seem worse than they are. The statute provided initially for separate urban and rural rates. And specific provisions for inner city and rural hospitals do not, of themselves, prevent PPS from working as a zero-sum system while they may make the rigors of cost containment tolerable. Yet, knowledgeable observers often speak of the danger that PPS will be "exceptioned to death." One point about this kind of incremental process is that it can gradually create more "slack" in the system so that the numerical update and recalibration computations have less and less validity as indications of what payments *ought* to be made. Moreover, as the RRC example illustrates, a lack of scruples about procedures can be a contagious and wasting disease, leading to yet more cynical, log-rolling deals.

Outlier Policy.   There are also ways in which PPS can be "tightened," i.e., made to articulate more precisely and according to the underlying "logic" or methodology of the system. One success story of this kind is outlier policy, where both the HCFA and ProPAC successfully advocated the decreasing of day outliers and moving toward cost outliers.

In the initial Administration proposal, to review some background, the HCFA had been extremely wary of outliers, approaching them somewhat as an apothecary does poison. Less than 1% of the total was allowed for them. The reason was that outliers, as the name indicates, fall outside the system and require a different method of payment, closer to cost-reimbursement. The greater the amount given over to outliers, the less the prospectiveness and the less the "system." Initially, the HCFA proposed that there be only "day" outliers, that is, cases that widely exceeded the normal length of stay. Advantages of this approach were that "days" could be easily counted and would not require the retention of the expensive and cumbersome Medicare Cost Report, as would "cost" outliers. Not surprisingly, these proposals seemed harsh and simplistic to the Congress, that provided for both cost and day outliers and that 5–6% of the total be allotted to outliers.

Except for the 5–6% limit on total payments and a provision for both cost and day outliers, the Congress left specifics up to the Secretary. Following its initial preference for day outliers, the HCFA allotted 85% of the pool to day outliers and 15% to cost. This division proved to be unsatisfactory. It underpaid hospitals that had short stays but costly patients. It overpaid some hospitals with long-stay patients, for instance, alcoholics or people needing skilled nursing facilities (SNFs), who might not be very sick but needed a place to stay. And it resulted in very unequal payments as between categories of hospitals and different regions of the country.[43] About the only justification for the existing method was that it provided another subsidy for urban, disproportionate share, and public hospitals. Here was an instance in which both interest and virtue coincided, and the HCFA, ProPAC, and the Congress all supported a move toward cost outliers.[44] This adjustment was made in the Secretary's final rule, changing the thresholds and payment formulas for FY 1989 so that roughly half the outliers would be paid as "cost" rather than 15% as before. It would be too much to say that tightening the system was the primary motivation. But it was a consequence. And the change was itself a result of seeing how the numbers played out and seeking a correction of the outlier policy that conformed to the underlying principles of PPS.

DRG Amendment and Recalibration.   Another success story has been the way in which DRG recalibration and amendment[45] have been implemented. For this success, though, little credit belongs to the original Administration proposal or the statute itself, both of which dealt with these issues casually and almost as afterthoughts. As for DRG amendment, procedures were left implicit and little was said about either the priorities or objectives that should guide the HCFA or ProPAC in amending the DRGs or recognizing new ones. Both the Secretary and the Commission were directed to "collect and assess factual information" and make "recommendations on relative weighting factors . . . to reflect appropriate differences in resource consumption in delivering safe, efficacious, and cost effective care." Beyond this, ProPAC was charged with "evaluating scientific evidence" with respect to new treatment modalities and technologies and making recommendations to the Secretary and the Congress. Much is left to the imagination and to discretion, especially about how responsive to be in recognizing new, state-of-the-art medical technologies or experimental therapies, and how to sort the differences between HCFA and ProPAC. Nevertheless, beginning with these vague statutory mandates, the HCFA, ProPAC, and the Congress have improvised a workable system that has produced generally good results, in the absence of any clear mandate or underlying philosophy in the statute itself.

PPS, with its employment of DRGs, represented a drastic change in payment policies for new therapies and medical technologies because it left such decisions initially up to the physicians and hospitals.[46] Under cost reimbursement, the HCFA decided whether a new drug or technology was covered and what the Medicare reimbursement would be. In contrast, DRGs bundle hospital services and pay a flat amount for the hospital admission rather than for the separate billable items. Therefore, it is up to the physicians and hospital administrators to decide on the use of expensive new therapies or technology incident to the hospital stay. For instance, hospitals adopt lithotrypsy[47] to treat kidney stones. In this case, the hospital will be using advanced technology and will be treating their patients in a less invasive way and with a lower probability of complications. The hospitals will also make money by saving on LOS and ancillaries. On the other hand, some high cost technology or treatment procedures do not pay for themselves: for instance, lengthy inpatient cancer therapy or magnetic resonance imaging. Here, the hospital is at risk. Progressive hospitals can adopt new methods—because they have a mission to give care of the highest quality, to beat out the competition, or to avoid malpractice suits—but added payment depends on getting a higher DRG weight assigned.

The distinction between DRG amendment and DRG recalibration is especially important with respect to technological innovation or substitution of new technology for other factor inputs. For instance, a hospital may decide to initiate magnetic resonance imaging or some very expensive treatment such as total parenteral nutrition. *If* the great majority of hospitals quickly adopt the new method of treatment *and* the data are quickly assembled and evaluated *and* recalibration takes place quickly, the hospital will make out reasonably well, except that the additional payment is delayed and may include a number of other factors folded into the new DRG weight. DRG amendment, on the other hand, is not only money up front, it is specifically payment for the additional resource use occasioned by the new technology or therapy. Understandably, health care providers and manufacturers of medical supplies and equipment care about this difference. And the pressure on the HCFA and ProPAC for DRG amendment is intense and persistent, including lobbying and PR campaigns on a scale usually associated with new breakfast cereals or weapons systems.

DRG amendment brings up one of the most difficult and persistent questions vexing American medicine generally and Medicare in particular: what priority to put on the ultimate in life-saving or life-enhancing technologies and how to enforce these priorities once determined. The statute speaks of "efficacious and cost effective care," charging ProPAC with "evaluation of scientific evidence." The problem, of course, is that our information base and methods for determining what is efficacious or cost effective and what are the trade-offs between them are crude and fragmentary. We know, for instance, that a dual chamber pacemaker works, but is it enough better than a single chamber one to warrant a DRG amendment?[48] Various kinds of plastic surgery are life-enhancing, but should Medicare pay for them? Should heart or liver transplants be generally available, despite the prognosis for the future life chances of the individual patient? For years, with cost-reimbursement such issues were buried under bureaucratic routine, but PPS has brought them into the open, and made them visible and topics for public debate. But how to resolve the basic question of what to pay for? The informally stated policy of both the HCFA and ProPAC is that DRGs should neither inhibit nor encourage the diffusion of technology. This formulation begs at least one question, of how "diffused" technology ought to be. If a dozen elite teaching hospitals make implantable defibrillators available to Medicare patients, should that DRG be amended to include this add-on? On the other hand, do 90% of hospitals have to adopt coronary angioplasty for that procedure to be recognized? One extreme would give away the whole store to a few high-tech hospitals; the other would penalize hospitals and deprive Medicare patients of quality care.[49]

Listed below are some of the major DRG reviews for the year 1987. Generally, the options are further study, reassignment,[50] a temporary DRG, amending the DRG, or a new DRG.

Benign prostatic hypertrophy
Cardiac pacemaker
Chronic obstructive pulmonary
    disease
Cystic fibrosis
Endocardial electrical stimulation
Heart transplantation
Implantable defibrillator
Inflatable penile prosthesis
Magnetic resonance imaging
Spinal cord injury
Total parenteral nutrition

Burns
Catheterization for myocardial
    infarction
Cochlear implantation
Dermatological disorders
End stage renal disease
Hemophilia
Inflammatory bowel disease
Lymphomas and leukemias
Malignant external otitis media
Tissue plasminogen activator

The list serves to illustrate the range of topics and how difficult the technical and policy aspects of decision-making are likely to be. Consider the complexities of trying to decide with respect to magnetic resonance imaging, for instance, its contribution to other Medicare DRGs, its cost-effectiveness relative to similar procedures such as CAT scans, inpatient versus outpatient utilization and costs, the rate of diffusion of this technology, the life-cycle of the equipment, the rate of entry of competing manufacturers, the probable rate of decline in unit costs for individual scans, and the best way of amending the DRG to achieve desired policy objectives. To be sure, the HCFA and ProPAC can avail themselves of expert testimony and consultants as well as the technology assessment capabilities of various governmental entities.[51] Also, with respect to medical technology, as with weapons systems, the word is out and there is a lot of technical lore (and scuttlebutt) on the street and in the scientific and trade journals. Still, the data and technical difficulties are enormous and on many new procedures or technologies, experts are often flatly opposed. As with much of government decision-making, the remarkable (and sometimes inexplicable) fact is that we often do well, notwithstanding.

As might be expected, ProPAC has generally been sympathetic to pleas for DRG amendment and the HCFA has been less so. Within the HCFA, there is a stronger priority put on prospectivity, and, consequently, a desire to stand by the existing rate, at least until recalibration. In BERC, where such decisions are initially made, program officials can also see pretty directly within this zero-sum system what the effects of amendment will be for other DRG weights and, derivatively, for other procedures. Therefore, the HCFA is doubly reluctant to change and likely to deny an amendment, argue for more evidence or evaluation, or compromise with a reassignment. ProPAC not only hears especially from the hospital industry but is charged by the statute with giving particular attention to new technology and needs for updating the DRG classifications and weights. Accordingly, ProPAC usually takes a lead in proposing a new or amended DRG or, as a less drastic alternative, a "temporary" DRG, a reassignment, or a reevaluation. Typically, the HCFA will refuse initially to go along, but will later relent, either as evidence accumulates or the technology diffuses more widely. Occasionally, Congress will intervene on particularly visible and expensive procedures, such as liver transplants or burn treatment. In practice, this procedure seems to work well. The HCFA's slowness acts as something of a brake on profligate hospitals. Yet ProPAC provides a useful theater for publicly airing the issues and for focusing attention on some big-ticket or precedent setting items. Both the outcome and the method seem to be rational.

A good example of the process at work was provided by the controversy over TPA[52] or Activase. TPA is a powerful thrombolytic agent, especially useful in preventing recurrences of a heart attack in the critical early hours immediately after the initial episode. It was produced by Genentech, the California "gene-splicing" firm. Genentech had not been especially successful with its other ventures and was looking hard for a big winner. TPA seemed to be that winner. Accordingly, it was hurried along through clinical trials and vigorously promoted in trade journal advertisements, with glossy and expensive information kits, and through sponsored, expenses-paid conferences of leading cardiologists.[53] Experts readily agreed that the drug was good, especially for the first 24 hours after a heart attack. But it was also expensive: $2000 for a treatment, with four or more treatments likely to be the norm. Furthermore, a close substitute, streptochinase, cost $200 or less, one-tenth as much. There was evidence that streptochinase plus aspirin might be just as effective as TPA. On the other hand, TPA was a gene-spliced, state-of-the-art drug and there were indications and much argument that it was more effective in the critical 24 hours after an attack. Furthermore, physicians were prescribing it and hospitals were reluctant to oppose them or to incur the malpractice liability if patients should die without it.

Under these circumstances, the media campaign and the lobbying for a DRG amendment were vigorous. The HCFA predictably took a conservative line: that the superiority of TPA over streptochinase was not proven and that hospitals that wished to be on the leading edge of technological innovation could absorb the expense and await a DRG recalibration. But hospitals, whatever their wishes about being first in the high-tech honors, were losing money because of TPA. Understandably, they saw this position taken by the HCFA as harsh; and ProPAC agreed with them. The Commission recommended an additional allowance, to be put into the discretionary adjustment factor (DAF), the logic of this being that TPA was an expense for new technology, but one that hospitals might well offset by economizing on nursing or other ancillaries. Neither the hospital industry nor the Genentech stockholders were happy with these decisions. About this time, additional findings reported in *Lancet*, the prestigious British medical journal, indicated that streptochinase with aspirin was as effective as TPA. This development destroyed much of the momentum of the TPA campaign, with the eventual result that the HCFA decision stuck.

The moral of this brief anecdote is not that there was or is a right decision. In retrospect, perhaps the HCFA had the better of this one. But the ProPAC solution was perfectly reasonable under the circumstances. The point is that the process is a good one for decision-making under conditions of complexity, uncertainty about the future, and fragmentary technical information. The TPA episode also shows how the contributions of *both* the HCFA and ProPAC can be valuable in assessing a complex issue and assigning an appropriate weight to the competing alternatives.

Recalibration is also a procedure for which details were left to subsequent implementation. When developing the initial Administration proposal, staff within the HCFA and DHHS were aware that updating, including recalibration, would create political controversy and so they approached it warily (Oday unpublished, 40). A number of options were considered, the final recommendation being that the Secretary appoint an in-house commission, whose advice could be taken or not. In the Congress, there were different views. In principle, Congress accepted the notion that the Secretary should have substantial discretion in implementing PPS and yet Congress created ProPAC, entrusting important advisory and monitoring activities to it, and legislated in detail with respect to some aspects of implementation. But recalibration was not among them. Here, the legislation provided, in general terms, that the Secretary should adjust the "classifications and weightings . . . for discharges in fiscal year 1986 and at least every four years thereafter."[54]

As previously noted, recalibration is a process by which DRG weights are reassigned for the whole array of DRGs to reflect changes in resource use for some DRGs or the inclusion of new or amended ones. If the DRGs associated with diabetes, for instance, involve longer or shorter lengths of stay or a different resource use over time, that difference will be reflected in new DRG weights that will affect all the other DRG weights, after the recalibration. Therefore, frequent recalibration is important to the hospitals, especially those where the technology or patient mix may be changing. The process was not intended to be strictly budget-neutral, since an allowance was made for "real case-mix change," for site substitution, and for technological advances, which can either increase or decrease relative weights.[55] In fact, the case-mix index for *all* PPS hospitals has increased about 3.2% a year, reaching 1.319 in 1989.[56] An important point, though, is that recalibration has always been zero-sum: the weights are "normalized" so that the sum of the parts does not increase. In other words, what one hospital gains another loses. Furthermore, the newly assigned rates form the basis for computing the individual hospital's case-mix index, which is one of the multipliers, along with the area wage index, in the computation of the ultimate payment. So recalibration is important for setting a prospective rate, but it also involves large amounts of money for individual hospitals and produces large annual redistributions of hospital income.

From one perspective, recalibration would seem to be an instance of PPS working as designed and near to perfection. The actual calculations, based on Medicare charge data, are made within the HCFA. Newly assigned DRG weights are announced, along with provider case-mix and area wage indexes in the Spring proposed rule. In the process of recalibration and assigning new case-mix indexes, the HCFA develops estimates of "real" case-mix change, making allowance for that part attributable to "code creep" and technical changes, such as new Grouper modifications. As originally intended, PPS sets a zero-sum prospective rate calculated to distribute total payments according to the resource experience within a DRG category and pay the hospitals for its typical or average experience through a revised case-mix index.

The recalibration process is sufficiently neutral and automatic that ProPAC and Congress have usually had little to say about it. The Commission proposed and the Congress mandated an annual recalibration, to keep pace with the dynamic evolution of the industry.[57] The Commission has strongly and repeatedly urged a shift from charges to costs, especially because of its conviction that the use of charges overpays the new and glamorous procedures and the high-rollers of the hospital industry, and that it contributes to big annual swings in payments. DHHS and the HCFA have expressed some agreement in principle but pleaded work-load and the trade-offs between timeliness of data and what it measures. ProPAC and the HCFA have also argued over whether the DAF (or PTAF) should reflect patient complexity (e.g., sicker) in calculating the allowance for case-mix change. In general, these would seem to be the kind of amiable disagreements one would expect, between the Commission that generally worries a bit more about equity for different hospitals and the HCFA that tends to favor prospectivity and efficiency incentives and that also has to develop the regulations and process the data.

Yet recalibration provides a good example of how automatic calculations, made year-by-year, can generate basic policy issues. In essence, recalibration came to be increasingly important in redistributing payments to hospitals. The annual update, which provided for overall urban and rural increases, was intended to be the main way in which payments would be changed. But as Congress took more and more out of the update, recalibration and the annual wage index, along with various other categorical add-ons assumed a greater importance. At the same time, the case-mix of hospitals was changing, mostly increasing, as patients were discharged sooner or treated on an outpatient basis, and as capital and labor costs increased. By 1987–1988, these two developments had considerably sharpened the unresolved tension in PPS between prospectiveness and fairness.

Confronted with this kind of development, one kind of thinking, close to the original conception of PPS, would say, "So, what?" The system was intended to reward those who respond quickly and effectively to the new environment and incentives, even though some hospitals do well while others languish or even shut their doors. The other argument, especially from ProPAC and favored in Congress, would say that hospitals should be made to suffer only for acts within their control and, especially important in the immediate context, not penalized by formulas that do not accurately represent appropriate resource use. The system is full of proxies and add-ons benefiting different categories, some analytically justified and others not. So, if hospitals are being squeezed until it really hurts, it is increasingly important that distributions through automatic, zero-sum calculations be accurate and fair. So, ProPAC has argued insistently for cost-based recalibration, more timely data, and increased use of the Medicare Cost Report. All of this makes a lot of sense, given the way in which PPS has been implemented, but it also represents a substantial change in emphasis, moving the system closer to an earlier system of cost-reimbursement.

Recalibration did provoke one political episode that may be a significant portent for the future. This had to do with the overall lowering of DRG rates in 1989. Because of the kind of evolutionary developments just described, DRG weights and hospital case-mix indexes tend to go up so that a periodic correction is appropriate. The HCFA had considered changing these overall weights retroactively in FY 1988, but decided that it would be fairer to do it prospectively in FY 1990. Unfortunately, this perfectly sensible measure fell afoul of the reconciliation process. Congress needed the $500 million involved to put toward its own budget savings. And so it took credit for itself in OBRA 1989 by directing the Secretary to make the reduction, that is, making it a matter of legislation. Subsequent recalibrations were to be made in a budget-neutral fashion, which had the effect of removing future discretion from the Secretary. Congress specified further that the Secretary include recommendations with respect to future recalibrations in the *Annual Report*, making it easy for Congress to include any potential savings in the update.

These changes may or may not have a lasting impact on recalibration, depending on what the Congress does in the future. Nevertheless, they are an example of how one of the relatively automatic, computational elements of the payment formula got moved to the political agenda. Such a precedent could be important for other indexes, such as the Area Wage Index, or a formula for including capital. A step of this kind has, furthermore, a self-defeating quality in that it makes even more essential some of the improvements in PPS methodology that could reassure the provider community[58] at the same time that it takes discretion from the Secretary and the HCFA, important for developing such measures.

Capital and DRGs. Given the changed political environment in which PPS has been implemented, major improvements in the methodology have proven difficult to achieve. One piece of unfinished business left over from the original passage of the legislation was the inclusion of capital payments in PPS. Despite repeated attempts, it is still unfinished business, and provides an illustration of how technical and political difficulties can work together to defeat a regulatory enterprise—at least until recently, when both ProPAC and the HCFA have taken up the issue of capital with renewed determination.

Neither hospital capital nor return on equity (RoE) was among the more contentious issues, either during the consideration of the legislation or later. In the aggregate, capital costs amounted to only 7–9%

(currently 10%) of Medicare payments to DRG hospitals, so that the absolute dollar amounts were not great. At the same time, they figured among the "add-ons" and "pass-throughs" of PPS, that could be in the aggregate a large item for some hospitals. Moreover, in principle, it would seem that capital *ought* to be included within the DRG methodology, not only to make it a "tighter" system, but also to build in additional incentives for economy and managerial efficiency.

Certainly, the original intentions were to include capital in PPS, though without anyone quite knowing how this could be achieved. As far as the HCFA architects of PPS were concerned, they recognized early on that there was no simple and equitable way to achieve this, at least at the time (Oday unpublished, 37). But, clearly, they hoped to do so. Within Congress, the House and the Senate differed in their philosophical approaches to capital, but both indicated a desire for eventual inclusion. The House wrote into PPS a so-called "1122 trigger" that provided for a reversion to the old Sec. 1122 capital planning requirements (established by the 1972 Amendments) unless a PPS capital payment mechanism was in place by September 1, 1986. The Senate, for its part, mandated a report with an 18 month deadline, calling on the Secretary to propose a method for dealing with "capital related costs" including return on equity.

Not surprisingly, neither of these deadlines had much practical significance. The "1122 trigger" was postponed and eventually repealed. And by the time that the Secretary's report on capital was eventually released, even though the report was quite sensible, it was pretty much irrelevant since Congress had by then developed its own way of dealing with the issue. This outcome was not the result of any lack of research or of good faith efforts, since capital payment was a popular topic in 1986 and 1987, producing research and reports on the part of the HCFA, ASPE, the OTA, ProPAC, and the hospital industry. More than a lack of effort, it was a case illustrating the difficulty, within the American political system, of achieving technical rationality and equity at the same time, particularly given the turbulence created by budget cycles, separation of powers, and interest group politics. A *pro tempore* resolution was eventually achieved, one that was fair and sensible, but at odds with the technical methodology of PPS.

The major difficulty has been about the kind of payment provisions to make. This had two aspects. One was providing for a transition, especially important for hospitals that had just made or might be planning major capital investments in the near future and, as well, for hospitals that had already largely depreciated existing capital.[59] While this issue was not obviously that difficult, it cut across types of hospitals in a way calculated to raise particularistic and parochial concerns to a high pitch.

It also got into arcane issues of capital cycles, relations between fixed and movable capital, and likely effects on the behavior of hospital managers. The other aspect of payment was how to fold capital into the individual DRGs: whether as an "index" like the wage index, which would simply be a multiplier of existing DRG weights; by calculating the capital intensity for specific DRGs; or simply by recalibration as the resource use for individual DRGs increased. With any one of these options, there would be a further question of what to do about the distinction between fixed and movable capital, an especially tough question not only because of the conceptual difficulty of devising an adequate and acceptable definition of these concepts, but also because of the cost-shifting incentives the distinction might create. In any event, each of these alternatives seemed to be lacking in an important way. To make capital simply a percentage add-on, for instance, would underpay capital intensive DRGs and might retard the introduction of life-saving technology. The recalibration option was undesirable for the same reason. But creating new weights based on the intensity of capital use for each DRG would prove administratively complex and burdensome to a degree. The hospital industry, for its part, favored the existing capital "pass through" (i.e., cost-reimbursement) since this represented for them a degree of freedom and some relaxation from the rigors of PPS. Not surprisingly, the industry made much of the conceptual or practical difficulties of other alternatives.

Capital looked like an issue that might well have taken forever, especially because it was technical, divisive, and had few political actors who cared much about it. Its political salience declined even more after the 1986 elections when Senator Durenberger (R., Minn.) lost the chairmanship of the Senate Finance Health Subcommittee. At about that time, however, budgetary politics intervened to accelerate the tempo of events. Early in 1986, the HCFA, acting on an EOMB passback, proposed a rule implementing changes in capital payment. These proposed changes were drastic and immediately stirred alarm in the hospital industry. Partly at the behest of industry spokesmen, but also in reaction to this flagrant bit of executive branch *hubris,* Congress interceded to block the rule. Congress, for its part, was of various minds about the capital issue. For one item, few within Congress or elsewhere saw any quick and elegant solution for the technical issues relating to hospital capital. At that time, especially with Gramm–Rudman, Congress had an interest in further Medicare budget reductions and ensuring that they, and not the executive branch, got the credit. Some members, losing a measure of patience, sought a way to "bring the hospitals to the table," that is, get the industry into a receptive mood and perhaps dispose its representatives to come up with proposals acceptable both to them and to the Congress. Accordingly in OBRA, 1986[60] Congress simply mandated annual across-the-board cuts in capital payments for DRG hospitals beginning at 3.5% in 1987 and rising to 7% in 1988 and 10% in 1987. And, liking this approach and hearing no serious capital proposals from the industry, Congress went further in 1987, setting new limits of 12% for 1988 and 15% for 1989, and prohibiting the Secretary from implementing any general rule in this area until expiration of that term.[61]

This way of resolving the question of hospital capital payments has been termed "rough justice":[62] that is, not technically warranted by the DRG methodology and not deriving from any economic calculation of horizontal or vertical equity but perhaps sensible and fair enough under the circumstances. As previously noted, the capital issue was technically difficult and lacked strong political thrust toward a solution. Therefore, the percentage cuts. The hospital industry, rather than responding with proposals of its own, preferred to absorb these increasing cuts. And Congress—even ProPAC—came to regard what amounted to a co-pay on capital investment as a tolerable solution, at least for the time being.[63] Given the circumstances, there would seem to be a rough justice in the outcome.

There was also a crude rationality in the compromise, inducing some attention to cost-effective behavior without unduly penalizing capital expenditures. At the same time, this result was fortuitous and came about not through intention but largely as an expedient: as a way out of technical difficulty and a response to the exogenous politics of the budget. It surrendered technical high ground to politics.

But there was one more development with respect to hospital capital expenditures, showing the importance of having tools for rational calculation and control ready for use in favorable situations. Neither the Congress, nor the HCFA, nor ProPAC gave up on the capital issue. OBRA 1987, that had initiated the method of "rough justice," also directed the Secretary to come up with a plan for inclusion of capital in PPS by FY 1992. Congress persisted with its across-the-board cuts each year, but expressed continuing interest in capital. ProPAC developed its own proposal. Then, in 1991, the HCFA, building on earlier efforts, proposed a solution of elegant simplicity that met earlier objections and provided a coherent method for including capital in the payment system.

The essence of the HCFA scheme was a compromise between vested interest and prospectiveness. Old capital would be protected by a 10-year transition. New capital would be paid on the basis of a national average FY 1992 capital cost per discharge, adjusted for case-mix, outliers, geographic location, and low-income patients.[64] During the transition, a "hold harmless" clause would allow hospitals with capital costs above the national average to make a one-time choice between the new federal rate or a blend, based on the transition schedule, of the federal rate and their own hospital-specific one. The HCFA scheme would mitigate hardship while encouraging the cost-effective use of capital. It would give the HCFA and the Congress leverage to control capital expenditure and yet would be consistent with and even strengthen the PPS methodology. It seemed to please every major party, except for the hospital associations, still attached to the capital pass-through, even in its rough-hewn condition.

For the faithful, these recent developments are a preferable way of achieving closure, bringing together a rational design, an additional provider incentive for efficiency, and an additional constraint on costs. A final rule from the HCFA is scheduled for October, 1991. On the merits, the HCFA proposal should succeed. It got both endorsement and praise from ProPAC.[65] This year, moreover, Congress seems disposed to act.

Improving DRGs. Another long-standing concern, and one that has had particular appeal to technicians and outside academic researchers, is whether to add some kind of modifier or adjuster to the DRGs that could improve their predictive capacity, especially for high-variation DRGs that are associated, for instance, with a severe illness or exceptional intensity of care. To recall some history, when PPS was enacted only the Yale group's DRG methodology had been extensively investigated and was ready for use. At that time, there were other approaches being studied that might serve to refine DRGs so as to make them better predictors of resource use, essentially by differentiating types of patients coming under a particular DRG as "sicker" or requiring greater resource use.

Improving DRGs is important, moreover, since quite apart from the outliers, the measure in which individual DRG weights predict resource use for specific diagnoses or procedures[66] can vary quite a bit. For an inpatient lens implantation, for instance, resource use is much the same for the overwhelming number of cases. For other DRGs, such as heart failure or a malignancy, the resource use can vary widely, so that, quite apart from outliers, the particular DRG will overpay or underpay a large number of cases and predict only a small part of the variance in resource use. By one kind of logic, a hospital's cost experience will average out *across* DRGs, so that with many different DRGs, winners offset losers. Aside from that fact that this approach treats hospitals like gambling casinos, it will not work for hospitals that treat a small number of patients (for instance, rural hospitals) or for those that have large numbers of patients within a *set* of high-variation DRGs (e.g., some public or inner-city hospitals). Furthermore, the hospitals themselves, pursuing the incentive structure for this system, can "specialize" in destructive ways, that is, to turn away or transfer patients likely to occasion excessive amounts of resource use.

A workable system of "patient classification" or a severity or intensity index appeals not only on grounds of economy and equity, because it would pay hospitals more accurately and fairly, but for technical reasons as well. For an item, it would help hospital managers to achieve cost-effective resource management, one of the original purposes of DRGs.[67] In addition, establishing such an index would be another way, much like a formula for capital, in which PPS could be tightened and made more precise, reducing the importance of various add-ons like the disproportionate share allowance and the indirect teaching adjustment. It might even, as Larry Oday has argued, reduce the incentives for hospitals to go to Congress to seek relief.[68]

Research on this topic has continued, with vigorous support from the HCFA. But there is also much accompanying skepticism. Some are concerned that SOIs or similar refinements will move PPS back in the direction of cost-reimbursement, minimizing the element of risk originally seen as important for changing the behavior of hospital managers. Others question whether some of the modifiers, like SOIs, would indeed contribute substantially to fairer payment and believe that they might even make matters worse.[69] And there is the further question of expense, since an index that could predict accurately and reliably would almost certainly require a number of additional variables and occasion substantial implementation costs.

One proposal that received a good bit of attention recently came, via the HCFA, from the Yale group itself. This would have involved increasing the number of DRGs, i.e., from its original 477 to more than double that amount. Simulations have shown that doubling the number of DRGs would increase their predictive capacity substantially. This approach has a further advantage that it could use existing "CCs" (complications and comorbidities) and codes. Yet ProPAC and others doubt that they would represent enough improvement to justify the political costs. PPS, as it has developed and now stands, has built into it, or onto it, many adjustments and proxies that would be affected, requiring a number of additional "fixes," so that the entire system would need redoing. Stuart Altman was frank to say, for one, that he doubted that there was political support for such a change, a view shared by others.[70]

Nevertheless, both the HCFA and ProPAC continue to work on DRG refinements. The latest prospect is a Grouper methodology developed by New York State, which involves a redefinition of specific DRGs rather than splitting them or adding modifiers. Since the New York system applies to the general population, it would require adaptation for Medicare.[71] But it adds predictive power to the DRGs without being as re-distributive and as politically upsetting as some other alternatives. So, this approach could represent the successful fulfillment of an important and long-standing charge to the HCFA and ProPAC. Yet it should not escape notice that one requisite for its success is that it would adjust or fine-tune an existing methodology without changing it in a way that would upset established routine or settled expectations.

Whether or not these attempts at DRG refinement prove successful, they illustrate ways in which PPS can be strengthened as a *system*. There is a continuing dialectic of rationality and politics, illustrated by the urban–rural issue and the various "fixes" for providers, on the one hand, and DRG refinement, recalibration, and amendment, on the other, in which ProPAC and the HCFA lose some, but there are other episodes in which the numbers and analysis are decisive or in which they significantly modify the outcomes.

Annual Update Factor. For all its technical rationality, PPS is a system that distributes the bulk of Medicare dollars, so that it inevitably gets swept into the politics of the budget, the reconciliation process, and, on occasion, confrontations between the Congress and the Administration. It is an integral part of a fierce struggle over allocations that repeatedly threatens to overwhelm the regulatory process or compromise its integrity. In this highly charged, political environment the most visible object of contention is the annual update factor. This is the percentage increase in the whole amount of DRG payments and, therefore, from the perspective of the hospitals, a vitally important number that largely determines the size of their annual margins. And for Congress and EOMB, this is where the budget savings are, especially since the really big entitlement in human services, Social Security, is "off the table," not to be considered. As a consequence, the annual update is a major area of controversy for the hospital industry, for the HCFA, the Congress, and the Executive Office of Management and Budget.

In the original legislation, the annual update received a considerable amount of attention and was one of the more elaborately crafted provisions in the bill. Ultimately, according to the statute the Secretary decides, but the intention was that the annual update would be largely a computed figure, based on the "hospital market basket," wage-related costs, case-mix changes, site substitution, and technological developments, with the recommendations of ProPAC providing some additional expert opinion. In fact, elaborate computations do go on within the HCFA and ProPAC, with each body calculating the various indexes and ultimate figures. But these computations bear little relation to the final update, which is a matter of high-level political intervention on the part of EOMB and two key committees of Congress, Senate Finance and the House Ways and Means. In other words, what was to have been a non-political, technical decision that followed the numbers has become highly politicized.

One of the major factors in politicizing the update factor has been the need for budget and deficit reduction, a driving motivation that became important even during the first two years of PPS when it was "budget neutral" with respect to TEFRA and the update set at "market basket plus 1%." Notwithstanding these provisions, Congress reduced the update to "market basket plus ¼%" in the Deficit Reduction Act of 1984 (DEFRA). Gramm–Rudman, late in 1985, gave additional sanction to this process by targeting Medicare as one of the candidates for sequestration, but this was a sanction hardly needed. From 1984 on and despite the statutory provision that the Secretary "shall determine" the update, Congress has each year since then determined this figure itself usually in the annual budget-reconciliation process.

A second important political influence was EOMB, that regularly passed back to the Secretary recommended figures for further reductions in the budget estimates before their submission to Congress. Within EOMB, according to a former Program Assistant Director,[72] their priority was "deficit-reduction and cooking money out anyway we could. . . . We would have taken anything, including atomic warfare to wipe out every other hospital." Since they learned that Congress would add 1% or 1.5% to anything they proposed, he added, they did the update with that in mind. With good reason, Congress believed that EOMB's top priority was budget reduction whether or not the hospitals or the Medicare program suffered. They also knew that the Secretary's figures did not represent the Department's best judgment since they were largely dictated by EOMB. Unavoidably, the update factor was a politically determined figure, and knowledge of this led Congress to distrust EOMB and give more weight to ProPAC's recommendations and its own priorities.

The legitimacy and weight of technically based recommendations for the update factor were also compromised by revelations of PPS overpayment and hospital margins, both of which turned out to be quite large. Far from PPS being "tight," it looked pretty sloppy, with dollars sloshing about from region to region and margins of 15 to 17% being earned by the hospitals. Since the news broke dramatically with a report by the Inspector General of DHSS late in 1985, it coincided with a period of intense concern about the deficit, and added force to arguments for paring the update.[73]

From the perspective of Congress, action was needed and it had to come from them. It was a time of "no new taxes" and a persistent domestic deficit. Congress distrusted EOMB and regarded Secretary

Heckler as ineffectual. At the same time, their own push for deficit reduction was strong, with the ardor of a new enthusiasm. Under these circumstances, Medicare hospitals, with their suspiciously large two-year margins and huge aggregate payments seemed almost chosen by Providence, and Congress set about the task using the tools that lay at hand.

The annual update was the method written into the statute as well as the most direct and efficient way to save large amounts of money. Congress began to move more aggressively with respect to the update factor, cutting it below the hospital market basket rate of inflation for the first time in the OBRA of 1986 (Figure 3.1). This policy was continued for the next two years, squeezing large amounts out of the Part A expenditures and gradually decreasing the hospital surpluses and operating margins. But as Congress ratcheted down on the update, these reductions affected hospitals differently, so that some were really in distress. To remedy this situation, techniques developed to ease the pinch for hospitals in particular districts or states: such as special rates for rural and big-city hospitals, tinkering with payment periods and wage indexes, and establishing special floors and ceilings, mysterious to the layman, but effective in delivering dollars to particular states or districts. With these practices added to the urban–rural swapping already in

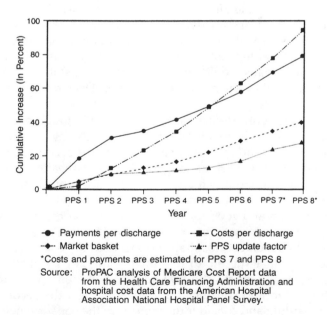

Figure 3-1. Cumulative Increases in PPS Costs and Payments Per Discharge, First Eight Years of PPS (In Percent)

vogue, what was rapidly emerging was a system of unacknowledged but quite brisk log-rolling, with hospital payments as governmental largesse rather than dams or military installations.

OBRA 1987 represented a breakthrough, or perhaps a breakdown, in the updating process, in part because of the crassness with which the log-rolling was pursued and because of the recognition, for the first time, of a three-tiered update: one for rural hospitals, one for urban; and one for the "large urban," i.e., core-city hospitals. Otherwise, OBRA 1987 continued an incremental, evolutionary process. Compared to the first years of PPS, though, it was like playing Wagner rather than Mozart: many more instruments and much more extravagant. Indeed, the comparison with an orchestra makes sense, for Congress began using pretty much every instrument available: tinkering with the DSA and the classifications of Regional Referral Centers and Sole Community Hospitals, reducing the capital allowance and the indirect teaching allowance, specifying the DRG weighting factor and the wage index methodology, abolishing forests and "deeming" hospitals to be in different counties, and so forth.

These developments were deplored both within Congress and within the health care constituency, with knowledgeable observers making dire predictions about the "regionalism," "micro-management," and exceptions on exceptions that threatened PPS as a viable system. Staff people in the HCFA and on the Hill were increasingly pessimistic about PPS, some saying that it was already no more than an "administered price system," with Congress largely controlling its administration. There was a cynical game invented called "guess the hospital," in which professionals and technicians would try to infer from the statutory specifications which hospital in which county had been selected for governmental largess.

One interesting counter-strategy was a "nice guy, tough guy" routine developed within the hospital industry. The "nice guy" approach was taken by Jack Owen and the American Hospital Association, arguing to Congress that PPS was itself endangered by this unhealthy business of lowering the update too much and then easing the pinch with special exceptions. The remedy, of course, was a more generous annual update, fair to the hospitals and good for PPS. This tactic was complemented by the "tough guy" approach of the Catholic Health Association, that mailed each of its member hospitals a computer tape enabling that hospital to develop data specific to it, showing the impact of PPS within their congressional district. The first approach invited the Congress to take the high road and consider the public interest; the second, to be more self-regarding and consider the welfare of the constituency and his or her own electoral prospects. Whatever may be the eventual result of this recent experience, there are indications that the HCFA and ProPAC are acutely aware of the dangers and that some members of Congress and their staff share this concern. To what extent the process can be reversed remains to be seen.

During 1988, a rancorous and inconclusive dispute about hospital margins reached a critical stage. The argument, so far as the facts were concerned, was inconclusive because of differences about how margins were defined and what the data actually showed. But however defined, margins were dropping, with more than half of the hospitals in the country losing money. A record number closed in 1988.[74] And the quarrels over this issue were leading to confrontations with the hospital industry that most policymakers wanted to avoid. There were angry public disputes between Representative Stark of the Ways and Means Health Subcommittee and Carol McCarthy, the new President of the American Hospital Association.[75] A group of 417 hospitals with large numbers of Medicare patients formed an Association of High Medicare Hospitals (AHMH) to lobby for additional payments; and other hospitals alleged that continuing underpayment of Medicare would inevitably lead to a two-tier system of patient care. Early in 1989, the American Hospital Association began a lobbying offensive in Congress, securing 257 signatures to a petition to block additional Medicare cuts. At the time, no one knew what the limits for PPS reductions were; but portents like these gave a clear indication that they were being rapidly approached.

Congress can retreat from the brink, however, as well as approach it. The motivation was complex, involving judgments about technical issues and beneficiary access as well as politics,[76] but ProPAC and Congress did respond, in a measure, to the hospitals' distress and their lobbying. OBRA 1989 eased the ratcheting-down process, making substantial concessions especially for hard-pressed rural and inner-city hospitals.[77] Part B, the physician payments, had to absorb two-thirds of the cuts in dollar amounts, even though representing only one-third of the Medicare program costs. According to one observer, most of this amounted to little more than targeting dollars at needy hospitals with little analytical justification.[78] In this manner, an uneasy and temporary accommodation was reached, though not one that policymakers were happy about.

III. PPS: THE FUTURE

While this visible and dangerous confrontation over hospital margins was taking place, a quieter process was developing within ProPAC that would lead, eventually, to a significant change in its role. Five years out in the implementation of PPS, the Commission was showing signs of aging[79] or, at least, of needing to move on to a new phase of maturing. It was well-established in its role of commenting on the Secretary's recommendations and in advising Congress on PPS changes and the update. Much of the creative, pioneering work of developing policies and establishing new procedures was complete. There was lots of unfinished business, on capital, DRG modifiers, and so forth, but relatively little new business. Work was becoming routine, and the staff and the commissioners wondered what should be next.

Regulatory policy, of which PPS is one variety, also has its limits, determined by a statute assigning jurisdiction, but also by the politics relevant to that activity and the limits of knowledge or a capacity for rational action. Each sphere of regulatory activity will differ, of course, with respect to what limits are and how they become effectively constraining. But by the fifth year of PPS, some of these limits were becoming increasingly clear to the members and staff of ProPAC and especially to its chairman, Stuart Altman and the Executive Director, Donald Young.

In essence, there were two related problems: a need for fresh challenge and the limiting constraints on policy. One way to get out of an impasse is to work around it, and that is essentially what the Commission did. In 1988, ProPAC began shifting its mission, seeking to broaden its jurisdiction and to establish for itself a larger role with respect to Congress. This process was incremental and piecemeal, not revolutionary or wholistic. And the Commission both responded to discerned trends and anticipated future ones; accepted and sought out new Congressional mandates. At the same time, the cumulative shift in focus of attention and practical activity has been substantial. It was a creative response to some inevitable trends, exemplifying imaginative and effective leadership.

The roiling hospital margins controversy of 1988–1989 helped in two ways to give increased prominence to one activity of the Commission: that of supplying Congress with reliable data and advice about PPS and its impact on hospitals and beneficiaries. One reason that such expertise was increasingly important was that there was confusion over definitions and the facts: over what should count in numerator and denominator, how great the decline in hospital margins was, and what effect PPS as such was having. The issue was also entangled in the budget reconciliation process, with EOMB and DHHS taking sides. Usually, the combination of uncertainty, big money stakes, and political passion means trouble, and this episode was no exception. Reason and data help; but as the Commission pointed out,[80] the reconciliation process has politicized the environment of advice-giving. Over time, their

Report went on to say, "analytic justification" from the Secretary has become less of a factor, so that the role of ProPAC in supplying credible expertise becomes more important, both as staff agency to Congress and to reassure the hospital industry.

One consequence of this kind of thinking was that the Commission sought to increase its own resources and capabilities to meet the need for "analytical justification" and to strengthen features of PPS that would tighten the system or increase its rigor. The Commission has pushed for additional and more timely data, for the merger of the A and B data files, and for a retention and increased use of the Medicare Cost Report. ProPAC has also strongly endorsed the efforts of the HCFA to enhance DRG performance and to incorporate capital into PPS—as well as continuing to work itself on these projects. Initiatives like these have behind them two controlling motives or reasons. One is to preserve a measure of neutrality and independence for the Commission, especially in its advocate capacity, by ensuring that it brings to this activity a high level of expertise.[81] Another desideratum is to ensure that the ratchet-down on payments or, alternatively, the concessions made to hospitals be fair and rational, and be seen to be so. This objective becomes increasingly important, of course, as "margins" decrease and cuts become harder to absorb.

A salient characteristic of the health care industry is its dynamism: it does not stand still while it is being regulated. And one way in which health care was changing was the steady movement of procedures and therapies out of the hospitals: to outpatient departments, ambulatory surgery centers, skilled nursing facilities (SNFs), rehabilitation facilities, free-standing imaging centers, and so forth. Part of ProPAC's responsibility from the beginning was to monitor site-shifting and it had done so; but by year five of PPS, it was clear that this process was taking place on so vast a scale that it required some adaptation in mission.

What this trend meant, for ProPAC and for the operation of PPS, was a loss of effective leverage. Somewhat like the earlier experience with "ancillaries" and the older Sec. 223 limits, the bundled DRG payments controlled less and less.[82] As patients and procedures moved out of the hospital, there was an "unbundling" in which Part B, or physicians' fees, now paid for items that were formally included in a global payment; and often, Medicare paid as well for a higher case-mix index for sicker inpatients remaining in the hospital. But as the Commission pointed out, there was little the hospital could do about it, because doctors make the decisions[83] about patient care, not the hospitals. Many of the hospitals, moreover were being hit with increasing numbers of uninsured, victims of urban violence, and "crack" patients and babies so that they were less and less able to control their own destinies.

One policy consequence of this development was to cast in doubt the regulatory enterprise itself. To Commissioners and staff alike, it seemed both irrational and unjust to "ratchet down" on the hospitals when they were unable to do much about their situation. Aside from an issue of fairness, PPS was becoming less effective as an instrument of control: the Commission was "running out of dials to twist,"[84] and "fine tuning"[85] the machinery produced little, if any, additional desirable results, so that there was a genuine skepticism about what to do. The Commission's recommendations for 1989 reflected some of this skepticism and helped moderate the PPS reductions in the budget reconciliation of that year.

A positive initiative on the Commission's part was to begin exploring the possibilities for closer collaboration between ProPAC and PPRC. This step had an obvious logic to it, because of the growing importance of site changes and cost shifting and a need to coordinate the regulation of Part A and Part B expenditures. One way of addressing this objective was to urge the HCFA to expedite the merger of Part A and Part B claims data, which would facilitate the monitoring of site shifting and the study of episodes of illness. In 1989, ProPAC and PPRC set up a liaison committee and the two commissions have increased both the scope and intensity of their collaboration since then.

For a time, there was speculation that there might even be a merger of the two commissions. There had been discussion between ProPAC and the Congress about a Part B responsibility before PPRC was created. And starting anew, there would be much to be said for such a merger. But in policy development, we are always where we are, which is to say, with separate policies and institutions, each with its own history, staff, and clientele. A merger provoked little interest in Congress.[86] And PPRC liked what it was doing and preferred to continue as it was. So the idea of a merger was dropped, for the time.

Another way in which ProPAC responded to the changing environment was by seeking to broaden its jurisdiction and the scope of its concerns. For instance, the excluded hospitals[87] had a separate update for which ProPAC submitted annual recommendations, but otherwise they were under cost reimbursement. A Discretionary Adjustment Factor (DAF) for these hospitals was also calculated annually along with some other important numbers. Beginning with 1988, the Commission began making specific recommendations on the DAF, just as it did for the PPS hospitals, and commenced other activities that would bring them under closer supervision. In 1989, with the blessing of Congress, ProPAC initiated a study of hospital outpatient services, recommending their inclusion in PPS in the November report of 1989.[88] A similar study recommendation was made for ambulatory surgery in 1989. The Commission also began including references to psychiatric hospitals, re-habilitation units, long-term care and home health services as part of the complex of problems relating to institutional care. By their actions, if not their avowed policy, the Commission was staking out a new role, as the advisory commission for all institutional care related to Medicare. This kind of development made good policy sense. Given that patient care was moving outside the hospital walls, this was a way of tracking and regaining some control over these Medicare dollars. It also represented an alternative to a Medicare Commission: have ProPAC take on *all* the institutional care, leaving the professional component to PPRC.

Congress agreed to this division of labor, ratifying it in OBRA 1990. Important for a number of new agenda items, OBRA 1990 directed the Secretary to develop PPS proposals for current non-PPS hospitals, out-patient hospital services, and skilled nursing facilities. For each of these proposals, the Congress specified that ProPAC submit "an analysis and comments."[89] ProPAC is given responsibility for advising with respect to these developments and, as well, for "new institutional reimbursement policies" related to PPS. The same statute made clear that Congress intended for PPRC to exercise a comparable role with respect to the professional component, assigning to PPRC a broad responsibility for advising on the implementation of the Medicare Fee Schedule, including its bearing on such issues as physician supply, quality assurance, and cost containment.[90]

A significant development in 1991 was a HCFA proposal for Am-bulatory Patient Groups (APGs) for payment of the facility component of hospital outpatient services. Since this initiative seems to be, to date, one of the most viable options for extending PPS, it merits some com-The report submitted to Congress in June 1991, was a response to a mandate of 1986. It was enthusiastically received in Congress, especially by Pete Stark (D., CA.), chairman of the House Ways and Means sub-committee, who saw in it a useful method for controlling the costs ballooning on either side of the hospital inpatient stay.[91] The develop-ment and implementation of such a system lies several years in the future, but the proposal itself raises questions about the future of PPS, especially as a *system*. The APGs build on some of the methodology of the original DRGs and were developed under a contract with the HCFA engaging some of the principals who worked on the earlier system. APGs are essentially a scheme for bundling services, with much discre-tion left to the payer as to the method of bundling, what extras to pay for, and how aggressive to be in discounting services or putting the provider at risk. ProPAC has endorsed the bundling feature, but given APGs a lukewarm reception. Hospital groups complain that the APGs would make them accountable for physicians' decisions over which they could exercise little control.[92] This amount of ambivalence points to some significant issues.

A policy issue raised by the APGs proposal is that of a conflict between principle and pragmatics. A prime virtue of the APGs is that they provide a method for controlling facility costs outside the hospital walls. APGs might be further adapted: combined with inpatient DRGs, used for other sites, or even to pay professional fees. This following of the dollars beyond the hospital walls realistically seeks out the cost containment problem where it is. But it weakens some features of prospective payment that were, historically, part of its greatest appeal, especially the setting of impersonally determined, objectively calculated, and assured payments. They would also put hospitals increasingly at risk for doctors' decisions over which they would have little influence, a tendency squarely at odds with ProPAC's policy of not holding hospitals for circumstances beyond their control. The APGs proposal brings to mind the various objectives sought by the designers of the original DRG methodology and the tensions that existed between these objectives. They serve as a reminder that you can't have everything, and that adapting PPS to extend its reach may also compromise its integrity.

With the approval of Congress, the Commission began in 1989 to expand its role in surveying and commenting on the status of hospitals, the health care industry as a whole, and the quality of care in America. The earlier history of this development was a 1984 mandate from the House Appropriations Committee to the Commission, directing it to review the impact of PPS on the American health care industry. This particular charge became part of the Commission's work plan each year, but was pursued in a modest way until 1989 and confined rather narrowly to PPS itself. That year marked a dramatic change, signalled particularly by the Commission's March report. In essence, the Commission shifted much of its attention from PPS alone to the health care environment as a whole, and to "major recent changes in health care of which PPS is a part but not necessarily the cause."[93]

The rationale for this shift of emphasis was that PPS was itself affected by various factors not discussed in the original legislation. One such development was the "ballooning" of expenditures in facilities other than the hospital: outpatient departments, ambulatory surgery, and a variety of alternative sites. Another was the special burden put on Medicare hospitals because of uncompensated care and various forms of cost-shifting. More broadly, there was a sense that the Medicare hospitals were but a part of the larger ills of the American health care system: victims of these pathologies and, in turn, contributing to them.

A result of the broadened concern with the afflictions of the hospitals was a re-examination of their "margins" and particularly how teaching, disproportionate share, and rural hospitals were faring and what to do to help them. The analysis showed, not surprisingly, that teaching hospitals were doing well, but that many inner city and rural hospitals were not, despite their differential updates and other special allowances. To meet their needs, ProPAC has recommended and Congress has followed a policy of "targeting" money more specifically.[94] Twice the formula for disproportionate share hospitals has been changed the subsidy increased dramatically.[95] Rural disproportionate share and sole community hospitals have also received additional amounts. In a related change, OBRA 1990 began a phase-out of the lower DRG rates (average standardized amounts) for rural hospitals, a levelling upward that would benefit them greatly.[96]

Targeting could be described as calling a spade a spade and then making one to do the job; but there is more. It represents a significant accommodation in ProPAC's advisory role. Targeting developed because of a recognition that some existing formulas, such as the disproportionate share and indirect teaching adjustments, weren't working as intended, i.e., to compensate hospitals for their added expenses. Despite various subsidies, moreover, inner city and rural hospitals were still going broke. ProPAC's analysis revealed some inadequacies in the existing formulas and documented unmet need,—need created especially by cost-shifting and demographic trends. Congress corrected its aim and fired for effect, substantially increasing its subsidies to these hospitals in 1990 and 1991.

What is notable about targeting is the decline in importance assigned to PPS numbers and system integrity and an increased emphasis upon an instrumental, means-ends conception of rationality: helping Congress to discern its own objectives more clearly and adapt various PPS formulas to reach them.[97] A second important point about this process is that it puts the inner city and rural hospitals on an independent basis, making it easier to justify their preservation in terms of beneficiary access and economic circumstance. It will be interesting to see how ProPAC's creative adaptation of its role plays out. Targeting has led not just to increased subsidies for some hospitals but also to the discontinuance of the separate updates, so that getting clear about means and ends can be important in influencing policy. Yet there is a saying that he who sups with the devil needs a long spoon. This development brings the Commission closer to political activities and a step farther from the original analytical discipline and some of the pro-competition objectives of PPS. And OBRA 1990, providing that ProPAC reports only to Congress, makes clear who will be sitting at the table.

Part of ProPAC's enlarged mission, especially since 1989, has been to look beyond PPS and its immediate impact to review the status of the health care industry as a whole. With respect to this particular responsi-bility, the March Report for 1989 marks a significant transition. One passage from that report is quoted at some length, especially as a com-ment on how PPS relates to the health care industry and the larger scheme of American government. In a chapter entitled, "The Prospec-tive Payment System: 1983–1989, the Report said:

> Despite the efforts of the health care industry, government, and the pri-vate sector payers to contain health care spending, the growth in aggre-gate expenditures has not changed. The consequences of an inability to moderate the growth in health care spending are difficult to untangle, but in many significant areas needs are not being met. These include paying for health services for millions of Americans who lack financial protection against the cost of illness, as well as for long-term care services.
>
> These more global considerations may suggest that the battle is being won but the war lost. Perhaps, having met many of the original goals of PPS, goals for cost containment need to be examined more broadly. This would require looking beyond individual pieces of the health care delivery system like the hospital.[98]

Three months later, the June Report added that "the challenges facing the American health care system may require a new set of organizational and financial arrangements."[99] In a sense, no more was being said than that a changing environment should lead to some re-examination of the payment scheme. Yet the prospect opening was vast. For a larger mes-sage communicated was that Medicare could not be isolated or quaran-tined while the rest of the health care neighborhood raged with an inflationary fever. Health care costs are passed on to Medicare benefici-aries, Medicaid recipients and the entire society through rising pre-miums and co-pays or lack of insurance and reduced access. But rising costs or reduced access come back to the hospitals, to business and insurance companies, and to state and local governments through per-vasive cost shifting practices. High costs impoverish patients and im-poverished patients create high costs. A Medicare Prospective Payment System is not enough; at best, it is part of a larger solution.

Subsequent statements and actions by ProPAC, the HCFA, and the Congress continue to develop these themes. The Commission reaffirms a need to improve its analytic base and to fine-tune PPS. It has recom-mended several major steps to increase the accuracy and fairness of case payments.[100] ProPAC and the Congress have also developed ways to ease the pinch for particularly distressed hospitals. Both the HCFA and ProPAC are at work on projects for extending PPS to non-PPS hospitals and to outpatient and other sites. Looking to the future, two themes stand out prominently. One is the need for substantial modification of the payment methodology if there is to be an effective containment of hospital costs, looking especially toward some kind of bundling of payment, possibly even capitation. The other is the inadequacy of a Part A or a Medicare solution alone and the importance of an approach that can effectively control cost-shifting.

What all of this may portend for the future of PPS is uncertain. It could well be that Congress will tinker and patch for some time, retaining PPS and the DRGs, and selectively relieving distressed providers. ProPAC and the HCFA may provide the leadership for a successful amendment or redesigning of the system. Or an impending collapse of the American health care system may produce a bail-out, for instance, a version of National Health Insurance. Whatever transpires, a cycle is drawing to a close, and it is time again to think about health insurance and payment policies comprehensively and, perhaps, radically as well. For this activity, ProPAC has anticipated developments and is well-positioned to advise Congress. With its current leadership and a strengthened sense of priority, the HCFA has emerged again as a significant source of actionable policy alternatives. The experience with PPS has enlarged and deepened the thinking of many in and out of government. Much more in the way of resources are at hand for a next phase in payment reform. Yet on a somber note, reasoned advice from whatever quarter is not likely to prevail without the political institutions that help it to do so. And there may be no way to create such institutions, given the differences between the President and the Congress over domestic policy, and the political and budgetary imperatives driving each of these separate branches of government.

CHRONOLOGY: IMPLEMENTATION

1. PPS officially begins October 1, 1983.
2. Deficit Reduction Act (DEFRA) (P.L. 98–369, July 18, 1984); Congress reduces the update factor.
3. General Accounting Office reports unexpectedly large hospital margins under PPS, May 1985; DHHS Inspector General's Report on hospital PPS margins, October 1985.
4. Margaret Heckler resigns as Secretary of DHHS, October, 1985; Otis R. Bowen, M.D., appointed as the new Secretary, November 1985; David Stockman, Director of EOMB, and Carolyne Davis, Administrator of the HCFA also resign.
5. Gramm–Rudman–Hollings (P.L. 99–177, Dec. 12, 1985), Balanced Budget and Emergency Deficit Control Act.

6. COBRA (P.L. 99–272, Apr. 7, 1986) Consolidated Omnibus Reconciliation Act of 1985; postponed transition for a year; legislated
   own version of the Disproportionate Share Allowance; established the Physician Payment Review Commission (PPRC).
7. SOBRA (P.L. 99–509, Oct. 21, 1986), Omnibus Budget Reconciliation Act of 1986; took away the Secretary's authority to set the
   update; reduced the update below hospital market basket rate of
   inflation; began percentage cuts of capital.
8. November, 1986. Republican Party loses control of the Senate.
9. OBRA 1987 (P.L. 100–203, Dec. 22, 1987) Omnibus Reconciliation
   Act of 1987; notable for the scope and variety of PPS amendments; established a three-tiered update: large urban, urban, and
   rural; Secretary prohibited from publishing any final rule resulting in more than $50 million PPS savings.
10. 1988, PPS fifth year. ProPAC June Report to Congress discusses
    changes in payment methodology and mission of the Commis-
    sion.
11. Hospital margins controversy, Fall–Winter, 1988–1989.
12. OBRA 1989 (P.L. 101–239, Dec. 19, 1989) Omnibus Budget Rec-
    onciliation Act of 1989; Congress sets update above the market
    basket rate of inflation for rural and large urban hospitals; in-
    creases subsidies for disproportionate share and rural hospitals;
    creates the Medicare Geographic Classification Board; takes
    away the Secretary's authority to reduce DRG weights by overall
    percentage; Medicare Fee Schedule passes.
13. OBRA 1990 (P.L. 101–508, Nov. 5, 1990) Omnibus Budget Recon-
    ciliation Act of 1990; Congress provides that ProPAC reports only
    to it; discontinues separate rural and large urban updates; initi-
    ates phase-out of different rural DRG rates (average standardized
    amounts); mandates development of PPS proposals for non-PPS
    hospitals, outpatient hospital services, and skilled nursing
    facilities.
14. The HCFA submits improved proposal for inclusion of capital in
    PPS and for Ambulatory Patient Groups (APGs), February and
    June, 1991.

NOTES

1. Interviews with James Bentley, American Association of Medical Colleges, November 11, 1987 and with James Scott, American Healthcare Institute,
November 5, 1987. In the light of subsequent developments, "tamper resistant"
might be a better term.

2.   Interview with Michael Bromberg, Federation of American Health Systems, November 24, 1987.

3.   Interview with Diana Jost, Blue Cross-Blue Shield, November 4, 1987.

4.   "Margins" in the case of not-for-profit hospitals.

5.   Including, for instance, not just the prescriptive rules, but also historic background, elaborate explanations, and data tables.

6.   Minus the percentage allowance for outliers, which falls outside the system, an amount not less than 5% or more than 6%.

7.   Special exceptions are made for Sole Community Hospitals and Regional Referral Centers. Sole Community Hospitals are paid largely on the basis of their own historic cost experience, and partially according to PPS rates. RRCs get special additional allowances.

8.   The "market-basket" figure is largely a technical computation, but there are many policy and judgmental decisions to be made about what proxies to use and how to weight specific factors.

9.   This is called the "discretionary adjustment factor" (DAF) by ProPAC and the "policy target adjustment factor" (PTAF) by the HCFA. It allows an increase for case-mix change and offsets this with estimates of scientific and technical advances, productivity increases, and "site of care substitution," changes that should lower costs per case.

10.   The first DRG weights, set in October 1983 for 1984, were based on 1981 cost data because at that time (1983), 1981 was the latest year for which complete data files were available. These figures were then trended forward to 1983. Recognizing that this procedure would inevitably lead to inaccuracies and distortions in DRG weighting, Congress provided for adjustments to the "classification and weighting" of DRGs in FY 1986 and "not less" than every four years thereafter. With better and more readily available data, ProPAC proposed going to annual recalibration in 1987, which is now the practice. ProPAC has also advocated using cost rather than the charge data for recalibration that is now used, a recommendation that the Secretary has entertained, but so far declined to implement.

11.   "Diffusion" in the technical jargon.

12.   Also called "code creep," billing for a service more intense than that provided. Both the HCFA and ProPAC recognized and expected a legitimate upcoding, resulting from increased familiarity with DRGs. This is to be distinguished from deliberate miscoding or persistently classifying doubtful or borderline cases to the benefit of the provider.

13.   Not surprisingly, this proposed amendment has not met with widespread acclaim, even though Stuart Altman, chairman of ProPAC, advocated it for years. Eventually, Congress did provide for a "volume adjuster," but only as an add-on for rural hospitals with small numbers of discharges.

14.   Informal rule-making. One important point is that much of HCFA regulation is carried out through memoranda, letters of transmittal, and so forth. Also, judicial review of PPS is limited. In particular, review of the rates set or the DRG classifications is precluded.

15.   At the same time, DHHS may also publish various rules or proposed rules for the exempt categories of hospitals and for CHAMPUS (Civilian Health and Medical Program—Uniformed Services).

16.   Such as whether Periodic Interim Payments (PIP) would be retained or not for sole community hospitals.

17.   HCFA has also had to deal with a large number of studies mandated by the Congress. With their reduced staff, the agency is heavily burdened.

18. Omnibus Budget Reconciliation Act of 1990 (P.L. 101–508, November 5, 1990), Sec. 4002 (g). Another effect of the legislation is to make ProPAC, like PPRC, a congressional agency.

19. The Office of Technology Assessment, a congressional agency, supervises the Commission and appoints the members, though with wide consultation, to be sure. Initially, there were 15 members, but the Commission was expanded to 17 in 1986 to broaden their expertise and representative base.

20. The "June Report," as it is known, has a curious history. Early on, the Commission requested an additional appropriation of $1 million for extramural research. It was told by Sen. Stevens (R., Alaska) of the Appropriations Committee that $1 million was not enough to do anything important, but too much to fritter away. And since he did not want ProPAC simply doing technology assessment, he directed them to work on a report that would deal with PPS and its impact on the American health care system. Interview with Donald A. Young, Executive Director, ProPAC, July 6, 1990.

21. RFP is a "request for proposal," an administrative device that enables the agency to solicit proposals and develop contracts or grants for targeted research, analysis, or other kinds of specialized activities.

22. Such as the HCFA, one of the well-known research and consulting firms, or an individual expert.

23. The present Executive Director, Donald A. Young, is a physician with past experience as a deputy director of BERC. As the first director, he was able to build the organization from the ground up, recruiting the staff for the personal qualities, skills, and expertise that he believed the Commission needed. As a result, the staff is efficient, expert, and high in morale.

24. A dictionary definition is, "influence or power derived from enjoying the confidence of another or others."

25. Deficit Reduction Act of 1984, P.L. 98–369, July 18, 1984.

26. P.L. 99–177, December 12, 1985.

27. Like some commandments, Gramm–Rudman may be taken seriously but still disobeyed. It seems to represent for Congress a severe remedy for grave distresses. Yet it was amended and weakened by OBRA 1987. Then, Gramm–Rudman was suspended, for the time being, by the five-year deficit reduction pact and "discretionary caps" instituted by OBRA 1990.

28. The catastrophic benefit (later repealed) being one of the few exceptions. P.L. 100–360, July 1, 1988.

29. The House Ways and Means Committee shares some of its jurisdiction with Energy and Commerce, and the Senate Finance Committee maintains some communication with Labor and Human Resources, but the tax committees are more important for budget reconciliation.

30. For Medicaid, the role of the House Energy and Commerce Committee is much more important.

31. Budget reconciliation has had both large and unintended consequences for the legislative process that are of some constitutional significance. With respect to the separation of powers it has meant that the Executive gained a Pyrrhic victory, winning on budget totals, but losing virtually any influence over substantive legislation in areas like Medicare/Medicaid. Another consequence has been the reemergence of old-style "power brokers" in some key committee and subcommittee posts: such as Stark and Rostenkowski of Ways and Means and Mitchell and Bentsen of Senate Finance.

32. Interview with Patrice Feinstein, June 9, 1988. This perspective is shared by Irwin Wolkstein, one of the "old hands" in the Social Security Administration, and an architect of Medicare and the Social Security Amendments of 1972.

33. Interviews with Daniel F. Bourque, Voluntary Hospitals of America, January 5, 1988; and James Scott, American Healthcare Institute, November 5, 1987.

34. An important point, though, is that PPS definitely saved on *government* outlays, since it reduced the amount on which the government paid in full. For a discussion, see Russell (1989).

35. For instance, miniaturization of equipment making possible outpatient procedures and changes in home healthcare allowances.

36. Such as Medicare Automated Data Retrieval System (MADRS) that would combine Part A and Part B data and facilitate the monitoring of episodes of care. Interview with Rose Connerton, Bureau of Data Management and Strategy, April 8, 1988.

37. Cf. Redbud Hosp. Dist. v. Heckler (N.D. Cal. July 30, 1984).

38. Deficit Reduction Act of 1984, P.L. 98–369, July 18, 1984.

39. Consolidated Omnibus Budget Reconciliation Act of 1985, P.L. 99–272, April 7, 1986, Sec. 9105.

40. As opposed to weighting-by-hospitals, which favored the larger hospitals.

41. Interviews with Edmund Mihalski, minority staff, Senate Finance Committee, February 10, 1988; and Edward Grossman, House Office of Legislative Counsel, February 4, 1988.

42. Another remarkable example was the "Packwood Amendment," part of COBRA, whereby Senator Packwood got an exception to the transition provisions for 1986 that applied only to the State of Oregon. It is only fair to point out, however, that the reason Packwood wanted an amendment was because the transition had been delayed, largely at the behest of Rostenkowski, Chairman of the House Ways and Means Committee. As one staff person observed, it was after all a kind of equity: one for Rostenkowski and one for Packwood. COBRA, P.L. 99–272, Sec. 9102.

43. *Medicare's Prospective Payment system: An Analysis of the Financial Risk of Outlier Cases* (Washington, D.C.: Congressional Research Service, 1987).

44. *Report and Recommendations to the Secretary, U.S. Department of Health and Human Services, March 1, 1988* (Washington, D.C., Prospective Payment Assessment Commission, 1988), p. 24, and Recommendation 18, pp. 48, 49.

45. "Amendment" is used non-technically to include such procedures as assigning new cases to a particular DRG, revaluing or changing relative weights, re-defining the DRG, or creating a new one.

46. Of course, only with respect to PPS hospitals, and then for the Part A portion of the payment.

47. Extracorporeal shock wave lithotrypsy to give it the full name.

48. This is, of course, one simple example among a vast number of rapidly developing and expensive technologies, new drugs, and pioneering therapeutic methods.

49. Another good example is artificial joints, for instance, hip or knee replacements. They are expensive but add much to the quality of life. Why shouldn't Medicare patients have them? Interview with Thomas Hoyer, BERC, May 31, 1988.

50. Usually to a higher DRG, though not always.

51. None of which may be of much help, considering that the comparative efficacy of state-of-the-art technologies and procedures is being reviewed.

52. Tissue plasminogen activator, a "clot buster" important for treating heart attacks.

53. *Barron's*, January 11, 1988, p. 8; for a recent account of this continuing drug war, see Andrew Pollack, "Tests Find Both Drugs Effective; Doctors Prescribe the Costly One," *New York Times*, June 30, 1991, pp. 1, 19.

54. P.L. 98–21, Sec. 601, April 20, 1983.

55. OBRA 1989, however, required recalibration to be budget neutral. P.L. 101–239, Sec. 6003(b)(2)(iii), Dec. 19, 1989.

56. *Medicare and the American Health Care System—Report to the Congress* (Washington, D.C.: ProPAC, 1991) p. 49.

57. Omnibus Budget Reconciliation Act of 1986 (P.L. 99–509, October 21, 1986).

58. Some of the hospital community was irritated by the recalibration episode, regarding it as an egregious bit of cheese-paring. Interview with Bruce Steinwold, Health Technology Associates, October 25, 1989.

59. Catholic, urban, and public hospitals often fell into this latter category.

60. Omnibus Budget Reconciliation Act of 1986, P.L. 99–509, October 21, 1986, Secs. 9302 and 9321.

61. Omnibus Budget Reconciliation Act of 1987, P.L. 100–203, December 22, 1987, Sec. 4006.

62. Interview with John Iglehart, editor of *Health Affairs*, July 15, 1989.

63. Note that the outcome is not too different from the method that prevailed under Hill-Burton and that now obtains in Canada: i.e., cost-sharing between the hospitals and governmental authorities.

64. *Medicine and Health, Perspectives*, May 27, 1991. "Prospective Payment System for Inpatient Capital-Related Costs, Proposed Rule, Health Care Financing Administration, *Federal Register*, Vol. 56 (41) p. 8476. Also, *Medicare's Capital Payment Policy* (Washington, D.C.: ProPAC, 1991).

65. At the request of Congress, ProPAC delayed its own proposal to give Congress the benefit of Commission comments on the HCFA proposal. ProPAC accepted the approach taken by the HCFA, called it "thoughtful and creative" and made relatively modest suggestions for amendment. Cf. *Medicare's Capital Payment Policy, ibid.*, p. 55; interview with Donald A. Young, Executive Director, ProPAC, June 20, 1991.

66. Surgery is based on the procedure rather than the diagnosis, a change made because it predicted resource use better.

67. A point made by John Thompson, one of the Yale group. Such indexes have been used effectively for management purposes, for instance, by a number of for profit hospitals and hospital chains. Cf. Nathanson *et al.* (1985, 66ff).

68. *Medicine and Health, Perspectives*, January 25, 1988, p. 2.

69. Skeptics argue that SOIs are really needed for only a few DRGs; also that they are likely to work differently for different hospitals (Nathanson, et al., 1985). One researcher argues that severity indexes may *not* reduce variance in DRGs, especially because each level of severity will also have associated with it a variation in resource use. (Cf. Allen Dobson and Elizabeth Hoy, "The Changing Nature of Hospital Profit Estimates under Medicare Prospective Payment," unpublished, 1988). Moreover, if severity indexes were added to DRGs without changing the indirect teaching adjustment and the disproportionate share allowance, they might well make hospital case payments more inequitable than at present.

70.   Interviews with Lisa Potetz, Senate Finance Committee, January 7, 1990, and Bruce Steinwold, Health Technology Associates, October 25, 1989.
71.   Telephone interview with Julian Pettengill, ProPAC, July 20, 1990.
72.   Interview with Donald Moran, Lewin-ICF, January 5, 1988. Other former EOMB officials substantially confirm this account.
73.   The issues here are both complicated and obscure. Hospital "overpayments" resulted from a number of factors, such as the failure to audit cost reports (on which the first year regional and national rates were based) and trending forward the 1981 cost reports to establish the initial DRG rates, without making adequate allowances for a decline in the rate of inflation, site shifting, and lower lengths of stay. Some would also consider the urban wage indexes and the doubled teaching adjustment forms of overpayment but they were not technically that, even though the teaching and urban hospitals reaped big gains. The issue of hospital margins is complicated because there is no agreement on how to define them, and the HCFA, ProPAC, and the hospital associations use different concepts so that the "margins" will differ by as much as 40% depending on what definition is employed. Obviously, the definition has great significance, especially for arguing about how hospitals are making out under Medicare. By one definition, Medicare hospital margins were currently about to cross the zero-line and turn negative and, by another, costs and revenues per discharge are still going up dramatically. In other words, the hospitals may be hurting, but not obviously so because of Medicare. In the same way, statements about huge margins in the early years cannot to taken at face value. Cf. Dobson and Hoy (1988, 126); Interview with David Abernethy, Staff of Health Subcommittee, House Ways and Means, January 21, 1988.
74.   *Medicine and Health*, January 23, 1989, p. 2.
75.   Stark accused her of "cooking" the data and staging a "public relations stunt." Washington insiders and many people in the healthcare industry were somewhat shocked by this unchivalrous "beating-up" on McCarthy. *Medicine and Health*, March 6, 1989, p. 1. Interview with Bruce Steinwold, Health Technology Associates, October 25, 1989.
76.   Bruce Steinwold, ibid.
77.   Another change was the creation of the Medicare Geographic Classification Board, a body to be appointed by the Secretary to hear appeals by hospitals requesting a change of geographic classification. Such appeals would be final unless overturned by the Secretary. The provision dumped on the Secretary an unwelcome responsibility, but did get Congress out of an increasingly disreputable and time-consuming activity of creating exceptions for individual hospitals.
78.   Lisa Potetz, Staff Finance Committee, January 17, 1990.
79.   A reference to the concept of the regulatory cycle. ProPAC is not, strictly speaking, a regulatory agency: it does not itself develop and promulgate the rules and enforce them. But its advice, combined with Congressional "micromanagement," comes pretty close to regulation, and its recommendations resemble informal rule-making enough to invite a comparison.
80.   *Report and Recommendations to the Secretary, U.S. Department of Health and Human Services, March 1, 1989* (Washington, D.C.: Prospective Payment Assessment Commission, 1989), pp. 13, 14.
81.   *Report and Recommendations to the Secretary, U.S. Department of Health and Human Services, March 1, 1990* (Washington, D.C.: Prospective Payment Assessment Commission, 1990), p. 12.
82.   As Donald Young, the Commission's Executive Director, described the

process, the "balloon" on both sides of the hospital inpatient stay kept growing and growing. Interview, May 30, 1990.

83.   *Report and Recommendations to the Secretary, U.S. Department of Health and Human Services, March 1, 1990* (Washington, D.C.: Prospective Payment Assessment Commission, 1990), p. 3.

84.   Interview with Sankey V. Williams, M.D., ProPAC Commissioner, July 11, 1990.

85.   Interview with Bruce Steinwold, Health Technology Associates, October 25, 1989.

86.   Interview with Lisa Potetz, Senate Finance Committee, January 17, 1990.

87.   Psychiatric, rehabilitation, and long-term care hospitals and related distinct-part units were excluded from PPS, but subject to a TEFRA rate of increase. Pediatric and cancer hospitals were also initially excluded, but later incorporated into PPS.

88.   *1990 Adjustments to the Medicare Prospective Payment System—Report to the Congress, November 1989* (Washington, D.C.: Prospective Payment Assessment Commission, 1989), p. 7.

89.   Omnibus Budget Reconciliation Act of 1990 (P.L. 101–508, November 5, 1990), Sec. 4002 (g).

90.   *Ibid.,* Sec. 4118 (j).

91.   Adopting the "balloon" metaphor given currency by ProPAC. Cf. Robert Pear, "New Cost Control Asked on Medicare," *New York Times,* June 9, 1991, pp. 1, 30.

92.   *Ibid.,* and Harold Larkin, "System Similar to DRGs up next for Ambulatory Care," *American Medical News,* May 27, 1991, pp. 11–12; *Design and Evaluation of a Prospective Payment System for Ambulatory Care, Final Report* (Wallingford, CT: 3M Health Information Systems, 1990).

93.   Report and Recommendations to the Secretary . . . March 1, 1989, Ibid., p. 20.

94.   For a discussion, see *Report and Recommendations to the Congress, March 1, 1991* (Washington, D.C.: ProPAC, 1991), esp. App. A.

95.   OBRA 1989, Sec. 6003 (c); and OBRA 1990, Sec. 4002 (b).

96.   OBRA 1990 dispenses with the separate updates but provides that the standardized amounts for rural hospitals will be gradually brought up to the urban level by large transitional update differentials for rural hospitals.

97.   Interview with Donald A. Young, Executive Director of ProPAC, June 20, 1991.

98.   *Report and Recommendations to the Secretary . . .* March 1, 1989, *op. cit.,* p. 21.

99.   *Medicare Prospective Payment and the American Health Care System—Report to the Congress, June 1989* (Washington, D.C.: ProPAC, 1989), p. 3.

100.   Such as improving the area wage index, case-mix measurements, and cost report data. Cf. Report and Recommendations to the Secretary . . . March 1, 1990, *op. cit.,* pp. 8, 9.

4

Physician Payment Reform: Background

Physician payment reform produced little that was radically new. The Medicare Fee Schedule, eventually passed in November 1989, built on traditional approaches, well understood and, for the most part, accepted by providers and by the Federal government. Yet the *scope* of change was great. And the *way* in which physician payment reform was achieved was novel. PPS, for all its innovative features, was designed within an executive department, much in the classic style. Physician payment reform was mainly the creation of congressional subcommittees and their own advisory body, the Physician Payment Review Commission. It required, above all, the step-by-step melding of political strategy and technical rationality. Like designing an airplane while in flight, the process can be both difficult and risky; yet it illustrates how much of health policy was made during the Reagan and Bush administrations, a time characterized especially by political antagonism between Congress and the President over domestic issues. And, like the example of the airplane, it reveals capacities for improvisation as well as ways in which important elements can get left out.

Physician payment reform during most of the Reagan Administration was a stepchild of policy, especially within the executive branch, receiving scant attention until other pressing issues had been dealt with. By that time, the big policy initiatives of the new administration were underway and resources committed to these, making a major Part B effort hard to develop quickly, especially one that was out of harmony with the established administration "pro-competition" theme. Physician reimbursement also came "late" in the cycle of presidential politics, after the Reagan Administration had achieved much of its "revolution" in domestic policy and was concentrating efforts on holding what had been gained. Characteristic of this second phase was a bitter and pervasive politics of the budget and OBRAs. Other typical second phase developments such as executive branch turnover, declining credibility on the Hill, and increasing White House preoccupation with the biennial electoral cycle added to the obstacles confronting any bold domestic policy initiatives originating within the executive branch.

One reason for a measure of caution, if not deliberate foot-dragging, was that this particular variety of policy seemed to be an example of a problem without a technical solution. There was no agreed on payment methodology, no equivalent of the DRGs. Instead, each of the principal alternatives—capitation, physician DRGs, or fee schedules—suffered from one or more major detractions, compelling enough to prevent a dominant consensus developing to support that alternative. Policy agreement about a topic as politically charged as physician reimbursement would have been hard to reach in the best of circumstances. Lack of a technical solution made the reaching of a consensus additionally difficult.

The driving initiative for Medicare physician payment reform came from Congress, mainly the Health Subcommittees of Ways and Means and Senate Finance. The chairmen and members of these committees relied for expertise on their committee and personal staffs and on Congressional agencies such as Office of Technology Assessment, the Congressional Budget Office, and the purpose-built Physician Payment Review Commission. This development, an innovation of constitutional import, was not one wished by the Congress. Quite the contrary, from 1984 on Congress prodded the administration for policy recommendations, seeking out the expertise of DHSS and HCFA, mandating scores of reports, and scolding EOMB for its intrusiveness in holding up departmental reports and recommendations. At first reluctantly, but then with increasing assurance and resolve, especially as Part B outlays and beneficiary premiums mounted, Congress set about to develop its own sources of data and policy analysis, aimed at producing a physician counterpart to PPS.

But the contrast in the way policy developed in these two areas is a large one. PPS is an example of a technical solution to a commonly acknowledged problem, based on extensive research, data and policy analysis, and field testing. It was developed within the executive branch, but with the active support of Congress and the most important interest group constituencies. Physician payment provides an example, by contrast, of policy development through short-term, piecemeal "fixes," with the development of a comprehensive proposal for reform coming only after some years of incremental legislative changes by Congress and micro-management of Medicare physician payment through the budget reconciliation process. Both the year-by-year amendments and the ultimate reform legislation developed in an environment of confrontation between the Congress and the Administration and of general disagreement within government and outside of it over what needed fixing, how badly it needed it, and how to go about it.

As an example of policy development, physician payment represents an extreme example of what Congress can do, with little help and some active opposition from the executive branch. It illustrates the kind of scenario we may expect in other areas of policy, assuming the continuance of the current partisan division between the President and the Congress. The constitutional separation of powers has also had a major impact on policy: the alternatives that were chosen, the choices that were preempted or ignored, and the effects of politics and administration on the substance of policy. As important as any aspect of Medicare physician payment policies is the way in which they were shaped by other domestic priorities of the Reagan and Bush eras and the budgetary skirmishes of Congress and the Executive.

The Medicare Fee Schedule was developed and enacted into law under severe constraints of decisions already made, mostly by the Congress, and of heavily defended institutional and ideological commitments, mostly on the part of the executive branch. In an important sense, it is a legacy of the past, of a series of incremental decisions made by the Congress and of the ideologies of the Reagan Administration. Physician payment reform is policy made by unintended consequence and ingenious adaptation. How this came about and how and why Congress took this particular route is the subject of this chapter.

I. MEDICARE: EARLY IMPLEMENTATION

The scheme eventually devised for reforming Medicare physician payment was a system of fee schedules with limits on "balance billing" to protect beneficiaries[1] and national "performance standards" intended to limit increases in volume of services.[2] Critics have pointed out that, unlike PPS, this "solution" leaves the provider and beneficiary incentives much as before. Consequently, they raise a doubt that fee schedules will have a lasting or substantial impact on rising Part B expenditures or provide an effective way of controlling health care costs more generally. Looking at the issue of Medicare physician payment historically, however, it is difficult to see how the outcome could have been much different. Physician reimbursement was a politically sensitive issue, indeed for a long time almost a taboo. Policy alternatives were difficult to develop, for technical as well as political reasons. Yet, effective short-term responses to both budget demands and the need for beneficiary protection were comparatively easy to make through the powerful and highly adaptive mechanism of the budget reconciliation process. Under constraints dictated by larger, exogenous political forces, House and Senate subcommittees moved expeditiously, mostly in the direction that policy had been inclined historically and without a careful or systemic examination of the alternatives or even of the implications of its own policy. What was lost in this process and how good the result will prove to be remain yet to be seen.

From the beginning of modern history, which is to say since the passage of Medicare, physicians had been given a special status, put in a different and privileged position in comparison with the hospitals. Unlike hospitals, physicians were paid their "reasonable charges," a reimbursement based on what they billed rather than their audited and "reasonable costs."[3] Unlike hospitals, that took what they were allowed as payment in full,[4] physicians were allowed to "balance bill," that is, bill the patient for their customary fee, over and above what Medicare allowed.[5] And physicians dealt with "carriers," rather than "fiscal intermediaries," the difference being that these third parties, typically private insurers such as Blue Shield or Aetna, were as a matter of law and policy meant to be even more independent of government than the counterpart FIs that reimbursed hospitals. Some said that these dispensations were made because Wilbur Mills still entertained hopes of running for President and hoped for the physicians' support. In any event, the American Medical Association made these items conditions of its acceptance of the legislation. According to Irwin Wolkstein, one of the principal architects of the legislation, the provisions for physician reimbursement were designed "overnight," following the AMA sponsored Byrne bill in outline and modeling the payment system on the Aetna Federal Employee Health Benefits scheme.[6] They were intended to ensure maximum acceptability on the part of the physicians.

Medicare–Medicaid was not itself a discrete event. Like other major statutes, it was tangled with other controversies and political differences that continued long after the statute itself had been enacted. With respect to Medicare in particular, a small number of DHEW[7] officials and congressional committee staff who felt that Medicare had given away too much were especially concerned with how the legislation would be implemented.[8] In 1966 and 1967, they began devising and promoting schemes addressing one or more of what have been subsequently identified as the important Medicare problem areas. Their proposals ranged from utilization review and hospital certificate-of-need through fee schedules and capitation and included almost all of the Part B (as well as the Part A) policy alternatives that have been seriously entertained since.[9]

During this period, the Social Security Administration began to tackle the issue of physicians fees, making their policy pretty much from whole cloth. The legislation specified "reasonable charges" and administration through "carriers." Initially, the carriers were told to do what they did with their non-Medicare providers, a policy that resulted in lax monitoring, payment of 90% or more of the claimed amounts submitted, and permitting frequent and immediately effective increases in fees charged.[10] But this was hardly a popular policy in the SSA. And, confronted with rapidly increasing Part B expenditures and a rise in Part B premiums, the SSA began tightening up, availing themselves of "notice and comment"[11] procedures and some of the general language in the statute.[12] One such measure was to set up an anniversary date for changes in physicians' fees, the effect of which was to lag fee increases. Another, often used by carriers privately and also mentioned in the statute, was to require a "prevailing charge" screen: pay at the 75th percentile of charges within the area covered by a particular Medicare carrier. Medicare would pay the lesser of a physician's "customary" or actual charge, the area prevailing charge limit, or the "reasonable" charge. And so was born the Customary, Prevailing and Reasonable (CPR) system of reimbursement, though with the category of "reasonable" yet to be implemented. Meanwhile, the SSA tinkered with other ideas, such as how an economic index might be devised that would tie Medicare Part B increases to resource costs and to increases in the general level of earnings.[13]

Social Security Amendments of 1972

An event that proved in retrospect to be of great importance for Medicare physician reimbursement was Title II of P.L. 92-603, the Social Security Amendments of 1972. One part of this statute, the smaller part, deals with Social Security and welfare amendments that were important initiatives of the Nixon Administration. Over half of the statute, more than 90 pages of text, contains the most varied and comprehensive array of amendments ever directed at the Medicare–Medicaid programs. This part of the statute came largely from the creative efforts of congressional staff, especially Jay Constantine of Senate Finance and William Fullerton of House Ways and Means. Aware that Medicare–Medicaid needed amending, both pervasively and fundamentally, they set about planning legislation that would help create the knowledge base and provide the authority needed for reform. The preparatory work extended over a period of years and entailed assembling types of data never gotten before, selecting among dozens of program initiatives, and working with administrative officials and committees of both houses to develop the final proposal. The 1970 Report to the Committee, written to prepare the ground for this legislation, is to this day a model for its conciseness, theoretical soundness, and documentation.[14] Title II of the 1972 Amendments rightly belongs high in the annals of legislation, a monument to the vision of a smaller number of public officials.

Including more than 90 different sections, Title II deals with almost every aspect of Medicare and Medicaid. It includes sweeping authorizations and the creation of new agencies as well as minute changes in coverage and reimbursement methodology. In broadest outlines the statute took two approaches to the amendment of Medicare. One was to create regulatory agencies and authority, aimed largely at cost containment, such as the Professional Standards Review Organizations, the Sec. 1122[15] limits on hospital capital expenditures, and a scheme for constraining physicians' Medicare charges.[16] The other was to move toward the development of alternative payment systems: by establishing a broad authority for research and demonstrations;[17] and by encouraging Medicare HMOs and "waivered" experiments.[18]

One provision of the Social Security Amendments especially important for the future of physician reimbursement was Sec. 224, which made legitimate, gave statutory authority, for the prevailing charge methodology that was already in effect. A second part of this section established the Medicare Economic Index (MEI) (cf. Dutton and McMenamin (1981). This provision was essentially a primitive update factor. The MEI went into effect in 1975. It tied increases in physician reimbursement to a base year, FY 1973, and an annually updated index. This index, employing "appropriate index data" allotted 40% to office costs and 60% to physician services, and indexed these to prevailing wage and salary rates and other proxies, such as rent and malpractice premiums.

Section 222 established a broad mandate to pursue "experiments and demonstration projects" with emphasis on alternative payment systems and prospective reimbursement. The Secretary was also authorized to waive compliance with Medicare and Medicaid requirements and to tap the Hospital Insurance and Supplemental Medical Insurance Trust Funds for project support. Although the emphasis of this section was on inpatient facilities, it included "other providers" of Medicare services. Moreover, under Sec. 224, which dealt with physicians charges, the Health Insurance Benefits Advisory Council (HIBAC) was directed to study methods of reimbursement for physicians' services specifically in order to evaluate "their effects upon (1) physicians' fees generally, (2) the extent of assignments accepted by physicians, and (3) the share of total physician-fee costs which the Medicare program does not pay and which the beneficiary must assume." HIBAC was instructed to report back to Congress no later than January 1, 1973, with recommendations as to the preferred method.

Another provision of the Social Security Amendments, with potential significance for Medicare physician reimbursement, was Sec. 1876, which provided for Federal government payments to HMOs that would enroll Medicare beneficiaries. Various HMO proposals had been under consideration, both during the Johnson and the Nixon administrations. Rising Medicare expenditures made them seem attractive as an option and one such alternative, a Medicare Part C, was proposed in a Social Security Bill of 1970. But the 1972 Amendments were the first experiment in direct Federal support of HMOs. The statute provided two types of payment, one for relatively new HMOs and another for ones with established records. The latter could enter into "risk sharing" contracts providing for annual payments of 95% of an "adjusted average per capital cost" for Medicare patients (AAPCC).[19] This approach seemed to hold forth some promise of inducing more cost-conscious behavior on the part of providers, both hospitals and physicians, without having to increase beneficiary out-of-pocket expenses. At the same time, this initiative was by no means universally supported, many fearing that those Medicare beneficiaries who joined HMOs would be medically "undeserved," and others dubious that the government would save any money. As events transpired, there proved to be much to support these fears. A number of Medicare and Medicaid HMOs delivered substandard care. And Sec. 1876 saved no money. But it did have an important impact on the future development of Medicare physician payment policy.

Economic Stabilization Program

A historic development of major significance was the Nixon–Ford Economic Stabilization Program (ESP), which lasted from 1971 until discontinued under the Ford Administration in 1974. ESP started with a general price freeze in 1971. But under Phase II, which began in 1972, hospitals and physicians requested and got a separate price control regime, responsive to the special characteristics of the health care industry. Although the experiment was a mixed success, it was important for learning about the practical and theoretical difficulties involved in trying to limit rising hospital and physician costs. Some of the most significant research and demonstrations on cost containment derived from this experience or from policy analysts who participated in it. (Zubkoff 1976).

Physician's fees and physician reimbursement received comparatively little attention during this period, since hospital costs were a much bigger and more urgent problem. ESP did substantially reduce the rate of increase in physicians' fees, though there was much "catch-up" pricing during the last year and after the program was terminated. A significant finding, however, was that controlling physician fees had a proportionately much smaller effect on either physicians' incomes or on the Part B expenditures per Medicare beneficiary.[20] Former Social Security officials recall this experience as their introduction to the "volume" issue: that is, that physicians faced with price controls can and will increase the volume or the intensity of the services provided to the individual patient. Along with the volume issue, they also grew familiar with related kinds of adaptive behavior on the part of physicians, such as upcoding and unbundling. Though aware of the problems, neither they nor the Cost of Living Council experts involved in ESP had theoretical concepts or practical techniques adequate to deal with them. Not surprisingly, another legacy of this ESP experience was skepticism that regulation was the right way to deal with Medicare costs.

During this period, important research and demonstration projects were begun, a number of them under the authority of Sec. 222 of the Social Security Amendments. Some of these projects contributed to the development of substantive theory, such as the famous RAND controlled experiment in cost-sharing.[21] Some, like the early fee schedule projects[22] and the Yale study of DRGs, were fundamental for later policy developments. Other studies aimed at building data bases: dealing with charges, office costs, participation behavior, and claims data.[23] The fundamental work begun at this point paid off in policy applications a decade or more thereafter, a testament to the foresight of those congressional staff members who designed the enabling legislation and the Social Security and DHEW officials who put it to work.

Low Priority

By the time of the Carter Administration, the first cycle of interest in physician payment reform had waned. Research continued on Part B data bases and various payment methodologies. And fee schedule proposals figured in the various National Health Insurance initiatives under the Nixon, Ford, and Carter Administrations. In the second half of the Carter Administration, price inflation and an increasingly conservative political mood in the country made clear that NHI was sure to be defeated. At that time, attention shifted to the second major Carter Administration initiative of cost containment, directed mostly at hospitals. Except for the Medicare–Medicaid Fraud and Abuse Amendments of 1977, little of consequence was done until the Reagan Administration and, then, only after the advent of the OBRAs and deficit reduction politics.[24]

Along with a shift of emphasis from NHI to cost containment, the Carter Administration was important for two other developments that ultimately affected physician payment as it did hospital reimbursement. One was a change in the scope of cost containment strategies, unavowed but nevertheless real, from an "all payers" to a Medicare-only approach. Also important was the growing skepticism that regulatory approaches worked, at least by themselves, and a casting about—within the Congress and the administration and among health policy activists of both political parties—for alternative strategies, especially "pro-competition" ones such as beneficiary cost-sharing, tax exemption caps, and HMO or "managed care" options.[25]

By 1980 and the advent of the Reagan Administration, some measures toward the reform of Medicare physician payment had already been taken. The introduction of the CPR basis for payment and increased surveillance of the carriers were early steps. The Social Security Amendments of 1972 provided a base for more stringent regulation as well as broad authorization for experiments and demonstrations aimed at the development of alternative payment systems. The projects initiated and the data collected during the latter half of the decade were of great value. Yet one point about these developments should be noted: that they built mostly on the existing fee-for-service payment method. HMOs and capitation were an exception, to be discussed later. But the important developments during this period, such as CPR, the MEI, the encouragement of "participation," and even the fee freeze, reinforced a positivistic assumption that the existing fee-for-service system, preferably with some incremental improvements and some more effective constraints on charges, was likely to stay.

A factor that reinforced this positivistic trend of policy was the difficulty of enlisting physicians in the "experiments and demonstrations" authorized by the Social Security Amendments of 1972. Various reasons have been ascribed: the difficulty of working with local carrier data, nomenclature and payment systems, physicians' edginess at getting into demonstrations that purported to change their modes of practice or billing methods, and the lack of cooperation from the medical societies.[26] One consequence of this lack of physician participation was to give increased importance to data collection and analysis: the claims files, participation lists, and office expenses. This is vital information, but most useful for making incremental changes in the existing system.

The preceding observation points up a strong contrast between physician payment reform and the development of PPS. For hospital payment, there was the strongest kind of presumption, both in the statutory authority and in the priorities for research and demonstrations projects that there would be a fundamental change in the method of payment, encouraging different incentives and new styles of hospital management. As for physician payment reform, the approach was positivistic and incremental. Section 222 of the Social Security Act of 1972 referred, in general terms, to "alternate methods of making payments" that would include "other providers" than hospitals, but left further priorities unstated. Attempts to develop policy alternatives through demonstrations met with little success. The existing data, the R&D prospects, and the low priority given to physician payment reform meant that any eventual attempt at fundamental change would begin with a constraining legacy from the past.

II. THE REAGAN ADMINISTRATION

Physician payment reform, as noted previously, was a stepchild of policy, meaning that it tended to be neglected while the more urgent problem of hospital costs was addressed. Issues of physician payment not only received less attention, they were taken up later. Within the Reagan Administration, this meant that they became serious agenda items after Richard Schweiker had departed the DHHS, in the aftermath of Stockman's initial assault on entitlements, after the size of the deficit became apparent, and after Congress and the Executive had settled into trench warfare over the budget. These historic factors shaped the making of policy with respect to physician reimbursement.

"Anti-regulation" and "pro-competition" were early themes of Reagan Administration and had an important effect on the development of physician payment policy—significantly greater than the impact they had on PPS. The notion of inducing competition into the health care "market"[27] was an increasingly popular idea, even during the Carter Administration, and led under Reagan to various proposals such as "caps" on tax-free employer contributions,[28] increased beneficiary cost sharing, voucher plans, and competitive bidding. Most of these ideas remained in the realm of unresearched proposals and ideology. But PPS was eventually sold in large part, especially to the administration, as a "pro-competition" strategy. "Vouchers" were popular for a time both in Congress and with the Reagan Administration. And Richard Schweiker ably promoted HMOs and capitation as "pro-competition" and "deregulation." This kind of practical activity reinforced by the pro-competition ideology helped give capitation and "managed care" a prominent place in the thinking of Reagan policy people, despite that fact that many in the HCFA, EOMB, and much of Congress remained cool to such proposals, especially as a solution to Medicare reimbursement problems.

TEFRA

TEFRA, that strange hybrid statute passed in the Spring of 1982, was important for physician payment as well as for PPS. The full name is The Tax Equity and Fiscal Responsibility Act of 1982 and most of its prolix titles were tax amendments or aimed at reducing the deficit. Title I, though, dealt with health and income security programs,[29] and was of decisive importance for hospital reimbursement. TEFRA dealt in the scantiest way with physician reimbursement, making some minor provisions with respect to payments for inpatient radiology and pathology and for assistants at surgery. Indirectly, though, TEFRA was of the greatest importance for the future of physician payment. It set in place the "anything but" TEFRA system of hospital reimbursement designed to help the hospitals perceive the desirability of the Secretary's soon-to-appear version of PPS. This step marked a provisional solution to the hospital reimbursement issue. PPS still had to be designed in detail and accepted by the Congress and the President, but the passage of TEFRA meant that the physician payment reform could now receive the kind of systematic attention and high priority previously reserved for the hospitals.

TEFRA represented a policy-making style that would characterize much of the future, so far as Medicare physician payment was concerned. For here, Congress acted very much on its own initiative, independently of the White House. TEFRA also combined major substantive amendments of health care policies with deficit reduction legislation, much like later[30] budget reconciliation and Gramm–Rudman procedures. Further, TEFRA provided an example of a tactic that became especially popular during the 1980s for making changes in Medicare physician payment: introduction of a proposal designed to soften up providers and "bring them to the table" with alternatives of their own. Thus, TEFRA was important as a historic transition, in shifting attention to physician payment, and procedurally in legitimating a style of legislation.

During the Summer of 1982, Medicare expenditures became a major target for budget savings, for two very good reasons. One was that the hospitals and physicians were popular victims: they were highly visible contributors to the mounting domestic deficit and they were not much loved by the voters. Another reason was that the Social Security entitlement was permanently "off the table," an attempt at reduction having led to the most disastrous political defeat of the Reagan first term. TEFRA, in attacking the deficit, included Medicare Part B expenditures, raising the issue of who was to pay, the provider or the beneficiary. Rather uncharacteristically for Congress, the statute came down on the beneficiary, writing in a temporary provision[31] setting the Part B premium to cover 25% of the Part B program costs. Another proposal, not adopted but indicating how the thinking with respect to providers was going, would have frozen the MEI for that year.

Executive Branch Initiatives

Meanwhile, the executive branch was developing its own approach to the physician reimbursement issue. Who was to pay, was also at issue within the administration, but with a much clearer preference for making the beneficiary the target. The Office of Management and Budget backed especially a reduction in the health insurance tax exemption and increased beneficiary co-pays, moderately sweetened with a "catastrophic" cap on beneficiary out-of-pocket expenditures. EOMB also targeted Part B for FY 1984. About this time, the HCFA formed its working group on physician payment reform. It was a time of transition and reordering priorities. Proposals for ceilings or "caps" and "freezes" in various indexes were popular during this season, a way of postponing some of the hard and obscure policy issues for a time.

As attention turned toward devices or techniques that might be used to restrain physician charges or change their behavior, no single option appeared obviously more attractive than another. But various agencies were formulating tentative views that later became entrenched policy positions. Congress began to look with favor on fee schedules, requesting of CBO estimates of savings that could be realized through fee schedules for surgery.[32] The White House, i.e., the Cabinet Council and the Health Policy Adviser, supported capitation. EOMB doubted that capitation would save any money and disliked fee schedules as too regulative, but looked with some favor on physician DRGs, especially for inpatient payments. And within DHHS and the HCFA, different groups supported fee schedules, capitation, variants of physician DRGs, and none of the above.[33] This kind of initial difference was already some indication that finding a happy solution might be difficult—indeed, that there might not be a solution.

As the various policy protagonists considered the options, the budget deficit continued to grow.[34] This meant, given President Reagan's strong position against new taxes, that Medicare hospital and physician payments were even more desirable targets. And this budgetary emphasis sharpened considerably the dilemmas between short-term, budget oriented, dollar-saving "fixes" and the design and development of long-term, systematic solutions. Driven by the rigid periodicity of the budget, both Congress and EOMB pressed for short-term solutions or for longer-term ones that were consistent with short-term budget savings. Given the structure of physician payment issues, this kind of budget-driven policy making would have made the development of a sound and considered long-term solution hard. It was doubly difficult in the absence, within the Reagan Administration, of health policy leadership that was either strong or unified. Without a mandate from above, the White House health policy adviser, EOMB, and DHHS each pressed for their priorities, and within those priorities, for the approach to physician payment reform that seemed best from their particular vantage point. As a consequence, the Administration was, at times, supporting three or even four different options. It is hardly surprising, in that situation, that no long-term policy solution was developed and that short-term, incremental, pragmatic expedients tended to determine the choices intimately made.

Much of the immediate demand for action came from Congress, for reasons that had to do both with policy and with immediate events. The policy issue centered on the question of "Who pays?" The Reagan Administration was reluctant to put the onus on the physicians, regarding them as political allies. Vouchers and beneficiary co-pays were consistent with administration "pro-competition" and private sector initiatives and also promised, in budgetary projections, to yield large savings. On the Hill, and especially in the House, controlled by the Democratic Party, these were viewed as unproved methods and, more to the point, unduly burdensome for Medicare beneficiaries. There was no OBRA for 1982, but both houses were talking fee freezes and physician assignment. An important step that addressed the issue of physician payment methodology was a mandate in the PPS legislation directing the Secretary to report back to Congress by 1985 on the feasibility of inpatient physician DRGs. Finally, at the Congressional Forum, of the Group Health Association of America, held in April 1983, Senator Dole, then Chairman of the Finance Committee, announced a "year of the physician." He said that, with PPS, Congress had "taken a pretty good whack at the hospitals" and that now it was time to "find out some way we can work with physicians to help us reduce the growth in Medicare spending."[35] The language was disarming; but the message was clear.

Physicians' Advisory Group: Policy Alternatives

At the same meeting of the GHAA, Carolyne Davis, the HCFA Administrator, announced the formation of a Physicians' Advisory Group[36] to consider approaches toward Medicare physician payment and especially whether to combine their payment with the DRG-based PPS. There were, of course, a number of policy options being considered within the HCFA and ASPE. Davis's objective was partly to canvass and discuss the alternatives, partly to gauge their acceptability within the provider community, and partly to inform the HCFA staff.[37] The group met informally, usually on Saturdays, for a year. A body of about 25–30, depending on who turned up, it included HCFA and ASPE staff, physicians representing separate specialties, and occasional drop-ins, such as William Roper, a White House policy adviser and later head of the HCFA.

In retrospect, the most important conclusion of the Physicians' Advisory Group was that it had no conclusion. The exploration of the alternatives, through staff option papers and weekend discussions, illuminated the structure of the physician payment issue, but it left the advisory group with three alternatives, each of them with some important advantages, but none of them satisfactory by itself.

Inpatient DRGs at first looked like a promising alternative. Aside from the symmetry of adding inpatient DRGS to the hospital DRG-based PPS, they held forth several attractions from a policy perspective. They would be "prospective" and "global," that is, set a fixed price for a "bundle" of procedures. By paying for a prescribed bundle, physician DRGs would allow the payer, ultimately the Federal government, to control both the price and the volume of services provided, an important advantage over fee schedules, which would not.

Inpatient DRGs also seemed at first inspection to be deployable in the near future, important because of the perennial short-term pressure to reduce the budget deficit.[38] For instance, nearly 60% of inpatient physician charges went for surgery and anesthesiology and these were already bundled. Radiology and pathology could be easily added. So, most likely, could a small number of expensive, high-volume procedures. Skilled nursing facilities, with a large proportion of routine services, were also likely to be amenable. Initially, there were grounds for optimism.

At the same time, there were important technical and practical problems with physician DRGs, revealing ways in which they were unlike hospital DRGs. One had to do with whether they would be clinically coherent and good resource-use predictors. On this vital question, there had been almost no research or experience. Even to do such research there needed to be a workable concept of a physician DRG and a data base developed to support such research.[39] Moreover, if roughly 55% of physician inpatient services were bundled, 45% were not, and the practical and theoretical difficulties of developing DRGs for these procedures would be formidable and not likely to be overcome quickly.

One of the most difficult practical issues was, "who to pay?" For instance, paying the individual physician, who typically performed a limited range of procedures, would put him or her at risk that those particular procedures were DRG winners. If they were losers, that provider would either lose money or learn how to select patients. Payment to a medical or surgical group would allow for some averaging. But members of such a group might have both the organized power and the incentives to collude with hospitals in gaming the system. At the hospital level, physician DRGs would presumably "average out," at least in theory, as they do with hospital DRGs. But this arrangement would put hospitals in the position of distributing payment among physicians, a conflict-laden responsibility at best, and one that most hospitals neither wanted to assume nor thought they could endure.

What to do about assignment raised another major dilemma, further complicated by a lack of knowledge about the predictive capabilities of physician DRGs. With hospitals, there was a tradition of assignment, long in use among private carriers such as Blue Cross, and predating even Medicare. Not so with physicians, where assignment was voluntary and rates of assignment varied widely by specialty and by region of the country. Moreover, the fact that physician DRGs would be bundled and paid at a fixed price would increase the incentives for physicians to recoup by billing the balance to the patient. This was bad in principle and would have been absolutely unacceptable to Congress. On the other hand, physician DRGs with mandatory assignment would put individual physicians at risk, especially those in the non-surgical specialities. But these were just the providers least accustomed to bundling and for whom physician DRGs would probably work least well, because of their inadequacy as predictors of resource use.[40] Not only, therefore, would there be an issue of fairness to the physician: more to the point, many of these physicians might withdraw their services, creating a nasty issue of beneficiary access to care.

Physician DRGs as an option lost popularity quickly, both within the HCFA and in Congress.[41] One reason was that they were not a solution. They provided no answer for services provided on an outpatient basis.[42] Inpatient DRGs, moreover, were unresearched as yet and presented some daunting, possibly insoluble, dilemmas to be confronted in their implementation.

Another option was capitation, implemented as a payment mechanism either through vouchers or some variety of government approved HMO or CMP.[43] Usually acknowledged as the most "elegant" solution, capitation fit well with the Reagan Administration's "pro-competition" ideology and had some support in Congress and DHHS. In principle, capitation had some major policy advantages. Paying an annual fee would enable the government to set an overall, prospective limit. Moreover, because it was a "per capita" amount, capitation created incentives to control inflationary tendencies inherent in CPR, such as upcoding or unbundling and increasing the volume or intensity of services per patient. And capitation minimized government regulation and supervision, giving the provider a large amount of freedom to manage in a cost-effective manner.

A major difficulty with capitation or the HMO was that they were not designed for and had never been systematically adapted to Medicare. Indeed, one result of reexamining physician payment was that it brought into bold relief the large gap in conception between the HMO as a device and the characteristics and the needs of the Medicare Part B population.[44]

One problem had to do with the AAPCC and whether it would work satisfactorily as a basis for payment. As provided by the Social Security Amendments of 1972 (as amended by TEFRA) HMOs or CMPs could contract for a prospective payment calculated on the basis of age, disability status, and "other factors" to be 95% of what would be paid by the government for comparable Medicare beneficiaries. The problem was that the AAPCC paid an *average* rate for the Medicare population in a particular county. The HMO, however, had to take individual enrollees from the Medicare population at large without the hedge of being able to choose particular firms or institutions where they would market. Nor could they raise their premiums in subsequent years, according to their own risk experience. A natural fear, well based in experience, was that "adverse selection" would occur, i.e., that sicker patients would take high-option plans and would not be adequately offset by healthy ones. Potentially, there were various ways this difficulty could be met, for instance, by identifying more precisely the high-risk enrollees and adjusting the AAPCC upward or by providing for a "catastrophic" reinsurance. However, the HCFA actuary took the position that the AAPCC was a fair payment and that health status or previous use adjusters would not solve the problem, which was really one of "administration" or "risk management" on the part of the HMO.[45] Others at the time said that the AAPCC was "broken" (couldn't be fixed); and many HMOs took a "you first" approach and waited for others to try out the "risk-based" option.

If there was a complaint on the part of the HMOs that they might not be paid enough, there was also a well-founded apprehension in government, especially EOMB, that Medicare HMOs would cost the program more money. Even though HMOs might be cost effective for the long term, so the argument ran, in the short term they were most likely to entail additional expenditure. One reason is that HMOs would divert patients, so that existing facilities would have unused capacity and higher unit costs. Much more important, though, was the tendency, evidenced by demonstration projects, for HMOs to enroll on average the healthier Medicare beneficiaries. Probably, the biggest factor was that older and sicker persons stayed with their present providers, mostly non-HMO. Whatever the cause, Medicare HMOs did lose money for the program: about $10 million a year for an unimpressive total of 190 thousand enrollees.[46]

Another problem with HMOs or managed care was that of beneficiary protection, an issue brought into prominence by the increased consideration being given to this option. Capitation and managed care essentially seek to save money by reducing the amount or the price of services provided, either of which could mean inferior care for the patient. Indeed, one of the most commonly employed devices, adapted from the Kaiser-Permanente[47] model, sets aside a bonus fund to reward providers for underspending the amount projected for hospital and physician services. Since HMOs were paid a capitation fee and did not generate the usual Medicare Part B claims, there was no big paper trail with which to document their activities. Moreover, periodic scandals involving either Medicare or Medicaid HMOs gave substance to these concerns and made even the strongest HMO supporters somewhat cautious.[48]

For the policy-maker, a major point with respect to capitation and managed care was that, however elegant they might be as an ultimate solution, they did not help much for the near term. Medicare HMO enrollments were increasing at an almost imperceptible rate: beneficiaries didn't join. There were quite possibly insoluble problems with respect to the AAPCC, adverse selection, and beneficiary protection. Even with a most favorable assessment of the prospects research and demonstrations were needed, and these were long-term projects.

Fee schedules had, by contrast, some big short-term advantages. Not the least of these was familiarity and acceptance. Both with traditional private insurance carriers and under Medicare, physicians already operated with a fee schedule—inequitable, irrational, and inflationary though it was. Physicians were accustomed to fee schedules and comfortable with them, warts and all. And Medicare itself was, in effect, a huge "demonstration" already under way with a vast accumulation of experience and data by the carriers and by the HCFA.

Fee schedules combined some long-term potential with a capacity for adaptation in the near-term. Based on a sound methodology, they could be used not only to amend the fee structure and make it fairer but would provide a good technical foundation for any future capitation or physician DRG schemes. For the immediate future, fee schedules lent themselves readily to partial solutions. They could be adapted piecemeal to adjust fees for particular specialties, add geographic multipliers, or reduce "overpriced" procedures. They could also be phased in with transition periods and percentage adjustments. As they were deployed, their effects on participation, access, and overall expenditure could be closely monitored through HCFA data files. Thus, they combined a possibility of incremental tinkering with a capacity for close monitoring. It is not surprising that they were a popular option in the HCFA and with Congress. During 1983, they were also picking up significant endorsements from other groups, such as the Medicare Advisory Council, the Grace Commission,[49] and the American Society of Internal Medicine.

Fee schedules might, however, be both inefficient and expensive. One anticipation, shared by many experienced persons, was that a maximum fee schedule would tend to become a minimum: that is, physicians who had previously charged less than Medicare allowed would tend to bill the fee schedule amount once it was established.[50] Furthermore, as with many new programs, fee schedules would probably entail an expensive "buy-in," in the form of an initial schedule that was set high to get maximum physician support. Unlike capitation or physician DRGs, fee schedules did not change the basic method of payment and therefore did nothing to change the incentives for physicians or the way in which they provided service. Specifically, nothing happened to make physicians practice medicine in a way that was any more cost-effective, except that fees for particular procedures could be changed and rates of increase lagged or set low through an annual update such as the MEI. But the physician would still be paid for piecework and would have even more incentive, with a fee schedule in place, to increase the volume or intensity of services rendered or to unbundle, upcode, or inflate claims in other ways. A possible solution, and the one eventually adopted, was to set an overall "target" or "standard," limiting volume globally, but that was not an option being seriously proposed in 1983.

With fee schedules under consideration, the issue of assignment bulks large. For some, the very notion of a fee schedule seemed to imply "that's the price," so that balance billing would be illegitimate. And it seemed a poor bargain if fee schedules saved the government money primarily at the expense of the Medicare beneficiaries. On the other hand, some physicians thought that the establishment of fee schedules made balance billing even more appropriate, partly as a matter of freedom for the practitioner, but also for those patients who wished to and could pay more for top quality physicians or special services.[51] Some who opposed mandatory assignment also pointed out that some physicians got only a small proportion of their income from Medicare and might simply withdraw from the program, creating a crisis of access.[52] There was a genuine policy dilemma, between risking heavy out of pocket expenditures for beneficiaries versus reduced access to care if physicians should withdraw.[53]

No single option did enough of the job. Fee schedules were easy to adapt for the short term, but volume was a killer over the long term. Capitation made sense as an ultimate goal, but issues of quality assurance and the payment formula would have to be resolved first. Physician DRGs could, at best, deal with some of physician reimbursement, but only a fraction of it. There was no "magic bullet," nothing that would provide a central ordering concept around which to build a coherent proposal.

Medicare physician payment could be described as a problem without a solution. More positively, though, it was a complex set of dilemmas requiring a long-term strategy and some short-term partial solutions. In the best of worlds, which was not this one so far as the DHSS and HCFA staff could see, developing a policy for Medicare Part B would require research and demonstrations to devise suitable methods and then careful monitoring of implementation to coordinate the approaches. This meant time, money, and purposive leadership. By 1984, each of these was in short supply.

A Failed Initiative

The Reagan Administration, committed to a "contractive" policy toward government and bent on achieving a maximum impact in the first years of the new regime, did not strongly support research or development in health policy. Disfavored especially were projects that would not produce a quick result or ones that were deemed inconsistent with Reaganite "deregulation" or "pro-competition" priorities.[54] As a consequence, the HCFA research budget declined by 1984 from $50 million a year to $30 million, a loss of 40%. Moreover, as a result of a quarrel with EOMB, the HCFA largely lost control of its own demonstrations. By then, Congress was mandating an increasing number of reports, often written within the HCFA by ORD staff. As a consequence, the HCFA had little to spend on research grants or contracts, a development of which the health policy research community was much aware. When the HCFA requested proposals on physician reimbursement for its 1984 grant cycle, for instance, not a single response was forthcoming.[55] At this critical juncture, the HCFA was singularly barren of ideas that could be implemented in the area of physician payment and in a poor position to develop any.[56]

Effective, purposive health policy leadership in the executive branch was lacking. The dilemmas of physician payment reform lent themselves to differences and there were plenty. Indeed, the Reagan Administration was notable for having at least four different approaches advocated within the executive branch at the same time. Within the HCFA, some favored working with the existing CPR methodology while others were for a fee schedule. The White House health policy adviser favored capitation, but with no specific remedies for its shortcomings. Meanwhile, EOMB was for physician DRGs, though mostly as a cost-saver and sometimes only for an arguing point. Probably the Reagan Administration's emphasis on ideology and on a contractive regime increased policy differences since both provided additional grounds for saying "yea" or "nay," and mostly the latter, without having to confront the practicalities of developing a specific policy proposal. Because of the complexities of physician payment reform, the HCFA was in the best position to propose something that could be actually implemented; but by 1984, the HCFA was short of resources and the will for new starts. The new Secretary of DHHS, Margaret Heckler, had no significant ideas of her own about health, nor was she an effective advocate for programs, either on the Hill or at the White House. Consequently, during her tenure,[57] no one spoke with authority for any one approach, as Richard Schweiker had done for PPS when he was Secretary.

By 1984, time was in short supply along with dollars and leadership. Congress had passed no budget reconciliation in 1983, having gotten entangled in an issue of "nongermane" amendments. Meanwhile, the deficit and Medicare Part B expenditures continued to rise. 1984 was an election year making providers, rather than beneficiaries, the preferred target, at least for Congress. In June of that year, with the unexpected acquiescence of David Stockman, the EOMB director, Congress legislated an 18 month fee freeze, important not only because it was an independent initiative on the part of Congress, but because it raised sharply the question of "what next?" As the name, "fee freeze," implies some day there has to be a thaw, and an issue of what to do then. Policies are made largely by choosing between alternatives. If the administration was to be influential with respect to physician payment reform, some entity within the executive branch needed to come forward soon with some actionable options.

One available policy vehicle was the congressionally mandated report on physician DRGs, due in 1985. This report was being prepared in the HCFA, primarily by Stephen Jencks and Allen Dobson of ORD. With the encouragement of Carolyne Davis, they proposed to expand the report, use it to explore the available alternates, and lay out a general strategy for physician payment reform. An important point that they would make is that there was no *one* solution. The most viable approach, in their view, was to aim at increasingly global control of physician payments, beginning with a fee schedule and moving toward physician DRGs and capitation. This strategy would begin with the familiar and move toward the unknown, allowing lead-time for research and for demonstrations testing physician DRGs and capitation schemes. Physician response and beneficiary access to care could be monitored as this plan moved forward. Especially, this approach would combine a long-term strategy with some options that could be implemented in the near future, an item important for the Congress. Dobson and Jencks estimated that a charge-based fee schedule[58] could be in place by October 1, 1986.[59]

The Jencks–Dobson proposal was not too different from the strategy ultimately adopted by Congress without benefit of significant executive branch participation. In that respect, had their proposal been endorsed by the Reagan Administration, it might have been of great historic importance. Especially promising was its melding of a long-range strategy with a proposal for immediate action. The HCFA could have begun work immediately on the fee schedules. And the Congress was going to act, with or without benefit of executive branch input. During the Spring of 1985, the Congressional Budget Office, acting at the request of Congress, had begun work on a report on physician payment reform, proposing a fee schedule and physician DRGs for inpatient services. Significantly, in the light of subsequent developments, the June draft omitted any discussion of capitation.[60]

The Jencks–Dobson proposal was prescient in identifying the difficulties confronting any single approach to physician reimbursement. The overall strategy made sense, particularly in the ordering of the development of alternative approaches. But there were loose ends. Especially, there were no answers for a number of troublesome unknowns and policy dilemmas. For instance, fee schedules and mandatory assignment were recommended, but with little attention to volume and access. Physician DRGs were presented in a hopeful light, but without discussing the all-important question of who gets paid. Capitation was recommended as the ultimate goal, despite serious questions about its feasibility, either technical or political. For most of these difficulties, the answer seemed to be additional demonstrations, although the prospects for any of these, given EOMB strictures, were remote.

The "Secretary's Report" itself, that had begun as a technical assessment of physician DRGs, was by now evolving into a vehicle for a major policy statement. It not only canvassed the options, it proposed a strategy. That point, by itself, is important, for a strategy relates and sequences a number of policies—in other words, set off a great many anxieties. Without advertising the fact, the Report being developed had major implications for the pro-competition, anti-regulation ideology of the Reagan Administration. It had major budgetary consequences. It could affect significantly the respective roles of Congress and the Executive in the making of health policy. And, not least, it would establish a set of relations and expectations with respect to providers that could well endure for the next generation. In a few words, it was a document pregnant with far reaching implications and laden with potential conflict. Early in 1985, it had already been through five iterations,[61] and the Jencks–Dobson proposals represented yet another.

At another time, these proposals might have had a reasonably good chance of adoption. But that would have taken high-level advocacy and leadership. 1985 was a dismal and inert year for DHSS and the HCFA. People from the first Reagan Administration were gone, were leaving, or had their bags packed. Carolyne Davis resigned in August. Margaret Heckler was embattled and expected to leave shortly. Almost no significant health initiatives were coming from DHSS.[62] Meanwhile, the policy vacuum was being increasingly filled by EOMB and the White House health policy adviser, both of whom took strong stands on physician reimbursement.

Not surprisingly, this version of the Secretary's Report was rejected. As it underwent the usual series of reviews within the HCFA, at the level of ASPE, and then by Roper's White House Working Group on Health Policy, opposition to various aspects grew, but most particularly to its "regulatory" implications. This was especially true after Carolyne Davis left in August. Eventually, Secretary Heckler took the Report to Edwin Meese's Domestic Policy Council, for a meeting at which Roper and other capitation advocates sat in. Back came the strong message that fee schedules, physician DRGs, and such short-term regulative approaches were out. The Administration policy was pro-competition: Medicare vouchers and capitation.[63]

At that time, Margaret Heckler said, in one of her last official statements as Secretary, that capitation was and had long been the favored option of the Reagan Administration. To implement, now, more radical immediate changes such as national fee schedules or physician DRGs would risk "clogging the system" and make capitation more difficult to implement at some future date. DHSS expected to launch several demonstrations in the near future to test the capitation idea. Meanwhile, she said, it was best to leave the old system of physician reimbursement much as it was, awaiting fuller implementation of the capitation alternative.[64]

A Capitation Alternative? The Administration's capitation proposal at this juncture may have made sense as a way of saying that no policy is better than one you do not like. But it did not address immediate political reality, at least from the perspective of Congress. Congress was busy with the deficit, developing both the Gramm–Rudman–Hollings deficit reduction legislation and putting together COBRA. The latter contained an extension of the fee freeze. It also included legislation establishing a Physician Payment Review Commission to develop a relative value scale, a preliminary to a national fee schedule.[65] For Congress, the urgent need was for a Part B proposal that could be acted on quickly. Capitation would take years: a new sequence of RFPs, demonstrations, evaluations, legislative drafting, etc. At this juncture, the Administration proposal seemed little better than a ploy. Coming from an Administration that had treated its own capitation policy largely as ideology, that had blown hot and cold, that had dallied with implementation, and that had, in general, bungled its own campaign, this latest initiative seemed almost impudent.

For the Reagan Administration, capitation was both ideology and policy, yet the relations between these two were never clearly sorted out. As ideology, proposals like vouchers and capitation sounded good as part of a pro-competition, anti-regulative theme that was especially prominent in the first years of the Reagan Administration and that would be periodically revived by true believers. But much of it was only ideology. Little was done to turn it into a viable policy by confronting the serious problems attending capitation as a payment methodology: such as what to do about quality assurance, adverse selection, and the AAPCC. At the same time, capitation was also being extensively implemented, especially by DHSS during the Schweiker tenure and by the HCFA under Carolyne Davis. But much of this was implementation without a sanctioned policy, and on this account ran into trouble, especially with the Office of Management and Budget. That agency effectively put a quietus on this activity, but in so doing weakened the option favored by its own Administration. Some of the details are interesting, for they illustrate vagaries of policy-making in the Reagan executive branch, as well as help to explain why Congress acted as it did.

One practice made possible on a large scale by the Social Security

Amendments of 1972 was the use of "waivers"[66] and demonstration projects to develop alternative ways of delivering health care or new methods of reimbursement for Medicare or Medicaid. The 1972 legislation was only the beginning, as a whole series of subsequent acts expanded this authority for specific kinds of activity, and authorized or mandated various studies and reports. This waiver and demonstration authority could be useful in demonstrating the feasibility of some untried methods—for instance, swing beds or incentive reimbursement—showing not only that they could work in practice and in various settings but also revealing difficulties that had not been anticipated in the theoretical analysis or modeling. In this way, demonstrations provided an important step from concept and analysis to practice.[67] They could also be used to increase the "visibility" of particular alternatives and develop support for them within the bureaucracy, on the part of State program officials and politicians, and within the Congress. Used ambitiously, they could help out faltering programs and build new ones, a potential that was exploited and abused both in the Carter and Reagan administrations.[68]

When Richard Schweiker took office as Secretary, he had four main agenda items. Two of these were primarily Reagan priorities: budget reduction and block grants. Two were Schweiker's: the drug approval process and health care cost containment.[69] Of these, cost containment was the more important and included, for Schweiker, some form of prospective payment for hospitals and strong support for capitation. Under the heading of "competition projects," capitation demonstrations for Medicare and Medicaid were agreed on by Secretary Schweiker and Carolyne Davis as a target objective[70] to be vigorously pursued, even though they lacked the legislative authority for such a program. These waivered demonstrations were pushed to a maximum, at times illegally,[71] without adequate monitoring, until the HCFA had half a million beneficiaries under waivered contracts.

EOMB uneasiness about waivers and demonstrations was long-standing and preceded the Reagan Administration. Under the Carter Administration, and especially when Patricia Harris was Secretary, the Office of Management and Budget had objected to expensive subsidies to inner-city hospitals and long-term care demonstrations which they saw as "back-door" agenda building. The Reagan EOMB was mindful of this history. Furthermore, it did not uncritically identify capitation with "competition." In fact, EOMB believed that capitation had serious problems and that resolving these might take years. Thus, it began with grounds for suspicion and especially with a view that capitation was not a short-term solution. By 1982 the deficit was urgent business, making any money-spending program out of conformity with Reagan priorities doubly suspect. For the EOMB, moreover, "top-down" policy-making was fundamental: a setting of priorities by the White House, with EOMB as central, and a development of departmental policies within these parameters. Under these circumstances, the Medicare–Medicaid demonstrations were a catastrophe waiting to happen.

Given EOMB's role under the first Reagan Administration as the premier staff agency and a key defender of the faith on domestic policy issues, many of its objections made sense.[72] One relatively minor objection was procedure: inadequate paper submissions and bad project management. At a more serious level, EOMB complained that the HCFA was straying into areas of policy such as long-term care and Medicaid waivers that conflicted with Reagan priorities. Money was a major item, especially failure adequately to estimate project costs or realistically compute the real costs to the government. And especially after the passage of TEFRA in August of 1982, EOMB could see no good reason why Medicare HMOs should be covertly subsidized through the Trust Funds instead of being put under the new risk-based contracts as speedily as possible.

During 1983, EOMB grew increasingly insistent about these concerns. The HCFA, for its part, argued that the waivered demonstrations were their program to manage and that it legitimately addressed Reagan priorities. Differences of opinion developed into a quarrel, leading to tactical skirmishing, and eventually to a major confrontation in 1984. The HCFA lost this fight, with the result that Brian Luce, the Director of ORD, was fired and humiliating peace terms imposed on the HCFA by EOMB. Because of the new criteria established, and particularly the requirement that all waivered demonstrations had to save the Federal government money, Carolyne Davis withdrew 12 HMO demonstrations then pending with EOMB. Practically, any further development of this program ceased.[73]

One effect of this demonstrations debacle was further to diminish the credibility of capitation as a policy alternative, to the point that it was little but ideology, an ideal aspiration of the Administration. To date, little research or policy analysis had been done on the payment methodology or quality assurance for HMOs or CMPs. Regulations for the TEFRA risk-based HMOs to implement the legislation passed in 1982 were delayed over two years and not yet published in final form. And EOMB had effectively shut down demonstrations in this area. After the 1984 elections, the Administration called for a revivial of pro-competition alternatives, with research and demonstrations on a broad range of alternative payment methodologies, including capitation, competitive bidding, vouchers, and PPOs.[74] But this pumped-up enthusiasm had little appeal in Congress, already skeptical of the capitation alternative and made increasingly so by perennial Medicare and Medicaid HMO scandals. The Administration initiative seemed mostly ritualistic, the recital of a creed, rather than an earnest of good works.

A cynical view would be that the Reagan Administration preferred this alternative: a policy option that filled space in the domestic agenda but was not to be taken seriously as a proposal for implementation. A more charitable interpretation is that the pro-competition ideology and the contractive theme of the Administration came into conflict. With no creative proposal, the Administration was left without a credible policy. Whatever its merits for other areas, "competition" as applied to health policy was largely a "buzz-word," energetically promoted by conservative think-tanks and some reputable economists, but not much researched or analyzed. In fact, the "competition" task forces within DHSS were soon abandoned as a waste of time. Moreover, the new political appointees within the HCFA were pushing for a maximum short-term impact and skeptical of research or schemes of the civil servants that had only a long-term pay-out.[75] Not surprisingly, little attention was paid to such low-visibility items as the AAPCC, adverse selection, and quality assurance in HMOs.[76] Instead, the DHSS and the HCFA pushed ahead to implement the capitation alternative without benefit of previous analysis or research and without a clear statutory authority or specific mandate from the White House. But EOMB insisted that an executive branch agency had no business spending large amounts of money for purposes not sanctioned in law or falling within Reagan Administration priorities. Given the EOMB's position as the "point" agency implementing the Reagan Administration's "contractive" policies and the continuing urgency of the budget deficit, this attitude made sense. But their actions, justifiable from one perspective, did not serve the Administration's needs for a health policy option. And by cutting off the waivered demonstrations for an agency already strapped for R&D money, EOMB's actions further diminished any prospect of developing a capitation proposal that could be taken seriously.

By the Fall of 1985, health policy in the executive branch with respect to Medicare physician payment was deadlocked, with no proposal commanding a consensus and each of the options opposed by one or more of the principals. The HCFA proposal for a fee schedule was vetoed, first by EOMB and then by the Domestic Policy Council. The "official" policy of the administration was capitation, but that was opposed by EOMB and had little support from the HCFA or within Congress. EOMB still pushed for physician DRGs, but largely at this point as a tactical maneuver. The Secretary's Report, long awaited in Congress, was mired in yet another rewrite.[77] In November, President Reagan appointed a new Secretary, Otis R. Bowen, an Indiana physician and former governor.

And in March 1986, he appointed a second physician, William L. Roper,[78] to be the new head of the HCFA. Secretary Heckler's statement of October 1985, specifically rejecting any alternative but capitation, ended this cycle of Administration efforts on a dismal note. The new appointments represented no change of policy, so far as physician payment was concerned. Bowen favored capitation. And Roper was a committed supporter of capitation, coming to the HCFA not to negotiate a change of policy but to uphold the established one.

III. ACTION BY CONGRESS

As early as the Spring of 1982, Congress began requesting from the DHSS proposals for what to do about Medicare physician payment. Not until the Secretary's Report, released in September 1987, did the Congress receive a reply, other than the periodic, ritualistic appearances before the subcommittees to recite once again the Administration's abiding faith in capitation. The Secretary's Report, finally delivered, was largely warmed-over hash. A plain fact is that the Administration never had a policy on physician payment, at least not one that deserved to be taken seriously by the Congress. Margaret Heckler's press conference of October 1985 tacitly admitted as much: there was nothing to be done for now; for the future, there was the Holy Grail of capitation.

But policy with respect to physician reimbursement *was* developed during this period, without an overall design, incrementally, implicitly, largely by the health subcommittees of House Ways and Means and Senate Finance, through the budget reconciliation process. In large measure, the eventual formula of a Physician Payment Review Commission and a national fee schedule was the logical extension of the incremental changes made through that process between 1983 and 1986.

That there *was* eventually a policy for Medicare physician reimbursement may have owed little to the Reagan Administration. On the other hand, the *way* in which that policy was developed owed a great deal to the Administration, and especially to its "contractive" budgetary goals and deficit reduction tactics, from the earliest consideration of physician payment reform down to the final legislation.

The Summer of 1982 was a season for strategic decisions that gave shape and direction to future Medicare payment policies. With Social Security entitlements regarded as a near suicidal object of attack, Medicare expenditures offered the next best opportunity. At this point, hospital reimbursement was much more important, but Part B expenditures also came up, with the question of "Who pays?" increasingly at issue.[79]

With respect to Part B, the Administration was both pro-competition and anti-entitlement, with policies designed to encourage cost-awareness as well as to save money. On the pro-competition side, the Administration proposed "vouchers" or "consumer choice" options and a cap on the tax deduction. These would be reinforced with cost-savers in the form of reduced Medicare benefits and increased co-pays and Part B premiums. Catastrophic health insurance would provide a kind of "safety-net," i.e., a cap limiting the total out-of-pocket expense. Whatever might have been the merits of the plan, it would have resulted in a substantially increased burden for the Medicare beneficiaries, and 1982 was an election year. Congress tends normally to favor the beneficiary, and more so in election years. Even so, no clear decision was reached that year. TEFRA, as previously noted, contained a provision setting the Part B premium at 25% of program costs. During the passage of TEFRA, the Congress also considered, but did not adopt, a freeze of the MEI. There was no budget reconciliation for that year, so the issue of "who pays?" was postponed for a time. But as the legislative season developed Congress, and especially the Democratic House, came to doubt more and more the attractiveness of the Administration's pro-competition package, and especially the propriety or fairness of the "beneficiary bashing" it entailed.

Fee Freeze

During 1983, the DHHS lost momentum. Richard Schweiker resigned early in that year.[80] Much of the time and energy of the HCFA staff, especially the leadership, was absorbed in the design and implementation of PPS. Despite Carolyne Davis's formation of the Physicians' Advisory Group, little that was new was undertaken with respect to physician reimbursement. For several years, though, a few specialists in beneficiary and reimbursement studies had been developing proposals for a "participating physician program" that would include a number of special incentives for physicians to take assignment: such as differential reimbursement rates, streamlined billing procedures, and the publication of an annual directory of "participating" physicians. The proposal was included as one of the recommendations of the DHHS Medicare Advisory Council for its June meeting, and became one of the more important contributions of the HCFA to the development of Medicare physician payment policy.[81]

This was the year in which the notion of a "freeze" became popular, at first as a compromise on spending and budget reduction and later, with respect to physician payment, as a substantive policy position. At the beginning of 1983, the Reagan Administration confronted the unpleasant reality that the recession was deeper and the deficit larger than anticipated. Another reality was a Democratic gain of 26 seats and the restoring of a working majority in the House of Representatives. At first, the notion of a "freeze" on nondefense, discretionary spending was mostly an EOMB expedient, partly tactical ploy and partly "blue smoke and mirrors," intended to protect the defense budget and avoid new taxes (Kirschten 1983). At the same time, it provided the basis for a short-term accord with Congress: a concession on entitlements, while holding the line on other domestic expenditures.

The notion of a "freeze" on Medicare payments to physicians as one application of this approach quickly caught on. It could be done. And there was something for everyone. From the White House perspective, and especially that of EOMB, a fee freeze would save some dollars and would likely pass Congress, while the more ambitious pro-competition package of a tax cap, co-pays, and vouchers was almost certainly doomed.[82] For Congress, a fee freeze helped with their pledge to reduce the deficit and, at the same time, kept the onus off the beneficiaries. For the physician, mindful of what had happened to the hospitals, accepting a fee freeze would be an earnest of their good intentions, important in a political climate that behooved providers to come forward with constructive proposals of their own.

During the Summer of 1983, the fee freeze proposal gained momentum. In June, the American Society of Internal Medicine came out in support of a one year freeze on the MEI. President Reagan, addressing the AMA annual convention in Chicago, advocated a one year freeze. The DHHS Medicare Advisory Council, coming to the end of its year's deliberations, endorsed a "participating physician program" and was looking with interest at proposals for a fee schedule. Both the House and Senate, at work on the budget reconciliation for the next fiscal year, crafted several variants of the fee freeze scheme.

Nevertheless, there remained the hard question of who pays: the physician or the beneficiary? No one had real difficulty with the notion that the Medicare payment should be frozen. But what about balance billing? Why wouldn't the physician simply bill the patients to make up for any income lost because of a fee freeze? And if the net effect of this budget reconciliation fix was to shift the burden to the patients, especially the elderly Medicare beneficiaries, what was the morality or political sense of that? One answer was mandatory assignment, strongly supported by the Democratic majority of the Health Subcommittee of Ways and Means. But mandatory assignment was opposed by the AMA. It was more coercive than anything tried to date. And it carried with it an unknown risk of withdrawal from the program, entailing a loss of access to physicians' services by Medicare beneficiaries and a political hassle of monstrous proportions. For this reason, and for substantive reasons of policy, the Senate Finance Committee, controlled by the Republican Party, opposed mandary assignment. So did EOMB and the White House, because of anti-regulatory policies as well as political indebtedness to the physicians.

The issue of assignment almost killed the fee freeze, despite the support for it that, by now, included an AMA endorsement of a one-year voluntary freeze.[83] In 1983, no reconciliation bill was passed.[84] In the holdover bill that went to conference in 1984, there was actually no freeze proposal from the House, mandatory assignment having been taken to the floor and defeated.[85] David Stockman suggested the essential compromise that emerged from the conference.[86] His proposal was to freeze physician *charges* at the 1984 rates, but allow balance billing for the difference between the Medicare payment and the frozen charges. This expedient avoided the issue of mandatory assignment, yet held the beneficiary harmless. At the same time, inducements would be offered to the physician to accept assignment through the participating physician program, just begun by the HCFA. Participating physicians could also bill their regular (non-Medicare) patients more, with the assurance that these increased rates would be built into their fee screen profiles for the post-freeze period. This compromise was readily accepted, though not without some astonishment that it could have come from David Stockman.

DEFRA[87] was not passed until July 18 of 1984, shortly before recess. It was a huge statute that combined a hodge-podge of revenue enhancements with the deficit reduction agreements that included the fee freeze. With respect to physician reimbursement, though, DEFRA had a much wider significance than just mandating a 15 month freeze. The freeze, initiated in Congress, was generally recognized in the health policy community as starting the reform of Medicare physician reimbursement in a serious way. It is important that that process began in Congress and that it began with a regulation of physicians' fees. In addition, Sec. 2309, "Study of Medicare Part B Payments," directed the Office of Technology Assessment, a Congressional agency, to conduct a study of physician reimbursement and report back to Congress by the end of 1985. It further directed that the study should consider inequities in payments as between "types of service, locality, and specialty, with particular attention to any inequities between cognitive services and medical procedures" and that the study should take into account the "overhead expenses" and the "relative time, complexity, and investment in professional training necessary to the provision of various procedures and services" and the "methodologies which could be applied in the development of fee schedules on a national or regional basis."[88] In short, Congress was not only moving in advance of and more rapidly than DHSS or the HCFA; it was moving in a specific direction.

DEFRA also went into many specifics of hospital and physician payment. In this respect, the statute marked a sharp gradient in the use of budget and deficit reduction as a technique for amending the statutory provisions for hospital and physician payment, periodically and in such detail as to control much of the process of implementation as well.[89] In DEFRA, there was much detail with respect to the newly established PPS. There were also provisions dealing with the coverage of and reimbursement for specific physicians' services, including such items as the treatment of mycotic toenails. More significant portents were contained in two other provisions. One was Sec. 2303, mandating fee schedules for clinical diagnostic laboratory tests. A second, Sec. 2304, directed HCFA to establish "reasonable cost" limits on physicians' services associated with the implanting or replacing of cardiac pacemakers. In essence, using the budget reconciliation procedures, Congress was beginning a piecemeal, incremental reform of the existing system of physicians' fees.

DEFRA was a remarkably good indication of what was to come. During 1985, Congress reached the conclusion that reforming Medicare physician payment was largely going to depend on initiatives taken by the legislative branch. As early as TEFRA in 1982, the Congress had invited proposals on physician reimbursement from DHHS. In the Social Security Amendments of 1983, enacting PPS, Congress specifically mandated a report on applications of prospective payment to physicians. Still lacking any sort of recommendation from the Administration, Congress directed the Office of Technology Assessment to prepare a report on physician reimbursement. Late in 1984, Congress moved up the date of the Secretary's Report from the end of 1985 to July of that year. Again, without avail: no report appeared. Instead, there was Secretary Heckler's statement that "only minor changes" were appropriate for now, with capitation a long-term possibility. From that date, Congress was to hear no recommendation from the Administration other than "vouchers" and capitation.

In the budget reconciliation legislation for that year,[90] Congress created its own source of expertise and advice, a Physician Payment Review Commission, similar in composition and structure to ProPAC for hospital payment (Iglehart 1988). One reason for this step was the clear indication that neither the HCFA nor DHHS was likely to develop any policy alternatives that Congress would wish to consider seriously. Another was the belief that Congress needed an advisory body to help make clear the long-term implications of its own actions and to moderate and legitimate its own decisions.[91]

The Commission was to make recommendations to Congress especially regarding changes in payment methodology for physicians' services. It was directed to take account of the OTA study of physician reimbursement that was under way and of the "Secretary's study," when and if it should appear. But the legislation gave a strong indication of the way Congress was inclined. The Secretary was to proceed with the development of a relative value scale, with July 1987 set as the date for completion. This was a first step toward a national fee schedule.

Years will be required before we can say whether this was the best way to go. But no actionable alternative was offered. Congress had repeatedly and insistently requested a considered proposal from the Executive branch, only to hear the familiar response that "capitation is the policy." Over time, the legislative subcommittees acted more and more on their own, through the reconciliation process. With no other choice offered, they took the one alternative that was actionable at the time.

CHRONOLOGY: PHYSICIAN PAYMENT: BACKGROUND

1. Implementation of Medicare begins, July 1, 1966.
2. Authority for R&D, experiments in payment reform, Secs. 222, 223, Social Security Amendments of 1972.
3. HMO Act of 1973, P.L. 93-222 (December 29, 1973).
4. Nixon–Ford Economic Stabilization Program, 1971–1974.
5. CHIP (1974), Nixon–Ford Comprehensive Health Insurance Proposal (H.R.12684, February, 1974) state fee schedules proposed; Kennedy–Mills Comprehensive National Health Insurance Act (H.R.13874, Apr. 1974) national fee schedules with global caps proposed.
6. Medicare Economic Index implemented, 1975.
7. Carter hospital cost containment effort, April 1977 to November 1979.
8. TEFRA, P.L. 97-248 (September 3, 1982).
9. PPS goes into effect, October 1983.
10. April 1983: Physicians' Advisory Group formed; Senator Dole announces a "Year of the Physician."
11. HCFA loses battle over "waivered" demonstrations, June 1984.
12. "Fee Freeze" goes into effect, July 1, 1984. Legislated by DEFRA (P.L. 98-369, July 18, 1984).
13. CBO begins a study report on physician payment reform.

14. Carolyne Davis leaves HCFA, August, 1985; Margaret Heckler leaves as Secretary of DHSS, October 1985.
15. White House (EOMB and Domestic Policy Council) vetoes the Jencks–Dobson proposal, September 1985.
16. Otis R. Bowen, M.D. appointed Secretary of DHSS, November 1985; William L. Roper, M.D. appointed Administrator of the HCFA, March, 1986.
17. COBRA (P.L. 99-272, April 7, 1986)—Congress creates Physician Payment Review Commission; mandates development of a relative value scale.

NOTES

1. Under Medicare, physicians have been allowed to bill patients for the "balance" of their expected fee, in excess of the amount paid by Medicare. There is some difference about terminology. "Balance billing" is the more traditional term, but PPRC, for instance, uses "extra billing." Obviously, how one feels about this semantic difference would depend on whether one was billing or being billed.
2. Technically, not "volume" as such, but increases in volume and intensity that led to higher overall Part B outlays.
3. Social Security Amendments of 1965, P.L. 89-97, Secs. 1833; 1814; 1861.
4. Usually called "mandatory assignment," meaning that they assigned their claim, took what was paid by Medicare, on a compulsory basis.
5. Both the American Medical Association and Wilbur Mills, then chairman of the House Ways and Means Committee, favored this provision. As a partial protection for Part B beneficiaries, the Medicare legislation provided that physicians could take "assignment" much as they did with private insurance carriers: that is, agree to accept as payment in full the amount the insurer allowed.
6. Interview with Irwin Wolkstein, Health Policy Alternatives, December 7, 1987.
7. Department of Health, Education, and Welfare—the predecessor of DHHS.
8. For instance, Robert Ball, Robert Myers, William Stewart, John Veneman, and Irwin Wolkstein in DHEW; William Fullerton of the House Ways and Means staff and Jay Constantine of the Senate Finance staff.
9. Hospital or physician DRGs were not among them. For a sense of the animating spirit of these proposals, see "Reimbursement Guidelines for Medicare," Hearing before the Committee on Finance, U.S. Senate, Eighty-ninth Congress, Second session, May 25, 1960 (Washington, D.C., Government Printing Office, 1966.)
10. Interviews with Irwin Wolkstein, Health Policy Alternatives, December 7, 1987; and Glenn Markus, Health Policy Alternatives, December 2, 1987.
11. Informal rule making.
12. The Social Security Amendments of 1967 authorized experiments aimed at cost-saving, but were not particularly helpful in this respect. More use was

made of inherent administrative authority and the language of the original statute.

13.   Interview with Irwin Wolkstein, Health Policy Alternatives, December 7, 1987; Dutton and McMenamin (1981, 137).

14.   *Medicare and Medicaid: Problems, Issues, and Alternatives.* Report of the Staff to the Committee on Finance, United States Senate, 91st Congress, 1st Session, February 1970.

15.   Cf. Sec. 221, Social Security Amendments of 1972.

16.   Secs. 223 and 224.

17.   Sec. 222.

18.   Waivers exempted particular providers or states from complying with the regular Medicare or Medicaid regulations so that they could engage in monitored experiments in alternate modes of service delivery or different payment methodologies. Sec. 226.

19.   Brown (1983, 205–207; 382–387 and chs. 5, 7, *passim*). The average adjusted per capital cost (AAPCC) was devised by the Social Security Actuary, using the best methods then available, to develop a satisfactory way to pay HMOs—complex organizations—a fair and financially attractive rate for providing health care to Medicare beneficiaries—a special and protected population. It is an actuarial estimate of the amount required to serve the non-HMO Medicare population within a geographic area (in practice, the county) adjusted for age, sex, institutional, and disability status.

20.   Interviews with Irwin Wolkstein, December 7, 1987; Glenn Markus, December 2, 1987. Also, Chris N. Theodore and Judith S. Warner, "Physicians' Fees and the Source of their Increase," in Zubkoff (1976).

21.   Newhouse et al. (1982); research begun in 1974.

22.   The Hsiao RVS project also benefitted from this authority, though more indirectly. Hsiao's first research was to investigate the effects of market incentives on the supply of physicians' services. From interviews with physicians, he became interested in the problem of devising a fair and technically sound method of physician payment and did a brief study. Independently, the HCFA developed an interest in fee schedules and let several contracts in 1980–1981, but results were inconclusive and mostly disappointing. Hsiao turned his attention to other research. Meanwhile, Massachusetts adopted a fee schedule for Medicaid, an experiment that proved to be both a technical and political disaster. Hsiao and his associates, now in Massachusetts, were asked to do what they could to improve the payment methodology. Shortly thereafter, interest within the HCFA revived, leading to another contract with Hsiao, which became the basis for the RBRVS. The parallel with the development of DRGs is significant, especially in showing the importance of lead-time, some freedom for investigators, and willingness to back promising leads. Telephone interview with William C. Hsiao, School of Public Health, Harvard University, July 8, 1991.

23.   Interviews with Bernard Potashnick, Medical Services Reimbursement, the HCFA, April 6, 1988; and Ira Burney, Office of Legislation and Policy, DHSS, March 3, 1988.

24.   P.L. 95-142, October 25, 1977; also, cf., *Forward Plan for Health* (Washington, D.C.: U.S. Department of Health, Education, and Welfare, 1975).

25.   Cf. Zubkoff (1976); "Proposals to Stimulate Health Care Competition," Hearing before the Subcommittee on Health of the Committee on Finance, U.S. Senate (Washington, D.C. Government Printing Office, 1980).

26. Interviews with Carolyne Davis, Ernst and Whinney, March 10, 1988; Karen Davis, Commissioner, PPRC, March 11, 1988; Brian Luce, Battelle, December 16, 1987; and Alphonse Esposito, ORD, the HCFA, April 10, 1988.

27. If it makes sense to think of it as a "market."

28. The idea being that by limiting the amount of employer contributions to health insurance that would be tax-free both employer and employee would have greater incentives to shop around for cheaper or more cost-effective providers.

29. Aside from the hospital payment scheme, TEFRA also reformed and strengthened the PSROs, redesignated as Peer Review Organizations, and created new opportunities and inducements for Medicare HMOs and Competitive Medical Plans (CMPs).

30. The OBRA of 1981 contained some substantive legislation on health, but only a few items, and those of relatively minor scope.

31. Since extended, with various modifications.

32. The *Blue Sheet*, February 16, 1983, p. 3.

33. Some claims data specialists believed that reform of CPR, encouraging participation, and targeting particularly high-volume and expensive procedures was the best option, especially for saving money and protecting beneficiaries at the same time. Interviews with Ira Burney, Office of Legislation and Policy, the HCFA, March 3, 1988; and Stephen Jencks, Office of Research and Demonstrations, the HCFA, March 30, 1988.

34. Along with recurring threats to the Trust Funds, occasioned by rising Part A and Part B expenditures.

35. The *Blue Sheet*, April 20, 1983, p. 31.

36. As it was most commonly known. Its official title was "Physicians' Discussion Group," so named to avoid Federal "advisory group" regulations on background investigations, financial disclosure, etc. Interview with William L. Roper, Administrator, the HCFA, June 10, 1988.

37. Interview with Carolyne K. Davis, Ernst and Whinney, March 10, 1988.

38. Interviews with Patrice Feinstein, former Associate Administrator, the HCFA, June 9, 1988; and Stephen Jencks, Office of Research and Demonstrations, March 30, 1988.

39. Interviews with Allen Dobson, Consolidated Consulting Group, February 15, 1988; and Stephen Jencks, Office of Research and Demonstrations, the HCFA, March 30, 1988. Also, discussion paper by Allen Dobson, "Prospective Payment System Construction Issues" (unpublished), May 1983.

40. *Ibid.*, Stephen Jencks. Also, Janet B. Mitchell, "Packaging Physician Services: Alternative Approaches to Medicare Part B Reimbursement," paper presented to conference sponsored by Health Industry Manufacturers Association, August 17–18, 1987. An earlier report of this research and analysis by Mitchell was influential in leading the HCFA to abandon the physician DRG option. Interview with Donald Young, Executive Director, Prospective Payment Assessment Commission, May 10, 1988.

41. EOMB was an exception, continuing to advocate this approach until the Bush Administration and the introduction of a fee schedule proposal in Congress.

42. There had been attempts to devise a way of paying prospectively for "bundled" services, notably "ambulatory visit groups" and "diagnostic cost groups" or DCGs, but these were as yet undeveloped and unproven.

43. "Competitive medical plan," a TEFRA contribution.

44. Interview with Glenn Markus, Health Policy Alternatives, December 2, 1987.

45. The adjusters were unrefined and would be costly and complex. In any event, the Medicare beneficiaries could still "select against" the HMO, whether or not an additional payment was made. Therefore, the AAPCC was the best payment device, as such, that was available. Interview with Roland E. (Guy) King, Chief Actuary, the HCFA, July 10, 1988; also "Final Report: Review of AAPCC Methodology for Implementing Prospective Contracts with HMO's," Milliman and Robertson, Inc., Consulting Actuaries (unpubl.), August 3, 1983.

46. This was less than 2% of the total of 30 million Medicare beneficiaries. EOMB estimated that the AAPCC overpaid providers by 5%. Losses for FY 1985 were estimated at $30 million, an impressive amount, especially with deficit reduction constraints becoming increasingly important. Cf. *Medicare Annual Report—Fiscal Year 1983* (Washington, D.C.: Government Printing Office, 1986); Interview with Lynn Etheredge, August 29, 1990.

47. Kaiser-Permanente is the biggest and one of the oldest HMOs in the United States.

48. Peer review for HMOs was mandated in COBRA, 1986. Consolidated Omnibus Budget Reconciliation Act of 1985, P.L. 99-272, April 7, 1986, Title IX, Sec. 9405.

49. The President's Private Sector Survey on Cost Control, 1983.

50. Interview with Ira Burney, Office of Legislation and Policy, the HCFA, March 3, 1988. Interview with Steven Sieverts, Blue Cross and Blue Shield of the National Capital Area, December 9, 1987. Burney's view was "why should the government pay the doctors more than they are asking?" Sieverts said that Blue Shield's fee schedules were one of their more closely guarded trade secrets, precisely because if they were known, physicians below the schedule would tend to raise their fees up to the limit.

51. An option, for instance, in some Canadian provinces.

52. If, for instance, the orthopedic surgeons or ophthalmologists in a few Texas counties were to withdraw, not a far-fetched possibility.

53. Making a point that demonstrations were needed.

54. Interviews with Patrice Feinstein, former Associate Administrator for Policy, HCFA, March 4, 1988; also with Donald Moran, Lewin-ICF, January 5, 1988.

55. Interviews with Patrice Feinstein, March 4, 1988; and with Carolyne K. Davis, Ernst and Whinney, March 10, 1988.

56. For instance, the HCFA had gotten only one demonstration on physician reimbursement under way by October 1984. *Medicine and Health*, October 22, 1984, p. 1.

57. From March 1983 to October 1985.

58. A "charge-based" system would use existing claims data to develop a "relative value scale," i.e., the value to be given each procedure, thereby avoiding the time-consuming though more "objective" method of estimating actual resource use for particular procedures. Since the "conversion factor," the multiplier of the value given a procedure, determines the ultimate payment, a charge-based system will work perfectly well to set prices. But it also builds into the fee schedule existing inequities and inappropriate incentives. In the Dobson–Jencks plan, a resource-based system would be gradually phased in; but the charge-based system had the merit of being quick to implement and easy to monitor.

59.   Interviews with Allen Dobson, Consolidated Consulting Group, February 15 and May 20, 1988. Also, Jencks and Dobson (1985, 1492); and Allen Dobson, "Briefing Notes on Physician Payment Report," unpublished, 1985.

60.   Though not the ultimate version. Interviews with Allen Dobson, February 15 and May 20, 1988. *Physician Reimbursement under Medicare: Options for Change* (Washington, D.C., Congressional Budget Office, April 1986).

61.   Interview with Patrice Feinstein, March 4, 1988.

62.   Most HCFA policy positions had been vacant for a year or more. The posts of Assistant Secretary for Planning and Evaluation, the Assistant Secretary for Health; the Social Security Commissioner; the head of the HCFA; and the head of the Health Resources and Services Administration were all unfilled. *Medicine and Health, Perspectives*, September 9, 1985.

63.   *Medicine and Health*, October 28, 1985, p. 2.

64.   Spencer Rich, "President Is Advised Not to Alter Doctors' Payments," *The Washington Post*, October 25, 1985, p. A25.

65.   Consolidated Omnibus Budget Reconciliation Act of 1985, P.L. 99-272, April 7, 1986, Secs. 9301, 9305.

66.   Waiving some of the usual Medicare or Medicaid requirement to enable States or private parties to experiment with alternative delivery or payment systems.

67.   Interviews with Alphonse Esposito, ORD, the HCFA, April 10, 1988. Karen Davis, Commissioner, PPRC, Department of Health Policy and Management, the Johns Hopkins University, March 11, 1988. Also, cf. Rivlin (1971).

68.   In theory, demonstrations were to confirm or disconfirm some proposition, such as whether the "swing-bed" option would save money for different kinds of hospitals. But demonstrations were not supposedly to support inner-city hospitals in deficit or build a new agenda of long-term care or "social HMOs" (S/HMOs). Since they could be charged to the Trust Funds, there was not only a discretionary fund available, there was also an issue about how extensively these beneficiary funds should be used.

69.   Interviews Richard Schweiker, American Council of Life Insurance, June 3, 1988; Robert J. Rubin, Lewin-ICF, December 13, 1987.

70.   Operating under MBO, or "Management for Objective." Interview with Carolyne Davis, March 10, 1988.

71.   There was authority for bona fide demonstrations, but not to use these demonstrations essentially to subsidize Medicare and Medicaid HMOs.

72.   There were also objections in other quarters: within the HFCA, ASPE, and the HMOS (Health Maintenance Organizations Service). Interviews with Brian Luce, Battelle, December 16, 1987; George Greenberg, Office of the Secretary, DHHS, February 25, 1988; Christine Boesz, Office of Prepaid Health Care, DHHS, April 1, 1988; Walter Francis, Office of the Secrtary, DHHS, February 16, 1988; Alissa Fox, Blue Cross–Blue Shield, March 28, 1988; and Barbara Cooper, CHAMPUS, March 22, 1988.

73.   Some of this quarrel is reported in *Medicine and Health*, especially May 7, 1984, p. 1, June 4, p. 1, and June 11, p. 1. There is a history reaching well back into the Carter Administration. OMB would routinely review such demonstrations, and had done so for some time. Under the Carter Administration, there were similar concerns about cost overruns and dubious program support masquerading as legitimate demonstrations. These and other practices were also a matter of some concern within the DHSS, especially on the part of the Department's own internal "staff" agencies: ASPE, the Department's own OMB, the

Inspector General, and the Office of the Secretary. With the Reagan EOMB, the mandate, the attitude, and the procedures were different. EOMB began more actively to query the purposes of these demonstrations, to request more information, better cost estimates, more explicit or candid project evaluations, contingency reserves, and so forth. An important action-forcing event was the passage of TEFRA, in August 1982, putting the risk-based Medicare HMOs on a new statutory basis. Another was the discovery by EOMB of the large number of HMO demonstrations (60) and the increase in the number of Medicare beneficiaries under waiver, so many that demonstrations seemed likely to undercut the new TEFRA option. In 1983, EOMB began requiring the HCFA to notify them in advance of all waiver applications and to estimate the total costs to the Federal government. Within the HCFA, the view was that EOMB was overstepping its role as a staff agency and trying to run a program that belonged to the HCFA. Whoever began the fight, it started: with the HCFA withholding information, challenging EOMB policies, and making end-runs to Congress. EOMB responded with demands for more information, challenging forms and procedures, and swamping the HCFA with exceptions and minutiae. Then, in June 1984, EOMB demanded submission of any waiver application involving more than $1 million in any one year. At one point, Carolyne Davis, the HCFA Administrator, leaked a memo to the influential "dope-sheet," *Medicine and Health*, that EOMB was asserting an authority that was "fundamentally inappropriate," but she chose not to carry an appeal to the White House. Ultimately, an agreement was reached whereby the HCFA would send 12 pending projects to the EOMB for discussion while Stockman and Heckler sought an interim agreement. These were sent to EOMB for return within two working days. Working around the clock, EOMB returned the projects with copious notes, exceptions, and detailed criticism. Davis capitulated. Among the terms of peace, she agreed to accept a system of internal review within DHSS, ceding control to the Assistant Secretary for Management and Budget and the Inspector General. Effectively, the HCFA lost control of the program. Thereafter, one or two demonstrations would be submitted each year, but without any hope they would pass. Cf. especially, *Medicine and Health*, May 7 and June 11, 1984.

74.   Preferred Provider Organizations, essentially agreements with a number of providers for discounts. On the Administration policies, cf. *Medicine and Health, Perspectives*, February 4, 1985, p. 3.

75.   Not an unreasonable attitude, though perhaps extreme in this instance. Research and development requires a long lead-time, often six to eight years from initial conception to the evaluation of results. Consequently, a new administration inevitably inherits R&D programs from a previous administration and faces, itself, the prospect that many of its R&D initiatives will be of use primarily to the next political generation. For this reason, among others, the initial Reagan appointees to the HCFA did not sponsor many long-term research or demonstration projects. They also came in with a determination not to be unduly influenced by the permanent civil service, an important theme in the early years of the Reagan Administration. For instance, Lyn Nofziger and the Heritage Foundation conducted training sessions instructing new political appointees on how to avoid being "co-opted" by the civil servants. Not only did such attitudes tend to inhibit communication between the "policy" people and the "technicians," many of the latter transferred or left the executive branch.

76.   Patrice Feinstein, Associate Administrator for Policy, said that, at that time, she did not know what the AAPCC was. She doubted that Richard Schweiker did, either. Her first inkling of trouble was scuttlebutt going around the

HCFA that the AAPCC was "broken." Interview with Patrice Feinstein, June 9, 1988.

77.   In the words of one of the participants, "It took five years, and still we couldn't produce a report." Allen Dobson, July 6, 1990.

78.   Roper had chaired the White House Working Group on Health Policy and was instrumental in getting the Domestic Policy Group to adopt capitation as White House policy. According to *Medicine and Health*, "His fingerprints were all over the Administration's 'competition' health policy," i.e., the revived, postelection version. *Medicine and Health*, April 14, 1986, p. 1.

79.   Unlike hospital insurance, Part B is voluntary and requires both opting in and payment of a premium along with with various co-pays and deductibles. It also allows balance billing on the part of the physician. Therefore, the issue of out-of-pocket expenses for the beneficiary and the fees and billing practices of the physician have a particular salience.

80.   January 11, 1983.

81.   *The Blue Sheet*, June 29, 1983, p. 7.

82.   *The Blue Sheet*, February 16, 1983, pp. 3, 4.

83.   According to some views, the AMA "voluntary freeze" was a decisive event in securing the needed support for passage: an opportunity too good to be missed. At the same time, Sheila Burke, chief health staff aide to Senator Dole, recalls Dole's instructions that she call James Sammons at the AMA convention to tell him that the fee freeze was one that could not be held off. So, the relation of cause and effect is uncertain. *The Blue Sheet*, February 29, 1984, p. 6. Interview with Sheila Burke, Staff of the Senate Minority Leader, March 8, 1988.

84.   During this period, Congress was struggling with deficit reductions proposals like the Gramm–Rudman–Hollings provisions ultimately adopted.

85.   An unusual situation. Andy Jacobs (D., Ind.), then Chairman of the Health Subcommittee, was so enamored of mandatory assignment that he and his committee members brought the proposal to the floor, despite lack of support for it in the full Ways and Means Committee. The proposal was defeated.

86.   According to one report, the basic proposal was developed by Stockman, Andy Jacobs, (D., Ind.) and Henson Moore (R., La.) either in the House Counsel's Office or as they walked to the Conference Committee meeting. Interview with Sandra Casber Wise, Staff of the Subcommittee on Social Security, House Ways and Means, January 12, 1988.

87.   The Deficit Reduction Act of 1984, P.L. 98-369, July 18, 1984.

88.   Much of the impetus for this provision came from Rep. Henry Waxman (D., Ca.), Chairman of the Health and Environment Subcommittee of the House Energy and Commerce Committee. He and his staff aide, Peter Bouxsein, who had earlier been a career civil servant in DHEW and the HCFA, thought that these provisions would be prudent, given the uncharted territory Congress was entering. A year later, Congress established the PPRC, so that this provision in DEFRA served as a preparatory step. Interview with Peter Bouxsein, August 16, 1989.

89.   Often called "micro-management." Some quarrel with this term, since Congress does not "manage," but writes detailed legislation. At the same time, such legislation is often accompanied by mandates, "come-into-agreement" provisions, and specified procedures, so that the practical effect is to control much of the administrative activity and available time.

90.   Consolidated Omnibus Budget Reconciliation Act of 1985, P.L. 99-272— April 7, 1986.

91.   Interview with Peter Bouxsein, Staff of the Health and Environment Subcommittee, House Energy and Commerce Committee, January 29, 1988.

5

Physician Payment: Designing the System

I. INTRODUCTION—THE PPRC

As noted in the previous chapter, physician payment reform was a case of making policy without benefit of much cooperation, even the usual sort of antagonistic cooperation, between the executive and legislative branches. This kind of policy-making came about in part because of the semi-permanent partisan division between the executive and legislative branches of the Federal government. As a consequence of this situation, the executive branch has become increasingly politicized over the last 20 years and, as one observer has commented, Congress has responded by devising its own bureaucracy.[1] In the field of health care, particularly, Congress has relied on various occasions on congressional agencies such as the Congressional Budget Office, the Office of Technology Assessment, the General Accounting Office, the Congressional Research Service, and ProPAC for expertise, policy assessment, and even policy proposals. In this respect, PPRC was one more in a growing array of congressional bureaucracies (Iglehart 1988, 863).

PPRC was unique, though, in being specifically devised to assist the Congress in the development of policy and even the design of legislation. One part of its mandate, as specified in COBRA, was to make recommendations "regarding adjustments to the reasonable charge levels for physicians services." This provision recognized and addressed the need of Congress to have expert advice on amendments, especially cuts, in the reimbursement for specific procedures, both as a cautionary provision and to temper the politics of the process.[2] A second COBRA provision directed the Commission to collect the data, do or contract for the necessary research, and present to Congress its recommendations for changing the system of physician payment, with special attention to the development of a relative value scale (RVS).[3] This recommendation addressed the other major concern of Congress, to have a way to develop proposals for systemic reform. As events transpired, these two mandates that seemed complementary conflicted at times. The first, directed at specific procedures, was useful primarily for short-term, incremental, cost-containing amendments. The second, dealing with payment methodology, was useful mainly for longer-term, systemic policy design. Congress, of course, wanted both, but on several occasions, cost containment won out as the dominant priority, with some detriment to the longer-term objective.

Commission Activities

The Commission of 11 members, soon increased to 13, was appointed in June, 1986, two months after the passage of COBRA. As with Pro-PAC, Congress used the device of having OTA appoint the members of the Commission and monitor its work. Even though not directed to choose a chairman, OTA did so, naming Dr. Philip R. Lee, a liberal Democrat who had served as the first Assistant Secretary for Health in the Johnson Administration. Since its inception, the Commission's executive director has been Paul B. Ginsburg, an economist, with experience in health care policy and research reaching back to the Nixon era. As mandated by law, the Commission members were broadly representative. About half were physicians (6), including a surgeon, two family physicians, two internists, and a psychiatrist.[4] Others came from a diversity of backgrounds, such as research, employee benefits, hospitals and teaching institutions, HMOs, public health, and nursing. Most regions of the country and a wide variety of institutions and constituencies were represented. Between them, the Commission members shared an impressive amount of practical experience and health policy expertise.

The task confronting PPRC was different from that faced by ProPAC. ProPAC's assignment was implementation: to apply a highly designed, technical statute for which most of the policy issues, if difficult, were yet well understood and annotated; and for which the basic technology, if imperfect, was still generally acknowledged as workable. For PPRC, on the other hand, the assignment was to develop a proposal for reforming physician payment in a situation in which little research had as yet been done; the methodology of reform was disputed; some of the most difficult policy issues had yet to be discovered; and the acquiescence of important provider groups was, at best, problematic. That a successful proposal was developed owes a certain amount to luck and circumstance. But it also owes much to the devising of an effective strategy.

Brought forth as it was, a congressional agency in the sixth year of the Reagan presidency, the Commission had, perforce, to plan accordingly. That circumstance meant, practically, that PPRC had to be responsive to Congress, both in developing an ultimate proposal and in advising the Congress on piecemeal changes in Part B payments. But the relations of Congress and the Executive being what they were in 1986, the Commission could not rely on the collaboration of DHHS or the HCFA in developing its advice to Congress, either about Part B amendments or a more basic reform of the payment system. Consequently, the Commission had to be prepared to assure itself on technical issues. Two major tasks confronted the Commission: developing a political consensus for a proposal that would inevitably be highly controversial and creating its own base of expert knowledge to support its advice to Congress.

One of the most important decisions, taken early by the Commission, was to work first on the development of an RVS. There was a compelling technical logic to this decision, since an RVS would be a necessary preliminary to reforming the existing CPT-4[5] and, arguably, a prerequisite for a move toward more far-reaching changes in payment methodology, such as physician DRGs or capitation. Furthermore, there was no assurance that the HCFA-sponsored efforts, of which the most important was the Harvard-based Hsiao–Braun study, would get done in a timely manner or prove to be usable.[6] From the beginning, much of the planning and the effort on the part of the Commission and the staff were aimed, therefore, at the eventual development of an RVS, either independently created or built on the Hsiao study or other work funded by the HCFA.

There were also some compelling political reasons for this choice. An RVS had been for some time identified by Congress as a priority. Moreover, work in this area would support the Commission's role in advising Congress about specific changes in payment schedules. A number of specialty groups within the provider community supported the development of an RVS, including the AMA that had endorsed this activity and was actively collaborating with the HCFA in a joint venture.[7] For the Commission, working on an RVS would be a good task for building consensus among the members. It gave them a clear objective. And technical issues, such as the measurement of work, could be addressed first, leaving for later the more contentious and political issues, such as what to do about specialty and regional differentials, annual updating, and volume controls.

First Things First

The Commission tended, for reasons relating to the structure of decisions as well as for political considerations, to pursue an approach of first things first. That meant in this context working first on the elements that were fundamental conceptually and practically and on which there was a good prospect for reaching consensus. Staff and Commission members, as well as informed observers, credit the conception of this strategy as well as its artful and successful implementation largely to the Chairman, Dr. Philip Lee, and to the Commission's executive director, Paul Ginsburg.[8] Though it is hard to imagine another strategy succeeding, appreciating that reality clearly and acting on it effectively proved to be of great importance. At the same time, this initial approach carries with it some dangers. One is that the consensus issues get resolved technically, but that this technical consensus proves inadequately compelling when the harder policy and political issues arise, so that neither rationality nor equity prevails. The other is that a heavy initial investment in the technical fundamentals, in this instance an RVS, tends to nudge the ultimate decision in a particular direction and preclude the systematic or effective canvassing of alternatives.

The most visible part of the Commission's activities are the bimonthly meetings that are devoted mainly to developing the policy statements that go into the annual report to Congress. These sessions are a kind of progress report on the reform of physician payment. Much of the work of the staff and its executive director goes into the planning for these meetings, doing or commissioning the research, writing the papers, and briefing the Commission members. At the Commission meetings, the agenda issues are publicly debated in morning and afternoon sessions over the course of two days. Technical presentations on issues pertinent to that session will be made by the staff or by consultants under contract with the Commission. These meetings are well attended by lobbyists from the various medical and surgical specialty societies and from other interest groups, such as the AARP[9] or insurance groups. They may make presentations of their own or comment during the open period. One or more observers from DHHS or the congressional staff are likely to be there. The sessions are lively, informative, and consequential. These meetings provide a way for the Commission to inform itself about policy issues and about provider sentiment. They give provider groups a chance to express their own views and to know what issues are developing and how they are likely to be resolved. And they afford a useful supplement to the typical Congressional subcommittee hearing, in providing a forum attentive to and competent to assess highly technical issues and in which self-interested parties can speak candidly, with less concern about making a public record.

Aside from the strategy of concentrating first on technical issues, some aspects of Commission procedure and structure are important. A decision, taken early in the Commission's history, was to have no committees—this in order to encourage greater collegiality. The Commission meets frequently in addition to their formal meetings, with staff members present, at evening sessions and at meals during their bimonthly sessions, and at planning retreats between these meetings. These informal gatherings reinforce a sense of common engagement in problem-solving and encourage both the Commission members and the individual staff professionals to transcend their particularistic perspectives. The commissioners are individuals with rich and varied backgrounds. Each represents, as it were, more than one interest or perspective. And they have developed a Commission ethos, partly through the prompting of the Chairman, of speaking as individual experts and Commission members more than as the representatives of a constituency or interest.[10]

Building consensus within the Commission had a counterpart in measures that helped to forestall opposition among provider and beneficiary groups. In addition to a strategy of deferring the more contentious issues, the Commission's first report was moderate in tone. In the priorities and goals that were set forth as guides for the reform of physician payment, fifth down the list, after financial protection for beneficiaries and equity among categories of physicians, was cost containment or "reductions in the growth of SMI outlays."[11] Aside from reassuring the provider community, this emphasis on avoiding conflict invited a wait and see attitude on their part with respect to the ultimate design. In addition, it prompted various groups, for instance, the American College of Physicians or the American Society of Internal Medicine, to come forward with endorsements and proposals of their own in hopes of influencing the evolving process. Even those groups that felt sure they would lose, such as the surgeons, thought it worthwhile, for instance, to make a case for a charge-based as opposed to a resource-based RVS.[12] In addition to postponing potentially disruptive conflict, the Commission's "low profile" approach brought providers into the process with proposals that entailed a shifting of position on their part, required a realistic confronting of issues, and were of some use to the commissioners.

Annual Reports

The Commission's first Annual Report, published March 1, 1987, was largely drafted by the executive director, Paul Ginsburg (Iglehart 1988). Among other purposes, the Report provided an initial survey of physician payment methodology and its reform, especially reviewing the existing Part B program, identifying the more salient problems, laying out tasks, and assessing some of the analytical and data requisites needed to accomplish these tasks. In the course of this survey, the Report also anticipated elements of the proposal ultimately adopted: a resource-based RVS, a geographically modified MEI, retention of the PAR program, and the use of "nonspecific caps or areawide budgets" to control volume.[13] Especially notable about the report is the strong inclination to build on or extend approaches already favored or being pursued by the Congress. The Report advocates continuing efforts to improve the Participating Physician Program (PAR). It approves the attack on so-called "overpriced" procedures through an "inherent reasonableness" process. And, most importantly, it endorses the creation of a national fee schedule, commenting that it is "generally considered the most feasible of alternatives in the near term."[14] To move from a relative value scale to a fee schedule is a natural enough progression.[15] At the same time, it is a commitment, like an initial dedication of a piece of equipment to a specific purpose. Other alternatives were alluded to and discussed briefly in a chapter entitled "Issues Deferred to Later Reports," but the only possibility clearly in focus was that of a fee schedule.

During the second year of its existence, the Commission and its staff did a vast amount of work on the components of a fee schedule, going step by step over the analytic and policy issues and planning toward an independent development of an RVS,[16] should this prove necessary. At the request of Congress, the Commission advised that body on specific cuts in physician payment and "overpriced" or "overvalued"[17] procedures, to help meet deficit reduction targets. In part at the prompting of Congress, the Commission, especially the staff, did examine some of the policy alternatives initially deferred, such as improving participation or utilization review, the development of practice guidelines and appropriateness review, and capitation in various modes of use. The consideration of these alternatives was largely at the level of analysis and literature review, without benefit of independent inquiry, while the great preponderance of their work and discussion went toward the development of a fee schedule.

One reason that the Commission devoted relatively little time or resources to the exploration of alternative approaches was a sense that Congress, and especially the House Ways and Means Health Subcommittee, chaired by Rep. Stark, was growing increasingly impatient and moving toward a commitment.[18] Such was indeed the case. Both in the House and the Senate, health policy leaders were concluding that decisive action was needed and that a national fee schedule was the only option available for implementation.[19] As a last gesture toward DHSS, the budget reconciliation act of 1987, enacted just before the Christmas recess, directed the Secretary to conduct a study of "changes in the payment system for physicians' services" that would be required for the implementation of a national fee schedule . . . on or after January 1, 1990."[20] No one had much hope that the Secretary would comply. Congress was preparing to go ahead, with or without cooperation from the executive branch, detailing specific instructions for routing the Hsiao study to PPRC for its recommendations.[21] With respect to the Hsiao study, Congress directed that the Secretary submit a copy of the report, together with supporting data and files, within 30 days of receipt.[22]

II. POLITICS AND THE DEFICIT

Though the issues are technical and medicine is a profession, decisions about health policy sometimes get made in an environment that is intensely political. PPRC was created in 1986, an election year. It was a period of almost continual deficit reduction negotiations and tactical maneuvers.[23] Moreover, it was the first year of the new Bowen–Roper administration: a time of transition, uncertainty, and adjustment in the relations between Congress and DHHS. During this year, policy with respect to physician payment developed in an environment strongly charged with politics and much affected by the budget deficit, the electoral cycle, and the constitutional separation of powers between the executive and the legislature.

1986 was also a year in which there was no comprehensive policy option that could win general assent. The administration was divided over capitation versus DRGS, with neither of these options popular in Congress.[24] Within the Congress, the House Ways and Means Subcommittee was inclining toward fee schedules, but not as yet sure and lacking wider support. Early in the year, the Senate Finance Committee held an important series of hearings, taking inventory of the policy alternatives, but reaching no general conclusion.[25] Aside from genuine uncertainties about the best approach, there was the additional cautionary calculus that an election year was not the best time for launching a novel or upsetting proposal likely to anger a number of powerful constituent groups.

A palpable reality, though, was that despite the physician fee freeze, Part B expenditures continued to rise, even more than hospital rates and only slightly less rapidly than they had before the freeze.[26] Gramm–Rudman went fully into effect with the consequences of making Part B expenditures a special target and emphasizing identifiable, specific cuts that could be appropriately credited. Rising Part B expenditures, of course, are a danger signal for Congressmen because they mean additional burdens for the beneficiaries,[27] important at any time to conscientious legislators, but especially so in an election year. As a consequence both of beneficiary concerns and cost containment imperatives, quick measures were important, even if incremental and piecemeal.

The MAACs

An action-forcing question for Congress was what to do after the fee freeze came to an end. This program, begun in July 1984 and initially limited to 15 months, had been twice extended and was now approaching its thirtieth month. By this time, it had gone stale and was generally recognized to be declining in effectiveness. During the 30 months and despite the freeze in physicians charges, Part B expenditures rose 10–15% a year, with the rate of increase accelerating as the freeze continued. Most of the rise in total expenditures was attributable to increased volume and intensity of services provided, indicating that the constraining effects of a price freeze were easy to avoid. Moreover, the freeze had already been ended for PAR physicians and the implications of the COBRA legislation of April 1986 was that the freeze would end for non-PAR physicians as well by January 1, 1987.

The program established to replace the fee freeze was known as MAACs, which stands for Maximum Allowable Actual Charges.[28] In effect, the MAACs lifted the fee freeze, but put a limit on balance billing. Physicians with high charges, i.e., more than 115% of the prevailing charge for nonparticipating physicians for the preceding year, could increase their total charge by 1% a year. Those who were below the 115% could, by a prescribed formula, increase their charges to that level by 1990. The practical effect was to put a limit of approximately 15% (+1% a year) on balance billing, but to allow physicians who had historically billed less than the 115% to catch up. MAACs were to last until December 20, 1990, or one year after the Secretary reported to Congress on a fee schedule. In fact, they were ultimately extended until 1992, when the Medicare Fee Schedule goes into effect.

The MAACs were a compromise, intended to protect beneficiaries at the same time that they gave physicians a respite and an opportunity to catch up, especially for some who had, allegedly, been pinched by the fee freeze. As additional background, there was general acknowledgment that something would need to be done about protection for beneficiaries when the fee freeze ended, but something, in any event, short of mandatory assignment, which no one was seriously proposing at that time. Immediately preceding consideration of the MAACs, the House Ways and Means Committee had agreed to reduce the differential in payments for PAR and non-PAR physicians from 5 to 4%, a concession to the non-PARs and a minor defeat for the more liberal, proregulation groups. In that context, Rep. Stark moved and secured the adoption of the MAACs as a beneficiary protection,[29] an instance, some would say, of getting megatons in exchange for kilotons.

While the MAACs were a compromise, they were also a good example of legislation by inadvertence, one in which some of the most important consequences were unintended. As originally proposed in both the Ways and Means and Energy and Commerce subcommittees, the MAACs would have been set by simply trending forward the MEI, taking an average of existing charges. That approach would have been simple and easy to administer. But it would have meant that some physicians would actually have found themselves getting *lower* fees after the freeze ended, an outcome that some within the House committees did not like and that was known to be unacceptable to the Senate Finance Committee. Therefore, the statute provided for differential treatment for those above and below the 115% of prevailing charges.[30] This deceptively simple provision turned out to difficult to implement: the regulations were prolix and complex, and enforcement of them frustrating to the HCFA and the carriers and baffling and infuriating to the physicians.[31] Subsequent to their passage, the MAACs were widely viewed as being like TEFRA, a regulatory scheme that would "drive the doctors crazy,"[32] and that would "make life so difficult"[33] that they would ask for and accept a more reasonable compromise, for instance a fee schedule.[34] This may be a case of discerning rational purpose after the event, but whatever the intent of the MAACs, they did persuade many provider groups that Congress, and especially the Health Subcommittee of Ways and Means, had in mind some nasty plans for them and was prepared to act on them unless they, the providers, could come up with some alternative acceptable both to them and to the Congress.

Overpriced Procedures

Another makeshift developed during 1986 was legislation for "inherently reasonable" charges and "overpriced" procedures. But where the MAACs were mainly for beneficiary protection, these initiatives were aimed primarily at reduction of Federal Medicare outlays and developed in a way that illustrates how separation of powers and budgetary politics served to drive policy toward procedures and substantive outcomes that neither the Congress, the HCFA, nor EOMB intended.

The prospect of enforcing "reasonable" charge limits for physicians' fees was one that had lain dormant for many years, even though the Social Security Amendments of 1972 gave this approach specific sanction.[35] Essentially, it is a concept of reducing payment for specific procedures for which the charge seems inflated or where those charges deviate, without appropriate justification, from amounts allowed to other providers. While this approach may seem an obvious one, administration determinations of "reasonableness" are difficult and time consuming, made even more so by the fact that Medicare physician payment is indirectly administered through carriers.[36] At the same time, a great deal of money can be involved in a relatively small number of codes: some that are expensive and high volume;[37] others that physicians are prone to exploit. Therefore, as Part B budget savings became increasingly important, especially after 1983, both the HCFA and Congress began looking more closely at such procedures.[38]

Within the HCFA, work on "overpriced" procedures—especially cataract surgery, coronary artery bypass grafts, and pacemakers—had proceeded slowly and circumspectly. Developing criteria and supporting evidence, even for a few procedures, entailed difficult conceptual problems and much labor-intensive, meticulous work with data. Subject to notice and comment procedures, the HCFA officials were, as one program analyst put it, "hit over the head by every lobbyist in the business" when they sought to develop a proposal.[39] It was not a popular activity and work on this program tended to be deferred.

Meanwhile, the HCFA was getting some prompting from two sources. One was from the Congress, where subcommittee staffs in both houses had been working on a variety of related items, including cataract surgery, payments for nurse anesthetists, and surgical second opinions, all potential savers.[40] One of the mandates in the budget reconciliation for 1985 (eventually passed in April 1986) was that the HCFA get on with this program and promulgate regulations specifying criteria to determine when physician charges were inherently reasonable. About that same time, EOMB had also been advancing the idea that "overpriced" procedures would be a good source for budget reductions, a proposition that gained added importance because of Gramm–Rudman, which required specifically identified cuts.

The HCFA took two steps that, under the circumstances, alarmed the provider community. One was to send out a letter of transmittal to the carriers in August 1985, instructing them to be alert to charges that were unreasonable; and a second was to publish, early in 1986, an NPRM[41] on "inherent reasonableness." Neither of these steps involved much preliminary consultation. They also came in the midst of a period of sharp tactical maneuvering over deficit reduction when EOMB was increasingly viewed as dictating DHHS and HCFA policy. Not surprisingly, they triggered a concern that the "inherent reasonableness" procedures would be used arbitrarily and primarily as a budget-trimming device.[42]

These developments set off some agonized protests to Congress, especially directed toward the Senate Finance Committee, then engaged in a wide-ranging consideration of proposals to modify the physician payment system.[43] This committee responded with a series of procedural safeguards for providers that became part of OBRA, 1986.[44] In this legislation, Congress ignored the executive branch and set forth criteria of its own, specifying in detail as well the procedures that would be followed in making a determination of "unreasonable."

One effect of the SOBRA (OBRA, 1986) legislation was to make the "inherent reasonableness" procedure so cumbersome as to be unworkable, a consequence not universally lamented in the HCFA. In this situation, Congress turned to the newly created PPRC, which among its other duties was supposed to advise Congress on specific "items and services" and, as provided by SOBRA, on reasonable charge limits.[45] With some trepidation, but also sensibly aware of their political status, PPRC did a "quick and dirty" study of some eight procedures,[46] using a number of RVSs, including some of the Hsiao material and the Ontario fee schedule.

The method chosen by Congress provided a quick way to dispense some "rough justice."[47] Not only was it quick, but by enabling Congress to make the cuts, it contributed to their deficit-reduction targets. And since it was done by legislation, it avoided the cumbersome notice and comment procedures of administrative rulemaking, with their attendant delays and risk of litigation. Some critics said that such a crudely instrumental use of PPRC so early in its institutional development compromised its credibility, especially with the provider community.[48] One effect of this procedure, though, was to involve the congressional subcommittees even more deeply in the activity loosely termed "micromanagement," meaning in this instance legislating on particular medical procedures and tinkering with ad hoc adjustments to the payment system. In this respect, the "inherent reasonableness" episode made palpable the need for a rational and comprehensive approach to reform, inasmuch as cutting Medicare Part B outlays procedure by procedure, even grossly "overpriced" ones, tended to ignore important long-term and systemic values such as regional equity, beneficiary access, and a provider sense of fairness.

Inpatient DRGs

A dramatic, if bizarre, set of maneuvers began toward the end of 1986, with the EOMB proposal for a system of inpatient DRGs, an option that many had comfortably believed to be dead. At this particular time, Secretary Bowen and William Roper, the new head of the HCFA, were developing a refurbished set of capitation proposals, while the Congress was moving rapidly toward a national fee schedule. In backing inpatient DRGs, EOMB took the position that the more global the payment, the better.[49] In their view, fee schedules would not control volume, and capitation still needed fixing. Inpatient DRGs would cover almost 60% of physician expenses and would be a logical step toward a more global system, such as capitation. The proposal made a certain kind of policy sense, but inasmuch as physician DRGs had by now been repeatedly passed over as an option deserving of serious consideration, the EOMB proposal was viewed generally as a tactical move. Effects it did have were to arouse consternation in the provider community and throw the HCFA-DHSS campaign into disarray.[50]

Ploy or not, EOMB put a demand for inpatient DRGs into its fall "pass-back" to DHHS. The Secretary balked, but eventually agreed to go ahead with the development of a more modest version: RAP-DRGs, or a DRG payment applied to radiology, anesthesiology, and pathology. Since this outcome was pretty much what EOMB had intended from the beginning, this course was acceptable.

The leverage that might be inherent in the RAP-DRG proposal was apparent not just to EOMB. Congressman Stark announced his support and said he intended to introduce legislation in the next session of Congress.[51] At this, the AMA and a number of specialty groups were perturbed, fearing that RAP-DRGs were a threat to be taken seriously and that they might be a first step toward a general system of physician DRGs. Senator Bentsen (D., Tex.) the new chairman of Senate Finance,[52] and generally more sympathetic to the provider community than Rep. Stark, disliked the RAP-DRG proposals and asked for an alternative, preferably a national fee schedule, which he had favored for some time. In this political context, the American College of Radiology broke ranks and approached the Waxman subcommittee to negotiate the parameters of a fee schedule for radiologists,[53] preferring a known irritant to a possible disaster. This development fostered disunity among the medical specialty groups and also greatly diminished the AMA's credibility as an umbrella organization and spokesman for physicians generally.[54]

Moving Toward a Decision

As Congress worked toward OBRA, 1987, an extraneous event that sharply increased their sense of urgency was the announcement in September by William Roper, the HCFA Administrator, that the Medicare Part B premium would rise by $7 per month, going from $17.90 to $24.80 a month, beginning in 1988. Not only would this be a substantial burden for Medicare beneficiaries, beginning in an election year, it also repre-sented an increase of 38.5% in one year.[55] Some of this amount was to cover Trust Fund depletion and other portions could be attributed to various accounting decisions, but about 60% was for physician charges, representing mostly increased volume.[56] Perhaps Dr. Roper, in releasing these figures, hoped to call the attention of Rep. Stark and others to the need for volume controls and capitation. What the legislators tended to conclude was that quick action was needed, most probably a fee sched-ule with some form of volume control added.[57]

OBRA, 1987 was replete with physician payment provisions, so much so that it resembled a christmas tree hung about with ornaments, to borrow the metaphor in use at the time. There were mandates to devel-op fee schedules. There were complex provisions with respect to the MEI update and, in particular, differential increases for PAR and non-PAR physicians and for primary-care doctors and those in undeserved areas. Limits were set for "overpriced" procedures and the MAACs amended. In addition, there were specific limits and regulations for particular procedures or procedures in particular settings. In other words, Congress was regulating physician reimbursement pretty com-prehensively and specifically but without an overall assessment of the consequences, either for providers or for beneficiaries. To continue the metaphor, more and more bells, whistles, and baubles were being piled on the tree without knowing what the tree would support.

By now, the House and the Senate had deployed so many of the elements of a national fee schedule that some such system, planned and coordinated, was needed to make sense of the actions taken to date. In its tinkering with the MEI, Congress was establishing an update and also using the MEI to provide incentives for participation and to redress disparities between regions and specialities. A fee freeze, followed by the MAACs, addressed left-handedly and inadvertently the issues of charge limits and balance billing. Reducing "overpriced" procedures invoked "inherent reasonableness" and the use of a variety of relative value scales. And Congress was well along in mandating fee schedules, having begun in 1984 with clinical lab tests and continued with nurse anesthetists, radiologists, and the rest of the anesthetists. By this time, Congress had developed a very effective technique of amending physi-cian payment, even though there was skepticism about the nonsystem being created. 1987 was a year of activism. With respect to physicians, the big Part B premium increase served as a triggering event.[58] Taking a major step, OBRA, 1987 called for a national fee schedule to be imple-mented by January 1, 1990.[59]

During the latter part of 1987 and throughout 1988, the PPRC was working with a clear sense of mission: to design a national fee schedule.

This was a task that involved, in broadest terms, two major parts. One was the work on a resource-based relative value scale. This entailed taking the results of the joint AMA–Harvard study[60] being done by Hsiao and associates or some alternative to it. In any event, the Commission and its staff had to be prepared to evaluate that study and move ahead from there, either to adopt the results of the study or to develop another option. But an RVS provides only an agreed on method for comparing services and procedures. It does not determine what shall be paid for them. Therefore, a second part of the Commission's task dealt with how the RVS should be applied: which is to say, with how it should be updated, what kind of regional and specialty differentials to allow, and, especially, what to do about assignment and volume. On most of these topics, the Commission had ongoing technical work either under contract or being done by its own staff. For some issues, they could draw on the data or research work of the HCFA staff.[61] The Commission itself held hearings and discussed substantive policy issues during the year, aiming toward the fee schedule deadline.

Despite all the preparations, little could be done until the Hsiao report was in hand. So, throughout much of the year, the Commission and its staff waited expectantly, like a prospective bridegroom of earlier times, eager to see what the marriage broker had arranged. Suspense was heightened by news that Hsiao was ill and that the report would be delayed yet another two months. Eventually it was delivered to the Secretary, on September 29, 1988, and, thereafter, within the statutorially prescribed month, a copy was sent to the Commission.

According to a procedure already established,[62] the Commission conducted an in-house evaluation, consulted with outside experts on its methodology and results, and held public hearings to gather and assess the comments of various interested parties. Although there were some important dissents, especially from the surgeons, and a good many areas identified where additional data collection and analysis would be required, the consensus was that the report was sound and provided a good basis on which to build.[63]

Even though the technical basis was established, there remained an enormous array of decisions, with relatively little time remaining before the March deadline for the 1989 Annual Report. Some of these issues were technical, such as the geographic MEI and malpractice costs. Others were complex: what to recommend with respect to practice guidelines, utilization review, or the PROs. Still others were hot political items, such as assignment or expenditure targets. In this phase of its work, it would have been easy for the Commission to bog down or split apart. Yet the Report was ready in time, and both coherent and persuasive. Aside from the one issue of assignment, there was no dissent. This outcome owed much to the abilities and hard work of the Commission members and staff. It also owed much to the initial strategy and the art of building consensus: setting a clear objective, choosing tasks that tended to unify, members and staff working as colleagues. The danger of consensus is, of course, that it avoids difficulty: it fails to confront technical problems or conflicts of principle. Events may prove that the Commission failed in this respect. In a final sense, only the future can tell. But for a more immediate appreciation, there is the Commission's own report and, as a background to that, the merits of the particular option they chose, a national fee schedule.

III. ELEMENTS OF A FEE SCHEDULE

A Resource-Based Relative Value Scale

For the Medicare Fee Schedule, the Commission chose a resource-based relative value scale, as opposed to a charge-based one, a decision that may seem obviously right and yet one that was subject to controversy then and continues to be so. The great advantage of a resource-based system, according to its advocates, is that it provides an objective measurement, at least one that is arguably so, and that can therefore be used as a fair basis of comparison of medical services and procedures.[64] On the other hand, a charge-based system offers two big, potential advantages. Since it is based on what physicians charge for their services, it reflects the market both on the down side as well as the up side. It poses less of a threat to beneficiary access. And it does not pay physicians *more* than they are willing to take for their services.[65] Furthermore, charge-based systems typically involve some element of negotiation.[66] For the physicians, this introduces a desirable element of participation and consensus. For the government, which is the sole purchaser for many Medicare services, it provides an important opportunity to use its market power to advantage in negotiation. These are non-trivial considerations and the choice between the two approaches was by no means foregone or obvious. In fact, the American College of Surgeons proposed an alternative fee schedule, largely based on charges[67] and DHHS briefly considered making a charge-based proposal of its own.[68] Within the Commission, the prevailing view was that existing charges were too grown over with past inequities and distortions to provide a basis for reform[69] and that if they were going to do this job, they needed to do it creditably.[70]

The basic idea of an RBRVS is fairly simple, even though the initial assumptions involved may be controversial and the actual process of generating the RVS complex indeed. There are also different versions of what an RBRVS should be, though the formula below represents the one developed in the Harvard study (Etheredge and Dobson 1984, 4):

RBRVS = total work × (1 + specialty practice costs) × (1 + opportunity costs of specialty training)

What this form says in an abbreviated fashion is that an RBRVS is developed by estimating the amount of "work" involved on the part of a physician in doing a particular procedure or providing a particular service and *multiplying* this by other figures that represent the practice costs for that specialty and the ".opportunity costs" of training for that particular specialty. Right away, one can see that the formula is deceptively simple and covers many complexities and points of controversy, such as what counts as work,[71] and how it should be estimated; whether practice costs should be *multiplied* by the work index or simply *added* to it; and whether opportunity costs[72] should be counted at all. In fact, on some of these points, the Commission rejected the Hsiao approach. But this formula can serve as a point of departure.

Work Values.   The basic device used to estimate work was to develop "vignettes" for which physicians would be asked to rank the magnitude of work and compare them with other procedures. Using groups of consultant physicians, vignettes were developed for 407 procedures ranging across the 18 selected medical and surgical specialty groups, with an average of 22 vignettes for each. After testing these vignettes in a pilot study, they were used in telephone interviews that were administered to 2,000 physicians. A goal was to have 100 physicians per specialty (Hsiao et al. 1988, 2361). The telephone interviews lasted about half an hour and covered 20 to 30 vignettes. A surgeon would be asked, for instance, to compare a "lower bowel resection for rectal carcinoma" with the selected standard procedure for general surgery, an "uncomplicated inguinal hernia repair." An internist would be asked to compare a "follow-up visit for a 55 year old male for management of hypertension, with mild fatigue, on a beta blocker/thiazide regime" with an "office evaluation of a 28 year old patient with regional enteritis, diarrhea, and a low grade fever, established patient" (Etheredge and Dobson 1989, 18). Respondents would rank the vignette in comparison with a standardized procedure (value of 100) as well as with others for which they would be willing to "trade" the vignette procedure.

The technique of using vignettes and telephone interviews depended heavily on the cooperation of physician panels, specialty groups, and the AMA to select representative procedures, develop the vignettes, and identify an interview sample. Thus, the RVS is very much their creation as well as that of the project designers and technicians. In this respect, organized medicine "bought into" the project and supported it strongly, which was an intended result. But there are also grounds for wondering whether the results do not also represent the physicians' long-standing and organized prejudices about what they deserve to get paid.[73] No doubt, the debate on this topic will go on for some time.[74] But two observations can be made about these results that have some political importance. One is that the work evaluations performed pretty well *across* specialties and also showed much common agreement about procedures that are consistently overvalued or undervalued (Etheredge and Dobson 1989, 23–24). Therefore, even if God has made all physicians "congruent fools," to paraphrase Descartes, an RBRVS may still provide the best foundation for policy decisions affecting them.[75]

Cross-Specialty Linkage. A second stage, termed "cross-specialty linkage," was both conceptually difficult and of enormous importance. Medical specialties notoriously differ about the value of their activities, and these professional differences are overlaid with generations of custom and prejudice. Comparing vascular surgery with the diagnosis of hypertension is like asking whether tennis is harder than bridge: each has its practitioners and its characteristic difficulties. At the same time, there has to be an agreed on method and a common scale, since an RVS is to be used for payment across specialties. Therefore, it is important that the scale devised be both fair and coherent: that is, seen to be right by the various specialties and paying amounts for individual services that are proportional to work. Furthermore, if the linkage process worked well, the RVS research would gain considerably in credibility as a valid base for a fee schedule (Etheredge and Dobson 1989, 33).

The technique employed nicely addressed these two constraints of perceived fairness and coherence. A first step was to ask a cross-specialty panel of 24 physicians to develop vignettes for services that were delivered by more than one specialty and that were either identical or equivalent. These "link services" were compared with results from the national survey, and some of them were eliminated. Additional linking services were identified through statistical analysis and more panel meetings. These procedures generated 82 cross-links, from 4 to 21 for each specialty, with an average of 9. The analysts then adjusted the link values so as to get the best fit across 18 specialties. The results seemed to show that a common scale was feasible and "made sense" in that the compromise values agreed closely with the original panel estimates and did not result in distortion of the existing intraservice scales (Braun et al., 1988, 2392).

This measure of success in cross-specialty linkage was important for the credibility of the RVS methodology as a whole, showing that a series of intraservice scales, like 18 separate lattices, could be linked together so as to form a mutually supporting structure. Even so, there have been pertinent criticisms, particularly from some of the specialty societies, pointing to a need for additional work or raising a question about underlying method. One reason for disquiet relates to the cross-specialty consensus process: that a single panel of 24 physicians may be too small to speak for 18 specialty groups. This objection gains point because of the wide variation in how adequately the specialties were linked. Some, such as family practice and internal medicine, were well-calibrated with 19–21 specialty links. Others, such as anesthesiology and pathology, had only 4 or 5. Moreover, some of the specialties that were well linked showed a higher than average percentage of difference between the links. Several of these specialties are of great importance for Medicare, such as internal medicine, general and orthopedic surgery, rheumatology, and urology (Etheredge and Dobson 1989, 35 ff); *PPRC, Annual Report* (1989, 322). These results could point to flaws in the method or gaps in the data that open the Report to serious challenge. As part of Phaze II of the study, a review of the linking values was prescribed, seeking comment from the specialty societies on the links and reviewing the results with Hsiao and associates, the AMA, and the HCFA. A new interspecialty scale was then constructed using the Hsiao methodology.[76]

Pre- and Post Service Work. Although physicians' services may seem like discrete units of activity that can be estimated separately, they are accompanied by varying amounts of pre- and postservice work that make up an important part of their ultimate value. Even a simple office visit, for instance, may entail a preliminary reading of a patient's medical record and subsequent telephone calls to a local pharmacist or to another physician to expedite a referral. Surgical procedures typically involve much more. For example, an intraocular lens insertion (IOL) includes a series of preoperative examinations and a number of follow-up visits. But the amount of work involved is difficult to measure because it is typically fragmented or mingled with other activities. Also, it varies greatly according to local practices (Dunn et al. 1988, 237). These differences are important especially for some specialties, because they can make up a large part of the total work involved, typically about half for most surgery and a quarter to a third for office visits or diagnostic procedures. Obviously, they can also be a source of considerable misunderstanding on the part of lay persons and policy makers as to whether Medicare is being overcharged for the services performed (Mitchell et al. 1987, 129). Accordingly, the third step for the Hsiao study group, devising a method to measure pre- and postservice work, was one of considerable importance.

The method used by the research group illustrates the practical difficulties of such endeavors as well as some of the pitfalls. Because of the enormous variability[77] of pre- and postservice activities and the mingling of these with intraservice work, a technique of direct measurement would be, at best, complicated, expensive, and of dubious reliability. It would also tax the patience and attention span of the physicians surveyed in the national telephone interviews. Therefore, the Hsiao group employed a technique that used sampling and estimation, asking physicians in the national telephone survey to estimate the time for a small sample of services and then using their own assumptions and the advice of clinicians to estimate the work per unit of time. Regression equations were then employed to extrapolate the same estimates to other services and procedures (Dunn et al. 1988, 2372–2373).

Unfortunately, their approach, perhaps well-designed to meet practical constraints, proved unsatisfactory on several other counts. For instance, the sample size and response rate were low for some specialities, such as thoracic and general surgery, creating one source of possible error (Etheredge and Dobson 1989, 44 ff). Variations in the estimates of time for some services were also high, a serious problem since these estimates were used for extrapolation to other unsurveyed services. Moreover, the regression formulas used for extrapolation contained multiple assumptions, plausible enough in themselves, but introducing additional possible sources of error.[78] Finally, the sample values did not adequately predict pre- and postservice times for the remainder of the 407 core services included in the national telephone survey.

Critical reviews of the Harvard study noted inadequacies in the pre- and postservice section as did most of the specialty societies submitting testimony to the PPRC. The Commission recommended further study of this problem including an "improved method that relies on direct estimates of work" and avoiding "extrapolations and assumptions" wherever possible.[79] Pre- and postservice values became a major project in Phase II. In the Phase II national survey, Hsiao and associates included estimates of total work in the EM vignettes. Both the Harvard group and PPRC worked on pre/post values for surgical services, an especially difficult and complex problem.

Extrapolation. Since the original survey applied to only 407 services out of the whole array of 7000 + CPT-4 codes, another requisite step was to get from this relatively small sample to the much larger group of unsurveyed services. This was done by a process of extrapolation, in which charge data from small "families" of about five closely- related codes were used. Each family had in it one or more "benchmark" procedures, i.e., one of the original survey group of 407. The assumption was that a small number of related codes would be relatively homogeneous and that the ratio of charges between them could serve tolerably well as proxies for the actual work values within the group. This process generated imputed values for approximately 1400 codes, only about one-fourth of the 6000 codes relevant to the study,[80] but accounting for roughly 80% of Medicare allowed charges.[81] In principle, filling in the undetermined numbers would not seem technically or conceptually difficult.

Although the process of extrapolation seems in principle sensible and sound, there were still a number of problem areas, most of them identified by the researchers themselves, that would need to be resolved before the RVS could be viewed as serviceable. First, and obviously, the "benchmarks" from which the extrapolations are made were of questionable validity since they used unreliable pre- and postservice work values.[82] Beyond this, the families varied considerably, some of them quite homogeneous and others showing great variation in mean charges for the services within the family, so that extrapolations from them would produce anomalous results unless further determinations of the specific work values are made. When a physician panel reviewed the extrapolated values, they found a relatively large proportion (15%) of the imputed values that they considered to be "outliers," i.e., deviating by more than 40% from their estimate of "true" values (Etheredge and Dobson 1989, 52). Furthermore, the extrapolation technique worked so poorly for CPT-4 visit codes that the researchers concluded that it was not a viable method. Since office visits are the largest single service group, accounting for 25% of all Medicare physician expenditures, this was a significant failing.

With 15% of the extrapolated values classified as "outliers" and technical difficulties with both surgical values and office visits, the RVS began to look like Swiss cheese: more holes than substance. Since much of the controversy over physicians' charges centers on "overvalued" procedures and specialty differentials, these defects were unacceptable if the fee schedule was to be useful as a tool for policymakers. Nevertheless, the attempts to fix the extrapolation procedure in Phase II proved unsuccessful and this part was left to a Phase III, with recommendations that small consensus panels be used to assign values to the unsurveyed codes.

Surgery.   One issue was surgery, in particular, the so-called surgical global services or global fees. Here, the problem was essentially that surgeons charge for a bundle of services—a surgical procedure(s) plus some number of pre- and postoperative visits and services. But different specialties have different practices and, even more, carriers pay differently.[82] In 1989, with the help of a consensus panel of surgeons and carrier representatives, the Commission had developed a policy for determining what would be included in a surgical global service. But this determination differed from the approach used in the Hsiao study; and the Phase I study had not predicted surgical values with a satisfying measure of accuracy. What the Commission had to do was to disaggregate the global values, use the Hsiao values for the surgical procedures, and add their own relative work values for the "evaluation and management" (E&M) or visit components, which had not been measured in the Hsiao study. This was hard to do, especially since there were no vignettes or direct measures for the bundled visits and, as the Commission noted, "few objective sources . . . available for comparison."[83] Essentially, the Commission relied on specialty societies to provide information about the visits and checked these values with claims and survey data and with carriers, group practices, and other sources. A validation study, employing a consensus panel of physicians, was concluded in the Spring of 1990. Since the global fees depend on the pre/post values, a completion of this project will require assembling and reconciling the various surveys and specialty panel reviews.[84] Time will determine how successful this approach will prove to be, but it provides an example of how the Commission was able to improvise, building on the Hsiao results. It also shows how an amount of slippage gets introduced, especially in reaching a consensus over such items as the definition of a surgical bundle, what particular visit codes are included, and how to value them.

Visit Codes. More radical was the Commission's method for dealing with the visit codes. This part of their work was especially important, for not only did visits represent the largest single category of Medicare physicians' services, both the Commission and the Hsiao study group acknowledged that the Phase I results were unsatisfactory. The Phase II assignment for the study group was to redo and expand this work: develop vignettes to estimate total work[85] and expand the study from 18 specialties to include all of the 32 specialties providing such services. To further refine these values, the Commission began a project of its own for introducing a direct measure of time involved in each visit.[86] Several elements were involved. One important step was to convene a consensus panel, chosen in consultation with the CPT-4 Editorial Board[87] and the AMA, to develop specific recommendations on how to incorporate time into the CPT-4 visit codes, and dealing with such issues as how to measure time,[88] how to relate these measures to visit classifications, how to count the services of nurses and physician assistants, and so forth. Through a separate study, the Commission sought to develop its own estimates of encounter time—using a survey as well as clipboards and stopwatches—for a sample of visit codes. To this element of time would be added "classification descriptors," that would differentiate visits by type of patient and site of service, thereby adding a more precise measure of "intensity" for visits. The concluding phase was to reconcile their estimate with the Hsiao results from Phase I and Phase II. All of this was an elaborate procedure, but by approaching the visit codes this way, resort to extrapolation was avoided.

These recommendations by the Commission were adopted in the legislation and made part of the implementation deadline, so that all of this work has to be complete by 1992. It represents a task of imposing magnitude and of great complexity. As Philip Lee, the Chairman of PPRC has observed, there is some risk of creating a system that is overdesigned and tuned too finely.[89] Events in 1991 showed that there was substance to this concern, when the HCFA declined to adopt some of the PPRC refinements in assigning values to particular HCPCS codes. With their many particular modifications, visit codes might also present another kind of problem: exposed to the political process, and inviting fix after fix.

Practice Costs.   To return to the basic formula for an RVS, the value of a service is made up primarily by the "total work" contributed by a physician and the specialty practice costs attributed to that particular service. "Practice costs" have long figured in fee schedules and there is a vast amount of data collected on them, especially by the AMA and the HCFA.[90] They constitute a large proportion of the total resource costs for physicians' services: an average for all specialties of about 48%, though ranging higher and lower depending on the specialty and the service. Unlike hospital overhead, moreover, physicians' practice costs have been accepted without much criticism as a cost of doing business, with little attention to whether they represent appropriate expenditures or not.

The method employed in the Hsiao study to generate an RVS practice cost index and allocate practice costs among services is not particularly relevant for the RVS that was ultimately adopted. This was so, in part, because the Commission disagreed, on policy grounds, with the approach taken in the study. Congressional mandates and the availability of new data from the 1989 HCFA survey of practice costs were also factors. Nevertheless, a brief examination of the Hsiao approach serves to illustrate some of the technical problems as well as helping to uncover some of the big value choices that can get buried under the data and technical expertise.

The approach taken by the Hsiao group was to construct a "practice cost index" and multiply this by "total work" to yield an ultimate value in the RVS. Unlike the calculations that went into establishing "total work," however, there were no independent surveys conducted to develop these practice costs. This would, of course, have been an expensive and time-consuming undertaking. What the study group did was use existing data, primarily the HCFA 1983 Physician Practice Cost and Income Survey (PPCIS), with some added reliance on the AMA's Socioeconomic Monitoring System. These data were used to calculate a practice cost factor for each of the 18 specialties. This factor was simply a percentage ratio of gross income to practice costs. This figure was then "standardized," using the practice cost factor for general surgery as a standard, so that each practice cost factor represented some percentage of the overhead costs for general surgery. That figure was then *multiplied* by the total work value and added to it, so that RV = TW (1 + PCI). That number represented the ultimate value for that particular service in the RVS, assuming that there were no further geographic or specialty adjustments.

The construction of the PCI illustrates the kinds of data problems sometimes faced by researchers in this field. As already noted, an independent, reasonably comprehensive, and systematic survey would have been a huge undertaking. At the same time, the HCFA practice cost survey was old (1983), samples for some specialties were very small, and many data elements were missing (Etheredge and Dobson 1989, 56–57; Becker et al. 1988, 2398–2399). Some of the data also appeared to be inconsistent: for instance, as the researchers drily reported, subtracting net income from gross income often yielded "expense totals . . . substantially different from the sums of the expense totals reported."[91] The AMA Socioeconomic Monitoring System is an annual survey, and therefore timely. It was used to develop some of the cost figures, but covered only 10 of the 18 specialties. Moreover, both of these data sets assigned specialists according to their own self-classification rather than the board-certified criterion used for the RBRVS study itself, introducing further discrepancies with unknown consequences.

It is important to note that the practice cost formula is multiplicative rather than additive: the practice cost index is *multiplied* by the "total work" rather than *added* to it. As the Harvard study researchers observed, they wished to have some way of recognizing the large variation in practice costs for services provided within specialties. They rejected time as a proxy, deeming it hard to operationalize. Instead, they made an assumption that "total work," already estimated, would be roughly proportional to practice costs. This choice seems at least plausible. A common accounting practice is to associate overhead with unit inpatient costs. Furthermore, high intensity work, for instance, laser photo-coagulation, is often associated with high overhead costs. But a multiplicative formula also greatly increases the effects of any changes made in the RVS and, thereby, their redistributive impact. For instance, a hip replacement under the RBRVS gets assigned a lower value than it previously had, affecting the surgeon's income not only by a lowering of "total work," but also by reducing the practice cost allowance, even though in real life the overhead remains unchanged.[92] Moreover, the formula has a further, hidden impact. Once the RVS goes into effect, it will change physicians' incomes. But the practice cost index, in the Hsiao version, is mathematically constructed so that it is proportional to income. Consequently, as income declines or increases, so does the practice cost index, once again magnifying the effect of any change in work values.

The Commission did not like the idea of a multiplicative formula. This is not surprising, considering the projections of changes the RBRVS would generate for some fees and some specialities: decreases on the order of 45–50% for surgical procedures and increases of 65–70% for office visits.[93] Aside from the fact that this kind of redistributive impact would destroy any hope for consensus within the Commission and the medical community, it would also profoundly upset a number of Representatives and Senators. Moreover, it seemed contrary to plain common sense and equity. In fact, the Commission never seriously considered the Hsiao study's approach to practice costs, and had already developed its own additive formula and estimates to go with it.[94]

Superficially, the notion of an additive formula for practice costs seems to make more sense, and it would certainly produce less of a shock to the expectations of physicians. But it still leaves open the question of how to apportion overhead expenses—amounting to roughly half of a physician's gross income—as between procedures that take very little time (IOL implants) and those that take a lot (multiple joint procedures) and between services that are labor intensive (endoscopies) and those that are capital intensive (magnetic resonance imaging). To address this problem, the Commission began work on a method to apportion practice expenses by categories of service rather than by specialty, eventually setting up six such categories, based on service type and site of care.[95] Meanwhile, the HCFA completed its own 1989–1990 version of the Physicians Practice Cost and Income Survey, so that a large, new data source was available. This was further supplemented with the Commission's own 1988 Survey of Physicians, the AMA's Periodic Survey of Physicians, and by supplemental data collected from solo and group practices and the Medical Group Management Association. The legislation itself provided for the cruder, historic approach of determining practice cost allowance by specialty, but in anticipation of further refinements included a broad mandate for the Commission to continue the study of practice expenses, reporting by July 1, 1991.

Add-Ons and Modifiers

A relative value scale, taken by itself, is only a part of the equation.[96] Like the hospital DRGs, it provides a technical element that can help to make the ultimate formula for payment more appealing on scientific or economic grounds, more equitable for provider or beneficiaries, and more instrumentally effective in achieving ultimate goals such as fairness, costs containment, or beneficiary access. According to the formula, FS = RBRVS × CF, where CF is the "conversion factor," the dollar amount that converts the RVS into a fee. With equations of this sort, what is left out are not only the various exceptions and add-ons that go into the ultimate payment system, but also the fundamental value assumptions about what gets included in the equation, how the parameters are set, how they get changed over time, and what institutional constraints are established. Here, as the saying goes, "the fun begins." In other words, the big and controversial decisions remain to be made: such as what to do about assignment and balance billing, how to determine the annual update figure, what regional and specialty differentials to include, if any, and what to do about the looming issue of volume. These were matters the Commission and staff had been discussing for the whole of their institutional existence and on which a consensus was, in most instances, steadily developing. Still, as they prepared the 1989 *Annual Report* containing the recommendations for legislation, much remained unresolved. And Congress was by no means a silent partner, stating some if its preferences forcefully.

One important question was simply what was to count as "work," a matter of large political significance as might be imagined. In the Hsiao study, it was initially seen as (1) time and (2) intensity. Work, in other words, should be measured by duration as well as by how "hard" it is. Now, time can be fairly well measured or estimated. But "intensity" is a pretty subjective notion. Therefore, to delineate this concept further, the researchers interviewed a small sample of 20 physicians about their own views of intensity and combined the results of these interviews with some further analysis, including multidimensional scaling (Hsiao et al. 1988, 2362). Ultimately, they put three other dimensions in place of intensity: (1) mental effort and judgment, (2) technical skill and physician effort, and (3) stress due to patient risk. This breaking up of the notion helps to bring the idea of intensity into sharper focus; but it also makes clear that it is a heavily loaded concept, giving much weight not just to "hard" work but also to the highly specialized and risky services and procedures—most of them already highly priced. In fact, street talk at the time was that "intensity" was simply a code word for "surgery," i.e., a formula to gain the acquiescence of the surgical specialties. However that may be, the Commission accepted the formula, warts and all.

Another contentious matter, similar to the controversy over "intensity," was whether to build into the RVS an allowance for the "opportunity costs" of specialty training. Physicians in the specialties—for instance, orthopedic surgeons or cardiologists—undergo long years of arduous training and reduced income to get to where they are. It is both equitable and makes sense economically to compensate them for their "opportunity cost." This is one line of argument, well entrenched in both popular lore and economic theory (Kaufman 1988). The Hsiao version of the RVS included such an allowance. On the other hand, specialists in the United States are already well paid. The difficulty is not in getting people to go into most specialties, but in keeping them out of them, i.e., getting a reasonable proportion to stick with primary care. Furthermore, "intensity" already implicitly recognized some additional payment for specialties. To the Commission, which tended to represent the primary care family and a beneficiary perspective,[97] this additional allowance seemed both unnecessary as an incentive and an unjustifiable kind of "double-dipping," already too familiar in professional and governmental circles.

One issue that the Commission debated over the course of many meetings was the question of whether to recognize "specialty differentials" or not. For instance, should the first visit with a family physician be paid the same as one with a rheumatologist, an EKG done by a nurse and one performed by a cardiologist, or the removal of a wart by a general practitioner and by a dermatologist? There are some good reasons for having such differentials, aside from the fact that they are established in the profession and recognized by most carriers. One reason for them is to ensure access: for example, an elderly patient in a rural area needing a specialist. Another is quality assurance: to make the practice of surgery less attractive to the underqualified. At the same time, recognition of a specialty differential would have projected the Commission into a truly formidable thicket of issues: such as how to define a specialty,[98] what to do about those already practicing as specialists though not formally qualified, how to set specialty differentials, and what kind of transition to devise.

On this issue, as well as others involving specialties versus primary care, the Commission stuck to its underlying philosophy of paying for work or, more inclusively, resource costs.[99] Thus, it recognized "intensity" since it was a way of defining work. On the other hand, opportunity cost would not be counted, since there was no more work involved. Nor would specialty differentials, except as they were implicitly recognized through work values or overhead costs. This outcome is the sort that brings joy to any policymaker, where expedience and principle coincide. By taking the Hsiao definition of work, including its notion of "intensity," some but not all of the claims of the surgeons and other specialists were acknowledged, an important political concession. Yet this same concept of work provided a principled ground for refusing both specialty differentials and a separate payment for opportunity costs. This was an outcome that seemed fair and avoided an array of difficulties.

Geographic Modifiers. A theoretically complex and politically touchy issue was that of geographic multipliers: what allowances or corrections to make for regional variations in existing fees, "doctor shortages" or lack of beneficiary access to services, and differences in practice costs. This was a topic that had to be addressed. Congress in the SOBRA legislation had already directed the Secretary of DHHS to develop a "geographic MEI" and indicated to the PPRC that such an index would be included in any eventual fee schedule.[100] But, to recall the experience with PPS, geographic formulas are highly charged issues and prone to political manipulation. However the Commission approached this issue, it was critically important.

Taking a very ambitious view of its mission and its capabilities, the Commission could have used geographic multipliers as part of a deliberate strategy to redress geographic maldistribution of medical manpower and services: setting differentials so as to move physicians within and between regions, to the rural areas and the inner cities. This was an approach popular with some economists. Something of this same approach had already been taken with PPS. Moreover, the Congress had specifically directed the Secretary, in its mandate to DHHS for a report on the fee schedule, to consider this particular method for attracting physicians to medically underserved areas.[101] At the same time, venturing this way would have gotten the Commission deeply into the politics of medical manpower, not an explicitly assigned part of its responsibility nor a subject about which either the Commission or its staff were particularly knowledgeable. In fact little was or is known about why physicians locate where they do or what impact such geographic differentials would have had, for instance, on balance billing, assignment, or patient access to services. In any event, the Commission would not have been in a good position to monitor the impact of its own policy. The Commission briefly discussed this kind of approach[102] but quickly and wisely abandoned it.

In the upshot, the Commission recognized regional variations only to the extent that they were part of practice costs, i.e., represented resource costs to physicians that differed by region.[103] Here, the Commission essentially adopted an approach developed by researchers from the Urban Institute and the Center for Health Economics Research, working under the contract with DHHS.[104] But there was an elegant, if small, additional contribution made by the Commission. For total practice costs, the two main components are physician inputs and nonphysician inputs. Including physician inputs sounds odd, since the physician is already paid for his or her "work." But physicians generally own their practices, either as individuals or members of a group. Therefore, their own management activities and other personal contributions to the practice are important and amount, as computed, to about 60% of the index. The remaining part, about 40%, is made up of employee wages, rent, malpractice insurance premiums, medical equipment and supplies. Obviously, there are many ways such as index can be modified or varied. And one small concession that would have made the Commission popular with many physicians would have been to recognize a "cost of living" adjustment for the physician component, in effect, an add-on for especially high cost areas such as Los Angeles and New York.[105] The Commission opted not to do this, choosing an "overhead only" index. This approach indexes the physician component to a representative mix of professional occupations.[106] Thus, the nonphysician inputs are regional, but the physician input, both for the work component and for practice costs, are essentially national. The underlying principle, central to the Commission and endorsed by the AMA as well, is that the net compensation to a physician for providing a given service should not vary from one locality to another.[107]

In making this decision, the Commission was adhering to its principle of paying only for work and other resource use. In part, this decision speaks to fairness, at least as perceived by the Commission: that physicians should not get an additional bonus, in the form of a cost-of-living increment, for choosing to practice in high cost areas—such as New York, San Francisco, or Honolulu. If they like the ambience, professional or otherwise, well and good. But they should not expect more pay for living there.[108] The Commission also indexed some elements of practice costs to national income figures for other professions, a common enough idea in other countries, but new to the United States and potentially of future policy significance. And by advocating one national rate of compensation for all physician inputs, they were not only underlining a potent political idea, but encouraging practitioners to move, and embarking on a limited experiment in the redistribution of physician incomes between regions.

How well this approach will survive the stresses of regional politics remains to be seen. In a manner reminiscent of the DHHS version of PPS, the Commission recommended to Congress a minimum of regional variations. As with PPS, providers from the large urban and rural areas have complained about anticipated redistributive consequences for them. Shortly after the publication of the Commission's 1989 Report, the HCFA came out with its own estimates of regional variations, showing in some detail how they would affect categories of providers.[109] The HCFA report had little if any effect in Congress, but was seen as a hostile gesture by the Commission. Furthermore, Rep. Henry Waxman (D.,Ca.), a health policy stalwart, dissented from this part of the Commission Report and was able to get from the Congress a partial cost-of-living adjustment. The legislation also mandates a series of studies that could lead to additional geographic modifiers, especially for urban and rural areas and malpractice insurance.

Balance Billing. One controversial topic deferred as long as possible was that of balance billing and mandatory assignment. Allowing physicians to bill patients for the "balance" of their expected fee was, of course, a long-established practice with private insurance companies such as Blue Shield, and had been accepted as a part of Part B reimbursement principles even though hospital payment was, from the beginning, on an assigned basis. From the earliest days of Medicare politics, though, one of the cherished objectives of a number of policy activists within the Social Security Administration and the Congress was to get rid of this asymmetry and establish the principle that the government fee should be regarded as payment in full. Also, as noted before, beneficiaries are dear to the Congress. It was the sudden rise of the Part B premium in September 1987 that quickened the Congress's resolve on a fee schedule. Since the original fee freeze in 1984, the issue of balance billing had been prominent, and several bills in Congress had sought to impose some form of mandatory assignment. Even as the Commission deliberated, for that matter, the physician community was groaning under the MAACs. Yet this was a hard policy choice, both on grounds of principle and as a matter of pragmatic politics. Over several months, as the Commission deliberated on its report, observers speculated on whether they would reach a consensus on this topic or not.

Given the underlying rationale of a fee schedule, which is to get to a fair payment for individual services, it would seem on grounds of principle that the Medicare fee should constitute payment in full. This was, in fact, the view of four commissioners expressed in a dissenting view— the sole issue on which there was a minority position in the entire 1989 Report. The majority recommended that there be a percentage limit on balance billing, but took no position on what that percentage should be.[110] They also strongly endorsed the participating physician program (PAR) and recommended that it be continued. It is hard to know how much their motivation was political, though it was partly that. "Fair" is, after all, largely a matter of how people perceive the decision rules. And the vast majority of physician specialty groups as well as the AMA opposed mandatory assignment.[111] Furthermore, as indicated by simulations, big city specialists and surgeons, groups that already stood to lose relatively or absolutely under the proposed fee schedule, would lose substantially more with mandatory assignment. A serious concern, therefore, might be the impact on beneficiary access: the possibility that a number of physicians would withdraw from Medicare or substantially alter the Medicare proportion of their practice. These were not considerations explicitly discussed in the report and may not, on balance, have figured as prominently as other policy grounds. Among these latter was the belief on the part of some commissioners that physicians ought to have some freedom about what they charged.[112] The Commission termed this a "safety valve,"[113] but it would seem to cover several other policy desiderata as well. One is the provision for some element of market responsiveness, which could be a useful way of rationing the services of physicians in high demand while still retaining them as Medicare providers. This option would also leave open to the physician the decision about whether to shift costs from needier patients to more affluent ones, an arrangement that carries with it some of the good and some of the bad of the American tradition of private charity.

As events developed, the Commission may have been prudent to take this approach to balance billing and mandatory assignment. Along with the "expenditure targets," these were the most controversial items in the proposed Medicare Fee Schedule. Over the summer, prior to the passage of the legislation, the surgeons made their own agreement with the Ways and Means Committee for a separate expenditure target (ET), and the American Medical Association threatened the withdrawal of its support for the fee schedule. To take a strong stand on balance billing might have overloaded the proposal with controversial features. Moreover, Congress regards itself as the protector of the beneficiaries and would certainly decide this matter in its own way, and that is how the Commission left the issue. At the same time, this resolution seemed to depart, in spirit at least, from the underlying rationale of "fair payment." In view of the fact that out-of-pocket expenses for some Medicare beneficiaries would actually increase,[114] this part of the Commission's proposals will not be remembered for its contribution to beneficiary welfare. It was the sole issue that split the Commission, and four members filed a minority report, urging the adoption of mandatory assignment as a goal of the payment system.[115]

Annual Update. Another topic that the Commission left largely up to Congress was the "update," that is the procedures by which periodic changes in the conversion factor and relative values in the fee schedule would be made. The Commission said it had considered four different approaches:

1. a formula, linking the conversion factor to an index of practice expenses,
2. use of the existing rule-making procedures of the DHHS (i.e., the HCFA),
3. use of an independent (sic) commission to advise Congress, and
4. negotiation between physicians and the Federal government.

The report went on to say that some combination of the above would be "most effective in the United States,"[116] and that updating should take place in much the same way that the fee schedule was originally developed. The Commission, with input from physicians and other groups, should advise Congress; and the Commission with the HCFA should monitor implementation. As the system was implemented, the Commission could explore ways for updating the RVS using consensus panels and differing methods for consultation with and possibly even negotiation with the medical profession and specialty groups. In other words, the specifics were left up to Congress: an approach that made good political sense, inasmuch as the update was a carefully guarded legislative prerogative and, besides, would need to be closely integrated with the substantive provisions of the legislation.[117]

The "Volume" Issue. The single most difficult question faced by the Commission was what to do about "volume." This is a term loosely employed to cover a variety of likely responses by physicians to a fee schedule: such as code creep and upcoding, unbundling, and increasing the intensity of service or the number of encounters. It is a problem inherent in fee schedules and third party reimbursement and every country that uses a fee schedule must cope with the "volume" problem. In the United States, Medicare officials and government policy-makers have been aware of this fact of life for a long time and at least as early as the Economic Stabilization Program in the early 1970s, when physician income continued to rise, much as before, despite price control. And from 1984 to 1986, overall Part B expenditures also rose, little affected by the fee freeze. So, this issue came as no surprise to the Commission members and was part of their agenda beginning with the Commission's earliest deliberations in 1987. In the same year, the Commission also received a letter from Reps. Stark and Gradison, indicating a bipartisan concern with this problem.[118] Not a popular topic, for a year and a half the Commission virtually ignored it, even though Paul Ginsburg, the Executive Director, would interject the "volume" issue from time to time into their deliberations; and as the Medicare Fee Schedule proposal developed, the Commission became increasingly aware that this one was a "make or break" issue that had to be resolved.[119]

But like taxes, the difficulty with a volume cap or an expenditure target may be at least as much with the specific provisions and with how it is implemented as with the policy itself. This proved to be true for the Commission, which largely agreed that some form of control was needed, but returned repeatedly to the issue of what kind of expenditure target to use and how to combine it with other incentives or controls: whether it should be national, regional, or state, and what withhold mechanism to use; what importance to give to specialty societies, professional leadership, and so forth. At one point, as the *Annual Report* deadline approached, the Commission considered a weak recommendation or none at all, an outcome that might have changed history quite a bit.

The eventual proposal was a strong one: a national expenditure target that would specify an annual maximum percentage of increase or "target" for Part B expenditures for physicians' services. This ET would be linked to performance, so that if the actual expenditure for the year was less than the target, an unlikely occurrence, then the conversion factor for the succeeding year could be adjusted upward. On the other hand, if the expenditure for a year exceeded the target, then the conversion factor for the year would be adjusted downward to recoup that excess, building in a penalty as an incentive for restraint. The Commission recommended that the ET be established first on a national basis, adding that regional, state, or substate areas might prove to be desirable and feasible in the future.

The particular version of volume control chosen was like that employed in the Canadian province of British Columbia, a lineage noted, with disapprobation, in the medical journals (C. Stevens 1989, 26). It was also an approach favored by the Ways and Means Health Subcommittee, and the Commission endorsement gave a small but positive impetus to the impending legislation.

In the Commission's approach to "volume," the ETs did not stand alone. Also recommended was a strengthened program of carrier and PRO review and an extensive program of effectiveness or outcomes research and the development of practice guidelines.

For obvious reasons, utilization review and ways of ensuring quality of care are integrally related to an expenditure target. A fee schedule sets a price. One way to game the price controls is by such expedients as upcoding and increasing the intensity and volume of service. But another approach, especially with ETs in place, is to save on the time and effort devoted to an individual Medicare procedure or service and divert these resources to private patients. So, both the ensuring of necessary care and the prevention of unnecessary care are important, and increasingly so if a fee schedule and expenditure target operate to control price and volume.

One way in which Commission recommendations addressed quality of care was through the endorsement of HCFA's endeavors to strengthen review of Part B claims and the existing carrier and PRO activities. The HCFA had already taken some steps in this direction, such as a new requirement that Part B claims submissions contain individual physician identification numbers and diagnosis codes for the services included. The HCFA was also engaged in an extensive program for improving the carrier and PRO utilization review capabilities. These endeavors the Commission supported. But it went further to urge that the PROs extend their review to care provided in the physicians' offices, a step likely to exasperate the physician community and test the outermost limits of the regulatory process, but one that seems strongly implied by the logic of the fee schedule and the expenditure targets.[120]

The Commission's most optimistic hopes were tied to the newly burgeoning enthusiasm for practice guidelines and research into the appropriateness or effectiveness of medical procedures. Briefly, the notion is that a lot of medical activity is unnecessary or even harmful. And if those medical services and procedures that are high volume, expensive, and unnecessary could be identified and physicians educated to reduce or eliminate them, patients would be better off and the government could save a lot of money (Eddy and Billing 1988, 18). There is a problem of how physicians are induced to change their ways (Eisenberg 1986), but the relationship of this activity to the general problem of expenditure targets and volume control is obvious: it represents a painless way of encouraging the same result and one that benefits the patient and that physicians might welcome. It was also popular at the moment, both in DHHS and in Congress, especially the Senate. Accordingly, the Commission recommended that the Federal government should support effectiveness research and practice guidelines through "funding, coordination, and evaluation." A second important part, not painless, was that practice guidelines be developed, disseminated, and utilized in PRO and carrier reviews.[121]

Together, the several Commission proposals for constraining the growth in volume had a coherent relationship. ETs were there as a warning and to provide a shared incentive. This global constraint could be made more specific, as need be, through regional or specialty ETs. Volume limitations were given some teeth and bite through increased carrier and PRO activities. But education would proceed, meanwhile, through the promulgation of practice guidelines and the findings of research on appropriateness or outcomes. The Commission did not specify in detail how these various strategies could be integrated, and a number of issues were left unresolved. But this part of the Report met with a strongly positive reception in Congress, both the House and Senate, and was adopted in its basic outlines.

IV. LEGISLATING THE MEDICARE FEE SCHEDULE

The PPRC's March 1989 *Annual Report* to Congress marked a transition in the development of the Medicare Fee Schedule, for by then it was reasonably clear within the Commission and among the Congressional subcommittee members and staff that the project was feasible, both politically and technically. Thereafter, the issue of whether there would be a Medicare Fee Schedule was taken as pretty much settled, at least by the Commission and the Congress. The report, moreover, contained a fully developed set of proposals for legislative enactment. Attention was now directed increasingly to perfecting the RVS methodology and improving data bases and analytical components. Also, with the decision about fundamental approach made, a number of politically charged issues about how the RVS would be packaged and implemented now became increasingly salient—for the Commission, the Congress, and the health care providers and their lobby groups.

Phase II and Beyond

One ought not, however, speak lightly of "technical work" or "refinement" of the Hsiao methodology, for the task remaining was both large in scope and challenging in complexity, entailing a Phase II and Phase III of the Hsiao study, extensive data collection and technical analysis by the Commission, and work with consensus panels that would extend over several years. Following an obvious division of labor, Hsiao and his associates worked to correct some of the methodological deficiencies identified in the earlier study, to revise work values, and to expand the RVS to include additional services and specialties. This activity entailed not only reviewing and revising previous work but expanding its scope to include 14 additional specialties. Closely relating its efforts to Hsiao II, the Commission began a visit survey[122] and a surgical global service project[123] that would help refine and validate some of Hsiao's work. It also continued its work on improvement of codes and coding practices, practice expense, professional liability expense (malpractice insurance), geographic adjusters, and the definition of payment areas—technical matters, but politically charged with distributive and redistributive decisions.

From this review of study phases and continuing activities, the process of refinement may seem not just endless but lacking visible mileposts. For that matter, refinements of the Medicare Fee Schedule will continue to be a significant part of the implementation activities, extending well beyond January 1992. That said, however, the Commissions third *Annual Report* (1989) deserves some comment not only for its scope and quality but for its historic significance. By the testimony of its chairman, Dr. Philip Lee,[124] it entailed an enormous amount of work, especially in reaching closure on so many issues. It was a large achievement, both in quality and scope and in its balanced discussion of the issues. At the same time, it closely tracked the thinking in Congress, a circumstance that contributed to the absence of controversy in the eventual passage of the Medicare Fee Schedule legislation. Coming as it did—the culmination of a series of steps leading in one direction—the Report probably contributed substantially to a sense in the government and the health care industry that the fee schedule was an inevitability. In any event, it certainly seemed to be the one live option, for notable by its absence was any counterproposal from the Administration or any of the specialty societies that was worth taking seriously.[125]

Preliminary Maneuvers

The fact that a substantial degree of consensus existed about *what* to do did not mean that there was a similar agreement about when to move forward legislatively. Some Congressmen saw the 1989 session as a likely time, pretty much on the theory that Congress always does *something* and that this proposal had momentum.[126] In the Senate, Jay Rockefeller had just become chairman of the newly created Medicare subcommittee of Finance, and was receptive to an attractive agenda item. On the other hand some of the important staff persons, who concern themselves with the specifics of agendas, were skeptical and thought maybe this year and maybe next.[127] Peter Bouxsein, then on the staff of the Health and Environment Subcommittee of Energy and Commerce reported inquiring of some of his staff counterparts on other health subcommittees and finding little interest, as of early Spring, for a bill that session.

Nevertheless, some groups did have a strong interest in the passage of a Medicare Fee Schedule, among them the American Association of Retired Persons, for whom the legislation represented beneficiary protection, and specialty societies such as the American Society of Internal Medicine and the American College of Physicians whose members stood to benefit from the higher payments for EM services. These groups lobbied for action that year. Others within Congress and HCFA were also interested. On the initiative of Bouxsein of the Energy and Commerce staff, a working party began drafting a bill early in the Spring of 1989. But this was, as yet, only one subcommittee and not one with specific jurisdiction over Medicare.

One of the most potent forces moving the Medicare Fee Schedule was, oddly, its most controversial feature: the expenditure target. This proposal was debated for months prior to the Commission's 1989 report and there was a growing conviction in government and within the provider community that the Commission would recommend an ET and that the Stark subcommittee would insist on it. As a foreboding matured into a near certainty, major provider groups began to take policy stands and come forward with counter-proposals. At one point, the AMA threatened to withdraw its support for the fee schedule if it included ETs as an integral part. More significantly, and more importantly for moving events, in February 1989 the American College of Surgeons offered its endorsement of the entire fee schedule proposal if it included a separate ET for surgeons. This was an important event, for it not only divided the opposition to ETs but brought in the surgeons, until then seen as a formidable opponent of the Medicare Fee Schedule. This welcome support, combined with the Commission's own endorsement of ETs in the 1989 report provided from the perspective of the Stark subcommittee a "window of opportunity" not to be wasted or trifled away. Not only was it valuable support but it held forth the prospect for relatively quick and uncontroversial enactment of the Medicare Fee Schedule—which probably could not have passed had it become politically controversial.[128]

In April, the Stark Subcommittee began working on its own version of physician payment reform, intended as a contribution to the budget reconciliation process for that year. Legislative hearings were held, though largely to let the lobbies know what was afoot rather than to solicit opinion. The payment reform proposal was pushed vigorously by Reps. Stark and Gradison, passing the Subcommittee on June 14 and the full Ways and Means Committee on June 28. Included were strong provisions on expenditure targets and balance billing and support for effectiveness research, an approach especially favored by Gradison.

Throughout the Spring of 1989, lobbying activity on the part of the AMA and the specialty societies was notable by its absence. There was the usual flurry of letters and appearances at the hearings, but nothing like the national campaigns and intense bargaining that preceded and accompanied the passage of the Prospective Payment System. The AMA was, in large part, already coopted and much concerned to preserve what remained of its image as a representative of and spokesman for the medical profession as a whole. The surgeons had already cut their deal. And the primary care physicians and those providing the "visits" or EM services stood to make out well under the fee schedule. Yet, as Samuel Johnson once observed, the prospect of being hanged has a wondrous capacity to concentrate the mind. In like manner, the strong endorsement of ETs produced a belated response from the medical groups, proposing alternatives and appealing to other forums, especially the Senate, for a method of controlling volume that would be less stringent.

One development that helped the bill in Committee and that was ultimately essential for the passage of the fee schedule was its endorsement by William Roper, the Deputy Assistant to the President for Domestic Policy.[129] Roper was philosophically committed to capitation as the right approach and had long opposed fee schedules because of their inflationary tendency. Yet, he was persuaded that this particular fee schedule proposal had developed great momentum and would be hard and costly to stop. While he supported the fee schedule, that support was conditioned on their being, as an integral part of the proposal, a stringent volume control: practically speaking, ETs. Once again, as with the ACS endorsement, this was an important development, since it amounted to support by the Bush Administration. Observers credit Roper, moreover, with persuading others: securing the acquiescence or support necessary for passage within the White House Office and, especially, the Executive Office of Management and Budget.[130] A few days later, Louis Sullivan, in his first public pronouncement as the new Secretary of DHHS, appeared before the Medicare subcommittee of Senate Finance to make known the Department's support. But Roper's support was especially critical, for had the bill been opposed within the White House Office, the delay and political controversy would almost certainly have stalled the legislation and prevented its passage in the 1989 session.

Meanwhile, the medical associations were searching for alternatives to the ETs. One possibility was to enhance the role of practice guidelines. This approach built on the growing support in both the House and Senate for a program that would sponsor research on effectiveness and outcomes combined with the development and use of practice guidelines. The proposal—put forward by the American Society of Internal Medicine and the American College of Physicians—was for increased funding to develop practice guidelines and the application of these guidelines by the Medicare carriers to key services, especially those that were high volume and that were scheduled for the biggest cuts under the Relative Value Schedule.[131] This endorsement of practice guidelines represented a radical change of policy on the part of these specialty societies, for they had long and vigorously denounced practice guidelines as unscientific, "cookbook" medicine. But given that the ETs had already passed Ways and Means and were supported by the Bush Administration, some constructive proposal seemed called for, however belated it might be. Accordingly, representatives from the specialty societies approached the more sympathetic committees in House and Senate. The proposal was also presented at the AMA annual meeting, accompanied with appeals for an anti-ET campaign by the state medical societies.[132]

In the Senate, support for the Medicare Fee Schedule was less strong, in part because of Senator Bentsen's belief that Texas physicians would make out badly with the changes in payment.[133] At the same time, both Senator Rockefeller (D., W.Va.), chairman of the new Medicare subcommittee, and Senator Durenberger (R., Minn.), the ranking minority member, were interested in the fate of the Medicare Fee Schedule and had held hearings in March and April 1989. The Subcommittee was not especially moved by the belated laments of the AMA and the specialty societies,[134] but the Senate often acts to mitigate house provisions, somewhat like a court of appeals within the judicial system. Moreover, there was more generalized sympathy for the physicians in the Senate than in the Stark Subcommittee and greater interest in effectiveness research and practice guidelines. Indeed, this particular approach to volume and quality of care had been an enthusiasm of Senator Mitchell (D., Me.), who immediately preceded Rockefeller as chairman of the Subcommittee.[135] Accordingly, the Subcommittee's bill, S1809, contained a long and elaborate section on "Patient Outcomes Assessment Research,"[136] that built on this earlier interest as well as addressing some of the concerns of the ASIM and ACP. In place of the ETs, the bill recommended "Volume Performance Standards" (VPSs). VPSs was a suggestion that originated from HHS, the one important substantive contribution coming from the executive branch. The terminology itself was less inflammatory, suggesting a group aspiration or collective effort rather than official penalties. But the difference was more than semantic, for a VPS was viewed as an advisory guideline rather than a specific target. In particular, it did not link prescribed penalties to the performance standard. Moreover, the Secretary's discretion in recommending an update would be narrowly confined, limiting this method of sanctioning as well.[137]

The Legislative Process

A remarkable feature of this particular legislation was the understanding, shared by the members and staff, that the Medicare Fee Schedule would be done as part of the budget reconciliation. In one way, this was a natural choice, since budget reconciliation had been the vehicle for most legislation dealing with payment reform, either for hospitals or for physicians. Moreover, Ways and Means did little in the way of substantive legislation except as an adjunct to tax bills or budget reconciliation.[138] But there was also the common awareness that the legislation *could* be enacted only through a procedure that largely bypassed the traditional legislative process: time was too short; and the bill too technical and controversial to survive minute examination and extended debate. In this respect physician payment reform represented a step beyond the Prospective Payment System in the "streamlining" of the legislative process: not just a "fast track" for one train, but an array of proposals and almost no time for Congress as a body to consider any of them separately.

Considering the Medicare Fee Schedule in isolation, one might be led to a comforting belief that its legislative progress would be easy and straightforward. Not so. Even though handily passed through the committee stage, physician payment reform thereafter was despaired of so many times that its proponents lost count. Much of the difficulty was occasioned by the OBRA process itself. Largely because it is such a powerful legislative vehicle, the OBRA gets loaded with controversial items and with a large number of extraneous and ill-assorted proposals. This feature of the budget reconciliation process creates its own problems—which in this 1989 session of Congress critically affected the legislative career of physician payment reform.

One important factor was time. Budget reconciliation is itself complex and requires an inordinate amount of sequencing and coordinating of committee deliberation and decision-making, in which the most difficult issues and the most laggard committees invariably slow or stall the process. By 1989, moreover, many of the most likely deficit reduction items had been worked over and squeezed hard, not once but many times, so that easy marks were hard to come by and tougher choices had to be made. Several big and contentious issues, such as the capital gains tax, slowed the process even more with the result that this year, committee reports were weeks and even months behind. As the weeks passed and Fall began, the Gramm–Rudman deadline of October 15 became important, since a triggering of the automatic sequester, which included Medicare, would have affected the prospects for physician payment reform, probably postponing it until 1990 at least.[139] The House passed its version of the budget reconciliation (HR3299) on October 5, but with several big issues unresolved, including the capital gains tax. Many in the Senate thought a reconciliation unlikely, and President Bush, along with most Senate Republicans, actually preferred a sequester to a reconciliation loaded with unwanted baggage.

Stripping. 1989 was also the year in which the steady burdening of the budget reconciliation process led to the separating of an unusual number of extraneous proposals including, at one juncture, physician payment reform itself. Along with the usual amount of extraneous minutiae, the House reconciliation bill contained several big and hot items, such as repeal of catastrophic health care insurance, Medicaid child health provisions, and a tax package combining capital gains, IRAs, and the top income-tax brackets. While some bluster and brinksmanship usually characterize the reconciliation process, this blockbuster item of taxes lifted the dispute to the level of high politics, threatening a major confrontation between the President and the Congress.

At this juncture, the Senate still had not drafted its version of the reconciliation. With the President threatening a veto and the Gramm–Rudman sequester approaching, the Senate Democratic leadership faced a tough decision and little time in which to make it. Their expedient, on proposal of the majority leader, Sen. Mitchell, was to "strip" their reconciliation proposal of all "extraneous" provisions, i.e., those not saving budget dollars in FY 1990. This tactic, it was hoped, would help meet the Gramm–Rudman deadline or, at least, make a sequester easier to repeal. It mollified the White House by removing the most controversial items from their reconciliation proposal. But it also stripped out physician payment reform from the Senate reconciliation package, requiring a hasty drafting of its own free-standing bill, S1809.[140]

On October 17, the 232 members participating in the reconciliation process began meeting and deliberating, but did little for the first two weeks while congressional leaders bargained and negotiated with the White House and between the House and Senate over top priority items, such as overall defense expenditures, taxes, tariffs and trade promotion, child care and catastrophic health insurance. President Bush continued to threaten a veto,[141] demanding in the alternative a clean reconciliation bill, with a number of the controversial and extraneous items eliminated. Without formally "stripping" the bill, the House leadership dropped many items, leaving child care and physician payment reform among the more contentious ones remaining in the bill.

With the reconciliation bill much reduced and Thanksgiving approaching, the House and Senate conferees began a negotiating marathon in the week of November 13, hoping that agreement could be reached in time for the recess. Further delay increased the probability that the Gramm–Rudman sequester would become permanent, as Congress grew weary and the Administration accepted this outcome as the best of a bad business. Rostenkowski and Bentsen, the key negotiators, pointed toward a Friday resolution, and congressional leaders took the unusual step of scheduling a Sunday session for floor debate.[142]

Meanwhile, physician payment reform had not fared well: indeed, it was almost swept aside by the high politics of budget reconciliation and the turbulence that generated. Versions of payment reform were approved by the two House subcommittees and included in HR3299; but they received scarcely a mention in the floor debates, which were devoted mainly to discussions of capital gains, income taxes, and the catastrophic insurance repeal. Immediately thereafter, payment reform was stripped from the Senate bill so that it went forward with no proposal whatever on the subject. Even though the Senate subcommittee staff drafted a bill,[143] some doubted that it was "conferenceable" and thought payment reform probably dead for this session of Congress. In any event, staffs within the House and Senate had little opportunity to negotiate the differences or talk them over with their principles, so that payment reform as a reconciliation item suffered from some serious liabilities.[144]

The Reconciliation Conference. The meeting of the Conference Committee on Friday, November 17, was a 15-hour high-stakes summit negotiation with Rostenkowski and Bentsen in charge. Prospects for the payment reform were poor, for there were still many hard and complex issues for which the reconciliation conference was an ill-suited forum. Indeed, the House conferees had already met to stake out their positions and were proceeding on the assumption that there would be no physician payment reform.[145] In the reconciliation conference, Ways and Means declared the payment reform "off the table" and refused even to discuss it without the inclusion of the ETs. To this, Bentsen said "no." For Ways and Means, Rostenkowski said "no." Late in the evening, payment reform was left for dead and its supporters told that no compromise could be reached on the three versions of the bill.[146]

Left for dead, though, was not the same as dead, and payment reform was revived a second time, largely owing to the efforts of Sen. John D. (Jay) Rockefeller, IV. As chairman of the new Medicare subcommittee, he had gotten deeply involved in the bill and was anxious to begin his tenure with a creditable showing.[147] He was told on Friday evening of the Conference results and urged to let the matter lie. But, according to report, he thought it intolerable to deal so summarily with an issue of this importance and took it on himself to convene a special Saturday morning meeting—within hours after the Conference—to seek an accord that would reconcile the three different versions of the payment reform. The meeting included Representatives and Senators most concerned with payment reform, personal and committee staff, and several from the Administration, especially William Roper, the White House Deputy for Domestic Policy. It was held, according to Rockefeller, in

Senator Durenberger's conference room because it alone had a table large enough to accommodate all the parties.[148]

After the meeting of the principles, staff worked throughout Saturday and into the evening on the details of a proposal. Provisional agreements were reached on a number of key items: the transition, MAACs and balance billing limits, practice cost differentials, and budget neutrality. On the most difficult issue, the Volume Performance Standard,[149] a partially "linked"[150] version was proposed: an increase in the update for good performance with a penalty limit of 2% below the MEI should Congress "default," i.e., not set its own update. In Representative Stark's opinion, this was a sheep in sheep's clothing, and he vetoed it, saying that he preferred no bill to this one. As for the physicians, he would get them through budget reconciliation and the update, just as before.[151] Once again, the prospects for a Medicare Fee Schedule seemed in doubt, at least for 1989.

Despite the impasse reached on Saturday, the various parties were close to agreement except for the issue of ETs or VPSs, which remained as the major obstacle. For most of the legislators, the other items, such as the transition, balance billing, regional differentials, etc., were relatively inconsequential and could be traded out or fixed in the course of implementation.[152] Yet the VPS, especially the issue of linkage, remained as a major sticking point. And legislative conferences, like other negotiating or brokering activities, have a tendency to "go sour" as time wears on.[153] On Sunday, committee staffs worked through the day, pulling together a proposal for a final attempt on Monday morning.

On Monday morning, conferees and their staff assembled in a Ways and Means committee room with the VPS and its linkage as yet unresolved. At this juncture, Wendell Primus, a principal staff aide to Rostenkowski,[154] appeared with a "piece of paper," developed by the Committee staff and backed by the Chairman. Whatever effect the intervention of Rostenkowski may have had, the working paper contained the elements of an agreement, including an acceptable formula for the Volume Performance Standard. The conferees met behind closed doors from 10:00 to 12:00 that morning and settled the outlines of a bill. In essence, they agreed to pretty much the same items that had been accepted on Saturday, with the critical addition of a Volume Performance Standard. The change was to link the VPS on the down side so that exceeding the performance standard would result in a penalty—a limited one—that would be superseded when, as would likely be the result, Congress acted to set the update itself. This seemed to satisfy most, except Stark himself, who withheld approval until the very end.

At 2:00, Monday afternoon, the various staffs assembled to draft a final version. This was in no way a purely technical or routine process, for specific numbers and language had to be supplied that would articulate the bargains and tradeoffs and give substance to sections and clauses settled only in principle. Decisions that entail swings of tens of millions of dollars for the Medicare program or for the physicians were made in minutes. Some provisions were negotiated meticulously and at length; others got settled because one house had better language.[155] Some parts of the bill were barely discussed in the conference process— for instance, the sections on outcomes research and the fee schedule provisions for the radiologists, anesthesiologists, and pathologists were adopted en bloc during the drafting session. The staff, some of whom had been working almost continuously for 72 hours, reached a weary conclusion between 3:00 and 4:00 a.m. Tuesday morning.

At 9:00, Tuesday morning, Senate staff delivered a final version to the House and waited for a response. They waited, and they waited—while one more installment of this serialized cliff-hanger was played out. The deadlock, obscure but critical, involved the referent for the term "index." The bill provided that the update would be adjusted, up or down, depending on whether the VPS was exceeded or not. But what was the "index" that served as a baseline? Was it a previous year's update? Or was it the MEI or some other "neutral" figure. This was a make-or-break issue. It would affect future reconciliation deadlines. And billions of dollars were at stake, enough to engage the Office of Management and Budget and even the Treasury in the dispute. The staff was split, Ways and Means insisting on the text as written, and Energy and Commerce protesting that the Conference itself had said that "index" meant "MEI." Motives were suspect: some believing that Ways and Means was reneging on the VPS and trying one last time to get its version of the ET. Telephone calls went back and forth and the day wore on into evening. The ultimate step of reconvening the Conference was considered, knowing that this would invariably open many issues and not just one. With Congress preparing for adjournment the next day, such a move would almost certainly have meant the postponement of payment reform for that session. Eventually, a telephone call to Wendell Primus brought the response that the index would be the MEI.[156] Still the staff on the Senate side waited. Finally, at 9:00 in the evening they received word that the House Conference had signed off and adjourned. A phone call from the Senate Finance staff for some final clarifications and the reconciliation conference was over.[157]

The Conference reported Tuesday night, November 21. Congress adjourned at 4:00, the next morning, having passed the reports less than eight hours after the conclusion of the Conference. Few members even saw the hastily assembled bill. It was a record, though not one to celebrate.[158]

V. APPRAISAL

Health policy legislation, particularly when done through the budget reconciliation process, can be likened to sausage-making: one may like the product and yet not care to examine too closely the way in which it is made. This could be said, with some justification, of payment reform. This legislation, along with the Prospective Payment System, was one of the most important Federal health care initiatives in the last quarter of the century. Yet it was passed not as a self-standing bill but as a comparatively minor element of the annual budget reconciliation. Because of this method of legislating, there was little opportunity for or resort to the kind of preliminary bargaining and persuasion, "coming to the table" and implicit commitment on the part of interest groups and legislators that, for instance, accompanied the passage of the Prospective Payment System. Committee hearings were perfunctory. Floor debate on the budget reconciliation act went off on controversial political issues: capital gains and repeal of catastrophic health insurance. And the reconciliation process, while successful, was hasty and pragmatic, dominated by the clock and tactical considerations, weary staff making early morning decisions with too little time and too little sleep. It was not, as Rep. Henry Waxman observed, a "procedure to be proud of."[159]

And yet, the budget reconciliation process may for some kinds of legislation make the best of difficult circumstances. No one thought or even seriously entertained the prospect that physician payment reform could have passed Congress following the ordinary legislative procedures. Budget reconciliation was the route other physician payment legislation had traveled. In addition, the activities of the PPRC, by creating a forum for interest groups and testing the winds with various trial balloons, provided an expert and relatively impartial substitute for the committee hearings and one that both Congress and the providers had come to trust. As a consequence of the Commission's activities and the year-by-year initiatives of the subcommittees involved in physician payment reforms since 1984, most of the alternatives had been canvassed repeatedly and discussed among the relevant specialty societies, members of the health policy constituency, and within government. The conference process, harum-scarum though it was, still produced a coherent and competent result that, in fact, drew only on the committee versions submitted to it and that was a balanced synthesis of and compromise between these versions. No doubt, the conference process, like a sausage machine, lacks some desirable elements of tidiness. But contemporary legislation is a time-constrained, difficult, and unpredictable process, frequently overwhelmed by large and supervening political events, in which some serious differences of interest and principle must be reconciled or avoided. For grinding out a reasonably acceptable product from such gristle, the reconciliation process may not be all bad.

One notable feature of the legislation, Title VI, Pt 2, Subpart A of the Omnibus Budget Reconciliation Act of 1989 (P.L. 101-239, December 19, 1989), is that it follows closely the major recommendations and the tenor of the PPRC recommendations, made in its 1989 *Annual Report*. In one sense, this outcome is hardly remarkable, since Congress created the PPRC, instructed it year by year, and got from it what it wanted. Yet the PPRC supplied for Congress a coherent vision, the rationale for proposals, and the data and specifics for individual provisions, so that much of the *Report*, with modifications, was adopted in the ultimate legislation. In this respect, the legislation itself stands as a recognition of and testimonial to the vision that in 1984 and 1985 led to the creation of the Commission, to the political savvy of the Commission leadership, and to the quick and skillful job done by the Commission and the staff in assembling data and policy proposals, especially in the critical first three years.

One item about which there was never much controversy or discussion was the Relative Value Scale and the Hsiao methodology. A major amendment that would have compromised the idea of nationally standardized work values came from Henry Waxman in the form of a geographic cost-of-living differential.[160] Congress finally acceded to this proposal, but allowed only one-quarter of the geographic differential. Otherwise Congress fully endorsed the RBRVS, mandating further refinements as recommended by the Commission as well as the development of relative values and fee schedules for radiology, anesthesiology, and pathology services.

Transition to full implementation of the fee schedule is important not just to providers' incomes, but also to the beneficiaries who receive the services and to the HCFA and the carriers who have to implement and monitor the program. The Commission had recommended full implementation in two years, between 1990 and 1992. On this one Congress, as might be expected, went back and forth, eventually putting together transition provisions that blended the several committee's approaches. Some stages of the transition began as early as 1990, though the major part of the transition was programmed for a four-year period beginning the first of January 1992 and ending January 1996. At the same time that Congress extended the transition, it also "front-loaded" the process, employing several devices. One was to allow a full MEI update only for primary care services. A second was to provide for reduction of payments for a list of 245 overvalued procedures, beginning April 1990.[161] Yet a third step was the reduction of up to 15% in the prevailing charges for services that exceeded the projected national fee schedule by more than 10%. With this approach, Congress could strike at excessive fees and ease the plight of beneficiaries at the same time that it extended the transition and increased prospects for acceptance of the MFS by providers.

Ever mindful of the beneficiaries' welfare, Congress took a fairly hard line on balance billing. The Commission, in its 1989 *Annual Report*, was divided on this issue, though it had recommended that the MAAC limits stay in place until they could be replaced by the fee schedule and that balance billing be limited to a fixed percentage of the fee schedule amount. Congress did just that, extending the MAACs for two years until 1992 and providing for a phase down in balance billing amounts from 25 to 15% between 1991 and 1993.[162] The legislation further ordered mandatory assignment for those Medicare beneficiaries eligible for Medicaid. Inasmuch as balance billing and mandatory assignment had occasioned much controversy earlier, one notable event, or non-event, was the lack of protest either from the AMA or the specialty societies with respect to these provisions. Several committee staff and other health policy observers noted this curiosity, offering the opinion that the medical providers were so distracted by and preoccupied with the ETs that this one went by the board even though, in the aggregate, the balance billing limits might well involve more money.[163] If so, they may prove to be one of those dormant issues that produce controversy in the future.

The Volume Performance Standard, neé Expenditure Target, was so controversial and so time-consuming that it is surprising that either it or any other item in the Medicare legislation was well done. And yet this particular item was a carefully crafted and precise compromise through which both sides got much of what they wanted. For Senate Finance and for Energy and Commerce in the House, both more sanguine about winning over the physicians rather than changing their behavior through sanctions, the emphasis on performance standards rather than expenditure targets was important symbolically.[164] Also, a partial linkage, with a bonus for good performance and a limited penalty for exceeding the standard, was livable, if not optimal. For Ways and Means, and especially Rep. Stark, the Volume Performance Standard was linked with a penalty feature, so that the principle was saved. The consequences of a default were sufficiently unattractive, moreover, that Congress would almost certainly be in the game of setting the update each year. This way, the annual baseline would be protected, and if prompt and/or drastic measures were required, they could be taken.

The legislation outflanked or contained several strategems intended to limit the reach or effects of the VPS. One deal made in the past was for a separate ET or VPS for the surgeons. A similar kind of exception, made later, was to allow "carve out groups,"[165] and other managed care plans such as HMOs or CMPs to have a special VPS of their own. Congress dealt with these differently, but in ways likely to put an eventual quietus on each. Generally, the legislation allows separate VPSs. It also directs the Secretary to recommend a separate standard for surgery each year and for 1992 a separate update. But there is no commitment on the part of Congress to act on a separate VPS, and the default formula specifies only national standards and updates, so that the surgery exception is not otherwise made an integral part of the legislation. Furthermore, the PPRC has already recommended that "surgical and nonsurgical VPSs . . . be evaluated further before they become a permanent part of the Medicare payment system."[166] The prospects for other specialty VPSs would seem doubtful, at best. For the COGs, HMOs, and other variants, such as sub-national VPSs, the legislation recommends study by the Secretary, with an option of submitting recommendations. Congress took the further step of specifically prohibiting the Secretary from implementing any separate performance standards without the express approval of Congress. And the Commission has moved preemptively, recommending against any more specialty performance standards and, for now, against subnational ones.[167] The Volume Performance Standard was nevertheless a compromise and some, within Congress and the Commission, preferred carrots to sticks, in other words, encouraging better medical practice to penalizing physicians for exceeding performance standards or expenditure targets. In part, this was a pragmatic calculus, that effectiveness research and practice guidelines were a better way to win the hearts and minds of doctors than hitting them over the head; in part, it was a matter of fairness, not punishing physicians in the aggregate for conditions over which they, as individuals, had no control.[168]

With respect to effectiveness research and practice guidelines, the legislation followed closely the Energy and Commerce version. These provisions are elaborate, calling for the creation, within the Public Health Service,[169] of a new Agency for Health Care Policy and Research, with an Administrator reporting directly to the Secretary of DHHS. Among its other duties, the Agency would have primary responsibility for conducting and supporting research on effectiveness and outcomes and disseminating the results of such research. As an integral part of this endeavor, the legislation creates a new Forum for Quality and Effectiveness in Health Care to help make the findings of such research known in the medical community and translate these results into practice guidelines, clinical standards, and review criteria. The Secretary, the carriers, and the PROs are directed, in various ways, to facilitate practical application to claims review and payments. Both elaborate and large in scope, the program represents a new kind of emphasis, not just in the United States but in the world. Authorizations were suitably increased for so ambitious a venture, rising to $185 million for FY 1994.

The four issues most important for physician payment reform were the RBRVS itself, the ET or VPS, balance billing and beneficiary protection, and effectiveness or outcomes research. With respect to these matters, Congress followed the tenor of the Commission's recommendations closely while also fashioning reasonable compromises between sharply opposing views in Congress. A prodigious amount still remained to be done prior to the beginning of full fee schedule implementation in 1992. For PPRC, the Hsiao group, and the specialty panels there were many issues and data problems with the relative work values, surgical global fees, practice expense, payment areas, and integrating the RAPs and LLPs.[170] The HCFA confronted a task similar in scope and difficulty to the initial implementation of PPS: policy decisions about specific applications of the statute; developing total values for each of the HCPCS codes; computing the modifiers; cross-walking values to the individual codes; folding in existing fee schedules and the non-physician practitioners; making the data computations and adjustments to achieve budget neutrality; responding to previous comments and negotiating differences with providers, PPRC, EOMB, and the Congress; writing manuals and soft-ware; instructing the carriers.[171] Somehow, it will all get done, though not with the kind of recognition such achievements deserve.

As an example of Congressional policymaking, physician payment reform is remarkable both for the sustained congressional initiative and for the creative employment of specialized political instrumentalities, particularly budget reconciliation and the purpose-built PPRC. As for its part in the process, PPRC worked fast and with outstanding competence to bring together a consensus proposal and develop the expertise to support their recommendations. It is hard to fault physician payment reform as an instance of policy development, except that some niceties of parliamentary procedure were omitted. Yet there remains a disquieting issue of whether PPRC and the Congress may have efficiently done the wrong thing or, perhaps, accomplished one task and ignored several more difficult ones looming ahead.

One prominent characteristic of the payment reform scheme is its ambivalent and potentially contradictory policy objectives. On the one hand, with an RBRVS and the prominence given to effectiveness research it looks toward objectivity, fairness, and persuasion. On the other, with the VPS and targeting of overvalued procedures, it emphasizes cost reduction and the reduction of Medicare outlays. A danger is that these two competing objectives will not be held in balance or employed so as to complement each other. Effectiveness or outcomes research takes time and works largely by changing attitudes rather than behavior, while cost containment is driven by the fiscal year calendar and the urgency of next year's deficit. Under such constraints, the short-term and the politically expedient are likely to dominate, even though policymakers try not to let them. As one member of the Ways and Means staff observed, with the Medicare Fee Schedule Congress has a policy tool that will focus attention and debate on redistributive issues and the consequences of the update.[172] Whether the availability of this new tool increases the respectful attention given to long-term consequences and side-effects or merely enables EOMB or Congress to cut the budget skillfully and target benefits more precisely remains to be seen. Past experience, for instance with respect to PPS, is mixed as best. And the deficit continues, as before.

A major crisis in the summer of 1991, preceding the 1992 implementation, showed concretely how this conflict in objectives might express itself. The background to this event was, again, deficit reduction. In OBRA 1990, Congress agreed to a five year reduction schedule that became a part of budget neutral calculations for the MFS. In addition the Bush Administration was calling for $3 billion in Medicare provider cuts for fiscal 1992.[173] These developments were themselves the occasion for uneasiness; but the HCFA proposed rule of June 1991, coming just before the AMA annual convention, provoked wide-spread protest in the physician community. In essence, the HCFA proposed regulations gave little and took much. For the primary care physicians, expecting much, the gains were disappointingly small. Surgeons and others would lose substantially. The other galling item, adding both insult and injury, was the proposed conversion factor, and especially the "behavioral offset" intended to compensate for volume increase. Not only was it large (50%) but all of it was loaded on the annual conversion factor and built into future updates.[174] Physicians were both disappointed and angry, complaining that promises made in 1990 were being broken in 1991 and that they, as a group, were being found guilty of cheating in advance, before the fee schedule had gone into effect. The right or wrong of this dismal episode is not the point. What is significant is the way in which overwhelming factors such as deficit reduction and the separation of powers can effect the MFS. This particular conjuncture of events may be fortuitous; but it is not a good beginning, especially if an important objective of the MFS is to win over the physicians.

Another concern is that the payment reform scheme, given the conflicting objectives of cost containment and persuading physicians to change their ways, will be too political in some respects and not political enough in others. Put another way, the burden of conflict resolution may be either too great or wrongly distributed. For its acceptance by the physician community and specialty societies, payment reform depends on its being perceived as fair and technically sound, for instance, in its work values, regional differentials, and outcomes research. At the same time, the fee schedule is a price set by an administrative and political process. The conversion factor and the volume performance standards are fundamentally and even visibly political. The MFS will, as William Glaser has observed[175] redistribute incomes among specialties and geographic regions in a fairly dramatic and visible way. Physicians adversely affected will have regard for this practical reality and not just for the putative neutrality and objectivity of the RVRBS. Nor are they likely to be adequately reassured by the advice-giving and consultative roles of the Secretary and the PPRC, especially when they can see for themselves the crass politics of the updates and the budget reconciliation. At the same time, those who are disaffected will not be constrained in their professional behavior by payment mechanisms such as capitation.[176] Neither will they have an effective means for negotiating their differences with the government. They can grumble, engage in various forms of professional *incivisme*, lobby and protest politically, or go on strike, but they lack provision for group action and collective bargaining. For this reason, some have thought that either state-wide or specialty VPSs might be desirable. In its present form, the MFS, relying as it does on rationality and fairness and yet readily adapting itself to budget-cutting and redistributive ends, could lead to a growing resentment that smolders until it erupts disastrously.

With physician payment as with PPS, elaborate legislative provision was made for the annual updates and the big numbers and yet comparatively little attention given to the procedures for on-going changes in the individual values and payments. As for the MFS, OBRA 1989 says that the Secretary shall revise the relative values "not less often than every 5 years" and to the extent that he or she "determines to be necessary" adjust them in the interim taking into account "change in medical practice, coding changes, new data on relative value components, or the addition of new procedures.[177] Given the politically charged nature of physician payment, this amounts to a large conferring of discretion. And since payment is now based on a fee schedule rather than charges, both the need for advice and the importance of specialized access are greatly increased. Sensitive to these considerations, the AMA has urged that the CPT Editorial Panel,[178] much influenced by its physician representatives, be given a key role in advising on code changes. Others in government and health affairs are determined to prevent this development, concerned about the importance of cumulative small decisions and the potential abuses of privileged access. Whatever the outcome of these particular moves, consultation and advice with respect to MFS amendment is likely to be a sensitive issue.

The Medicare Fee Schedule, like the Prospective Payment System, is a beginning. And like PPS, it focuses on one title of the Medicare payment scheme: in a word, attacks part of a total problem of health care costs. Inevitably, this payment reform will invite new and creative ways of unbundling claims, of substituting one factor input for another, and of cost-shifting from the public to the private sector. ProPAC has, for a parallel example, devoted an increasing amount of its attention to the way in which similar problems are affecting hospitals and health care in both Medicare and the private sector. Just as Congress added to ProPAC's agenda, so it has assigned PPRC, in OBRA 1989 and OBRA 1990, a clutch of new topics for investigating and advising: Medicaid physician payment; state-based volume performance standards; payment incentives for physicians in underserved areas and specialties; the supply of physicians; cost of health insurance for businesses; and budget recommendations made to the President that affect Medicare physician payment.[179] Part of the drama and fascination accompanying physician payment reform will be to see how these issues develop and how they are managed as the Medicare Fee Schedule is implemented in the next few years.

These comments are not meant to deny credit for a great accomplishment. Rather, they point to some unresolved tensions and possible fault lines within the system that will, most probably, affect the development of physician payment in the future. Indeed, the MFS may well be only a first step toward larger changes in the future, for instance, capitation or managed care schemes, all payers legislation, or more comprehensive health insurance. Without doubt, the MFS is an elaborately crafted tool; whether it is the right one or not will depend on our future needs and the stresses to which it is subjected.

The determination and vigilence with which the MFS is implemented will be of special importance. In contrast with PPS, implementation will be pretty much "politics by another name." One reason is that the redistributive mechanisms in the MFS are more visible and more blatantly political. The provider community is already alarmed and mobilized, so that the implementation process begins with little if any store of good will. Because the MFS is less an interdependent system, add-ons and exceptions will be easier. Involving as it does decisions about thousands of codes rather than 490 DRGs, it will inevitably require much resort to consultants and consensus panels, risking through this kind of delegation an encroaching control of specialists and private consultants. It will be a time for public virtue to be not only shrewd but determined and politically skillful.[180]

CHRONOLOGY: PHYSICIAN PAYMENT: DESIGNING THE SYSTEM

1. Congress creates PPRC, mandates a Relative Value Scale, COBRA (P.L. 99-272, April 7, 1986).
2. PPRC begins meeting, November 1986; First Annual Report, March 1987, calls for creation of a Medicare Fee Schedule.
3. MAACs legislated, OBRA, 1986 (P.L. 99-509, October 21, 1986).
4. Legislation on "inherent reasonableness" and "overpriced" procedures developed, OBRA, 1986; and OBRA, 1987 (P.L. 100-203, December 22, 1987).
5. Increase in Medicare Part B premium announced, September 1987.
6. OBRA, 1987 calls for a Medicare Fee Schedule by January 1, 1990.
7. Harvard Study (Hsiao Report) delivered to DHHS, September 29, 1988.
8. American College of Surgeons endorses Medicare Fee Schedule with a separate Expenditure Target, February 1989.
9. Third *Annual Report* of PPRC, March 1989, submitting comprehensive set of proposals for a Medicare Fee Schedule.
10. A version of Medicare Fee Schedule passes Ways and Means subcommittee, June 14, 1989; Full committee, June 28, 1989.
11. Reconciliation Conference convenes October 17, 1989.
12. DHHS sends Congress its proposals for physician payment reform, October 20, 1989.
13. Medicare Fee Schedule passes Congress, November 22, 1989.
14. Hsiao Phase II Report, September 1990.
15. Model Fee Schedule published by the HCFA, September 1990; Proposed Rule published, June 5, 1991.

NOTES

  1. Interview with Donald Young, Executive Director, Prospective Payment Assessment Commission, May 24, 1988.
  2. Interview with Peter Bouxsein, staff of the Health and Environment Subcommittee of the House Energy and Commerce Committee, January 29, 1988. Bouxsein was largely responsible for the design and adoption of this device. He was a member of the HCFA staff from 1979 to 1982 in the Bureau of Program Policy (now the Bureau of Eligibility, Reimbursement, and Coverage) and since then a staff aide to Congressman Henry Waxman of the House Energy and Commerce Committee. A particular concern of his and of Waxman's was that Congress be advised in the steps it was taking, especially about some of their possible consequences.

3.   Consolidated Omnibus Budget Reconciliation Act of 1985, P.L. 99-272, April 7, 1986, Sec. 9305. COBRA directed the Commission to submit its recommendation with respect to an RVS by July 1, 1987 with recommendations for implementations to follow by July 1988. COBRA included inpatient DRGs as one of the changes in payment methodology to be considered; but the primary emphasis was on an RVS. Notably missing was capitation.

4.   Specialty groups, including surgeons, have objected that the Commission overrepresents primary care.

5.   Fourth edition of the Current Procedural Terminology, a coding system developed by the American Medical Association and used as the basis for the HCFA Common Procedures Coding System (HCPCS).

6.   In fact, the study was more than a year late, and there were some efforts within DHHS to terminate the project before it was completed.

7.   Whereas in the past, physician groups had been reluctant to cooperate in any research that might entail a modification of the payment system. *Medicine and Health,* October 22, 1984, p. 1.

8.   A judgment that observation of the Commission's public proceedings confirms. Paul Ginsburg, an economist with an academic background, has a remarkable capacity for identifying technical issues needing Commission discussion and presenting them cogently and dispassionately. Philip Lee, a seasoned medical politician and policy broker, is especially good at anticipating contentious issues, rephrasing them in a way that blunts controversy, and finding common denominators that help build consensus. Together, the two complement each other and make an exceptionally effective team.

9.   American Association of Retired Persons, one of the most powerful of Washington lobbies, especially on Medicare issues.

10.   For instance, the one surgeon was also an emeritus head of surgery and professor at the Mayo Clinic; the "public representative" was a professor and researcher of health policy; one of the internists was a professor of medicine and active in health care research; the Blue Cross–Blue Shield representative was a professor of hospital management, and so forth. Members spoke as representatives of their own profession or constituency; but this identification was much modified by the multiplicity of roles and the Commission ethos.

11.   *Medicare Physician Payment: An Agenda for Reform* (Washington, D.C., Physician Payment Review Commission, 1987), pp. x, xi. The entire list of "priorities or goals" was (1) access to care, (2) quality of care, (3) financial protection of beneficiaries, (4) equity among providers, (5) reduction in growth of SMI outlays, (6) understandability, (7) orderly change, and (8) pluralism. The reader is invited to examine this list to see in it the group assurances and appeals the Commission was making. Cf. Iglehart (1988).

12.   A charge-based RVS would be developed largely from existing Medicare submitted or allowed charges. It would, therefore conform closely to existing specialty and regional differentials, which would favor surgeons. Advantages of a charge-based RVS are that it could be implemented quickly and that it would not redistribute income or alienate any major group of physicians. From the Commission's perspective, though, a charge-based RVS would fail to achieve one of the most important objectives being sought in the development of an RVS, which was to make possible a "fairer" schedule of payments. Indeed, one of the major appeals that the Commission could make to the provider community was that an RVS would help to create a "level playing field," i.e., provide a technically sound basis for redressing inequities in payments as between various specialties and regions.

13. *Medicare Physician Payment: An Agenda for Reform* (1987), especially "Executive Summary" and Ch. 3, p. 43. Also, Lynn M. Etheredge, "The Volume of Medicare Physician Services," in Holahan and Etheredge (1986).

14. *Medicare Physician Payment: An Agenda for Reform* (1987, 7).

15. A relative value scale is a measure of or proxy for effort or "work." As such, it might well figure in payment methodologies such as capitation or physician DRGs. Going from a relative value scale to a fee schedule, however, requires a multiplier or conversion factor that converts the relative value into dollars. Into the conversion factor are built various modifiers determined by policy choices with respect to such matters as regional and specialty variations, assignment policy, practice costs, and so forth. The point is that these modifiers are used to redistribute income and create incentives. By endorsing a fee schedule so strongly, the Commission was not only moving toward closure on this issue, it was creating expectations that would be difficult to deny, at least without arousing strong sentiments of unfairness on the part of providers.

16. Hoping, of course, that the Hsiao study would be in time and would prove satisfactory.

17. Congress used the language "overpriced" while the Commission preferred "overvalued."

18. Interview with Marilyn Field, Associate Director, PPRC, October 13, 1987.

19. *Medicine and Health*, September 21, 1987, p. 1. Interviews with Stephen Bandeian, Health Subcommittee of the House Ways and Means Committee, February 3, 1988; and William Vaughan, staff of Rep. Fortney H. (Pete) Stark (D., Ca.), January 25, 1988.

20. Omnibus Budget Reconciliation Act of 1987, P.L. 100-203, December 22, 1987, Sec. 4055(c).

21. The study was being performed under a contract with the HCFA. By this time, many legislators and congressional staff believed that DHHS and EOMB were delaying reports deliberately to prevent further action on them being taken, especially by the Congress. For instance, the report on physician DRGs, mandated early in 1983, appeared in September 1987, over a year and a half late. By the end of 1987, more than 19 reports that Congress had directed DHHS to submit were overdue, with another dozen or so soon to be in arrears. *Background Material and Data on Programs within the Jurisdiction of the Committee on Ways and Means, 1988 Edition*. Committee on Ways and Mean, U.S. House of Representatives, 100th Congress, Second Session, 1988.

22. OBRA, 1987. P.L. 100-203, Sec. 4055(b)(3).

23. Both COBRA and SOBRA (OBRA, 1986) were passed in this year. 1986 was also the first year operating under "Gramm–Rudman," The Balanced Budget and Emergency Deficit Control Act of 1985, P.L. 99-177, December 12, 1985.

24. More later on EOMB. Within the Congress, capitation was now viewed as a worn-out tune, played because the Administration had nothing better. Early in 1985, moreover, the IMC scandal broke. International Medical Centers was a Florida-based HMO, the largest under the Medicare voucher program. It had 36% of the 550 thousand beneficiaries enrolled in the entire program. The plan had been granted a number of special dispensations not accorded other Medicare HMOs and generally regarded as bad policy. Aside from managing badly, IMC also engaged in such practices as screening and compulsory disenrollment of elderly beneficiaries, nonpayment of providers, and paying big fees for former Reagan appointees or campaign staff to act as lobbyists. Like some of the bigger "thrifts" or savings and loans banks, IMC was too big to cut off and

various rescue schemes were tried. At the time, the episode greatly diminished enthusiasm for the HMO option. Over the years, moreover, there had been several scandals involving Medicare and Medicaid HMOs, including links with organized crime. *Medicine and Health, Perspectives,* May 19, 1986.

25. Until the 1986 election, the Republican Party had a majority in the Senate, and was less favorable toward the fee schedule option. See, *"Proposals to Modify Medicare's Physician Payment System,"* Hearing Before the Subcommittee on Health of the Committee on Finance, United States Senate, 99th Congress, Second Session, April 25, 1986.

26. According to one study, based on a 100% sample of four states, Part B expenditures rose by 29.5% over the three years between 1983 and 1986, with the rate of increase declining very slightly after the freeze was in effect. Since prices rose little, clearly volume increase was a dominant factor. Mitchell et al. (1989, 21).

27. Rising Part B expenditures, whether they result from higher fees or from greater volume or intensity, can affect beneficiaries' out-of-pocket costs in several ways. If the physician's fees increase, so do the Medicare beneficiary's co-payments, 20 cents for every dollar. Similarly, with increased volume or greater intensity: the beneficiary is paying 20% of whatever is billed. If the physician is nonparticipating and bills proportionally as the fee increases or to cover a decline in Medicare allowance, the out-of-pocket for the beneficiary also goes up. Finally, Part B premiums since TEFRA have been tied to overall Part B expenditures—now set to cover 25% of program costs, though from 1984 to 1988, they were indexed at 50%. Since beneficiaries feel the effects of increased physicians' charges pretty directly, fee freezes, a fee schedule, and ways to encourage assignment are visible and popular ways to ease costs for them.

28. Omnibus Budget Reconciliation Act of 1986, P.L. 99-509, October 21, 1986, Sec. 9331.

29. Interview with William Vaughan, staff of Rep. Fortney H. (Pete) Stark (D., Ca.), January 25, 1988.

30. Interview with Stephen Bandeian, staff of the Health Subcommittee, House Ways and Means Committee, February 3, 1988.

31. One of the major problems was that the statute specified charges for a specific procedure for an entire year. This required the establishment of a profile of charges for that procedure and raised difficulties about any changes in procedures or coding during the year, physicians who moved, physicians with multiple carriers, how to weight averages, unintended vs. known violations, and so forth. A member of the House Council staff said that they "filled whole blackboards," trying to establish how the MAACs would work (Edward Grossman, February 4, 1988). One of the HCFA officials who had to worry about implementation described writing the regulations as "a series of lost weekends" and said that, generally, the implementation and enforcement of the MAACs was "not our finest hour" (Bernard Potashnick, Medical Services Reimbursement, HCFA, April 6, 1988).

32. Diana Jost, Blue Cross–Blue Shield, November 4, 1987.

33. Interview with Edward Grossman, House Legislative Council, February 4, 1988.

34. Interview with William Vaughan, staff of Rep. Fortney H. (Pete) Stark (D., Ca.), January 25, 1988.

35. The original Medicare legislation refers to "reasonable charge" limits for physicians. Though this part of the legislation was not implemented as such, the Social Security Administration did begin developing a CPR system largely mod-

eled on payment systems then in use by the carriers for their private insurers. The Social Security Amendments of 1972 set forth in some detail "reasonable cost" and "reasonable charge" provisions, but relatively little was done with the Part B sections, except for CPR and the MEI.

36. A determination of "reasonable" is subject to the usual "notice and comment" procedures for rule making, which consume time and take data gathering and research. These procedures also provide opportunity for legal intervention and bringing of law suits. For physicians' services, moreover, what is a "reasonable" payment can be difficult to say, just as it would be for inpatient DRGs—in contrast, for instance, to routine room and board per diem charges for hospitals. In addition, carriers were reluctant to get involved in this process, which would entail changing their forms, their data processing methods, and probably, also, their amicable relations with providers with whom they also did business, independently of the Medicare connection.

37. For example, the procedures identified and reduced by OBRA, 1987 were coronary artery bypass surgery, total hip replacement, cataract surgery, transurethral prostatectomy, suprapubic prostatectomy, dilation and curettage, carpal tunnel repair, pacemaker surgery, bronchoscopy, upper gastrointestinal endoscopy, knee arthroscopy, and knee athroplasty. Omnibus Budget Reconciliation Act of 1987, P.L. 100-203, December 22, 1987, Sec. 4045. Other procedures can, of course, be added. Among less expensive procedures, but ones for which the cumulative billings amount to a lot are lab tests, x-rays, and EKGs.

38. Interviews with Henry Desmarais, Health Policy Alternatives, December 16, 1987; and Bruce Kelly, staff of the Senate Finance Committee, February 1, 1988.

39. Interview with Bernard Potashnick, Medical Services Reimbursement, HCFA, April 6, 1988.

40. Interview with Bruce Kelly, staff of the Senate Finance Committee, February 1, 1988.

41. Notice of Proposed Rulemaking.

42. Interview with Richard Trachtman, American Society of Internal Medicine, November 10, 1987; also, statement by the American Society of Internal Medicine in "Proposals to Modify Medicare's Physician Payment System," op. cit., p. 381. HCFA staff denied that there was such an intention, saying the "inherent reasonableness" process was too difficult to use. At the same time, it was a year of scrounging for all sorts of Gramm–Rudman savings that included proposals, for instance, to amend the MEI calculations for office rent, freezing the DRGs, postponing hospital payments, and doing away with the Periodic Interim Payments (PIP). This kind of itchy quest made such allegations credible.

43. Ibid. The Senate still had a Republican majority, so the Senate Finance Committee provided a more sympathetic forum than the House and Ways and Means.

44. Omnibus Budget Reconciliation Act of 1986, Public Law 99-509, October 21, 1986. Sec. 9333.

45. SOBRA actually provided that the Secretary should submit recommendations to PPRC, indicating that Congress still wished to see such recommendations. In this context, Gramm–Rudman became important, for if the Secretary merely recommended and Congress took action, the savings could be counted by the Congress.

46. Five different relative value scales were used. In essence, a few "index procedures" were used to "link" or standardize the RVSs, then the values at-

tributed to the target procedures were compared with Medicare charges to see if the latter were "overpriced."

47. The term is borrowed from John Iglehart. Interview, July 15, 1988.

48. Interview with Diana Jost, Blue Cross–Blue Shield, November 4, 1987. In any event, how one views this development depends on what one means by "credibility" and with whom "credibility" is sought. Certainly, PPRC gained credibility with Congress and also acquired a reputation for being able to react quickly and produce a credible product, whatever may have been the reaction among some providers.

49. *Medicine and Health*, November 30 and December 8, 1986; and *Special Report*, December 8, p. 1.

50. Ibid.

51. *Medicine and Health, Perspectives*. January 26, 1987, p. 1; Rep. Henry Waxman (D., Ca.) also supported the RAP-DRGs. Interview with Peter Bouxsein, staff of the Health and Environment Subcommittee, House Energy and Commerce Committee, January 29, 1988.

52. As a result of the election of 1986, in which the Republican Party lost control of the Senate.

53. The Stark and Waxman subcommittees were viewed as having developed, intentionally or unintentionally, what amounted to a "tough cop–nice cop" routine in which one would soften up the suspect while the other could be approached with pleas for mercy or appeals to reason. Stark was a tough-minded, confrontational banker with a reputation for never avoiding a good fight. Waxman was a soft-spoken lawyer with a talent for finding acceptable compromises. Furthermore, Peter Bouxsein, a chief staff person for the Health and Environment Subcommittee, was the primary designer of the PPRC legislation and especially knowledgeable about reimbursement policy. On a number of issues, these subcommittees shared jurisdiction. For these reasons, providers often sought out the Waxman subcommittee when some mediation was desired. On this particular issue of RAP-DRGs, Bouxsein recalls querying Waxman's decision to support them. Waxman continued to do so, pretty clearly having in mind the kind of "coming to the table" result that developed. Interview with Peter Bouxsein, January 29, 1988.

54. The AMA was outraged by this "betrayal" and sought to retaliate by getting Congress to limit the radiology fee schedule in a way that would be disadvantageous to the radiologists. *Medicine and Health*, August 10, 1987, p. 1.

55. *Medicine and Health*, September 21, 1987, p. 1.

56. For a somewhat skeptical account, see McMenamin (1988, 94).

57. Interviews with Stephen Bandeian, staff of the Health Subcommittee of the House Ways and Means Committee, February 3, 1988; Bruce Kelly, Senate Finance Committee staff, February 1, 1987; and Anne Weiss, staff of the Senate Finance Committee, January 11, 1988.

58. Cf. Iglehart (1988); *Medicine and Health*, September 21, 1987.

59. The Commission decided against a charge based RVS, though not without some protest. Cf. Appendix 3, "Minority Statement," p. 53, *Physician Payment Review Commission, Annual Report to Congress* (Washington, D.C., 1988).

60. This project was begun in 1986 and supported by a grant from the HCFA. The agency also supported some of Hsiao's earlier work.

61. Even though there was little official support from DHHS or the HCFA, Commission staff reported that, at the staff level, technicians in the HCFA and DHHS were often very helpful and generous with their time and the results of their work.

62. *Physician Payment Review Commission—Annual Report to Congress* (Washington, D.C., 1989), p. 34.

63. Ibid.; Also, *Annual Report* (1989).

64. Though why "resources" are a better basis than a regulated market is not obvious. Buried underneath this whole issue of "resource-based" versus "charge-based" is, of course, the old controversy about "just price" and the gild versus the market. Cf. Holahan and Etheredge (1986), chs. 3, 4.

65. Interviews with Ira Burney, Office of Legislation and Policy, DHHS, March 3, 1988; and Stephen Sieverts, Blue Cross–Blue Shield of the National Capitol Area, December 9, 1987. A number of critics of the resource-based system fear that the fee schedule will become not just a prospective maximum but a minimum as well: that is, physicians who customarily charged *less* will now charge up to the maximum the fee schedule allows. Sieverts, of Blue Cross–Blue Shield, observed that one of their most closely held trade secrets was their fee schedule, precisely for this reason.

66. Charge-based systems start with historic charges, either submitted or allowed. They may use several procedures, such as a chest X-ray or an appendectomy, that are technically stable and homogeneous to serve as benchmarks. But they rely mainly on consensus panels and negotiation to set the final value.

67. Cf. "Statement of the American College of Surgeons to the PPRC," presented by W. Gerald Austen, MD, FACS, February 8, 1989 (Chicago: American College of Surgeons, 1989).

68. Interviews with George Greenberg, Office of the Secretary, DHHS, May 11, 1989; Ira Burney, Office of Legislation and Policy, DHHS, March 3, 1989; also, cf. Rosenbach et al. (1989).

69. Interview with John Eisenberg, PPRC, July 10, 1989; also, cf. PPRC, *Annual Report* for 1988 (p. 53) and for 1989 (p. 35n).

70. Of course, the jury is still out as to whether the RBRVS is technically adequate and as to whether this was the right choice to make. An important political factor was that the AMA backed this approach and cosponsored the Hsiao study. In addition, one of the most effective ways of attacking any proposal they do not like is for the AMA or physician specialty groups to claim that the methodology is "flawed," the scientific data "inadequate," or the conclusions "unsound," and that, generally, "not enough is known" to proceed. Cloaked with the aura of science and authority, this tactic has worked well for the medical associations for at least 50 years.

71. "Work" was measured by "time" and "complexity." The latter was especially important, including (1) mental effort and judgment, (2) technical skill and physical effort, and (3) stress due to patient risk. In the views of many, "complexity" was just a way to build in the indexes that would support surgeons and other specialists at their accustomed income level.

72. "Opportunity costs of training" is a concept from labor economics. Used in the present context, what it implies is that physicians should be compensated both for the direct expense of their specialty training and for the foregone income or "opportunity costs" during these years of training. Those who object to this idea say that it amounts to "double counting" since specialists made more money because of that training. So, why should they be paid an additional bonus for undergoing the training?

73. As critics have pointed out, any kind of index uses various proxies. And a notion of "work" that includes something as subjective as "complexity" may make no more sense than "allowed charges." Interviews with George Green-

berg, Office of the Secretary, DHHS, May 11, 1989; and with Dena Puskin, ProPAC, October 12, 1987.

74. A good discussion of the methodological issues can be found in the series on the RBRVS published by William Hsiao and associates (1988) and in Etheredge and Dobson (1989).

75. Whether or not physicians are "congruent fools," the survey results may depend on the questions asked and how the response data are manipulated. With respect to the all important work and time values for visits, for instance, PPRC has suggested that some of the discrepancies may have resulted from the long, complex vignettes used and from estimations based on individual physician responses rather than mean response values for the particular evaluation and management (EM) vignette. *Annual Report to Congress, 1991* (Washington, D.C.: PPRC, 1991), esp. Ch. 2, pp. 26–42.

76. Ibid., xv, xvi. In a review of Phase II, though, a consultant for PPRC reports that, despite using several methods, they were unable to replicate the interspecialty scale, the re-runs scoring typically better than Phase II. If that is so, how much confidence should there be in the Phase II results? or in any specific interspecialty results? Interview with Allen Dobson, Lewin-ICF, June 20, 1991. PPRC continues it review of the linking process, though acknowledging "the lack of any 'gold standard' to indicate that a particular cross-specialty alignment is correct." *Annual Report*, 1991, p. 50.

77. Pre- and postservice work varies not only by service but also according to the specialty group providing the service and the location in which it is performed (Dunn et al. 1988, 2372).

78. Two key assumptions were that pre- and postservice work consisted essentially of evaluation and management, i.e., were much like the services physicians performed in office visits, and that the work per unit of time correlated positively with values for intraservice work.

79. PPRC, *Annual Report* (1989), pp. 325–326.

80. 6000 was the operative figure rather than the 7000 + codes of CPT-4 because only 18 specialties were represented in the study.

81. PPRC, *Annual Report* (1989), 327.

82. Ibid., p. 330.

83. As the Commission indicated, each individual surgical code could represent any one of 44 different combinations of component services, depending on the carrier area. *Annual Report*, Physician Payment Review Commission, 1990.

83. Ibid., p. 50.

84. *Annual Report*, 1991, pp. 43–48; also, *Pre- and Postoperative Visits Associated with Surgical Global Services*, No. 91–2 (Washington, D.C.: PPRC, 1991).

85. The initial study had not included pre- and postservice work in the vignette procedures.

86. *Annual Report*, Physician Payment Review Commission, 1989, p. 330.

87. A 12-member panel that includes representatives of various medical specialties, and from the HCFA, the Health Insurance Association of America, and Blue Cross–Blue Shield. The panel meets four times a year to consider changes to the codes. These changes are included in an annual update of CPT. Ibid., pp. 45 ff.

88. For instance, face-to-face time, scheduled time, or including face-to-face and nonface-to-face.

89. Interview with Philip R. Lee, M.D., October 20, 1989; also Jamie Reuter, staff, Health Subcommittee, House Ways and Means Committee, May 30, 1990.

90. The AMA, though its Socioeconomic Monitoring System services, publishes an annual survey. For the last 10 years, the HCFA has also sponsored a similar survey known as the Physician Practice Cost and Income Study, which is quite exhaustive but published less frequently. A new HCFA study was published in 1989, but the last one before that was 1983.

91. A finding possibly of interest to the Internal Revenue Service, but bothersome to the researchers (Becker 1988, 2399).

92. A multiplicative formula would also introduce inequities between procedures that were especially labor intensive (e.g., endoscopies) and those that were capital intensive (e.g., magnetic resonance imaging).

93. *Medicine Health*, March 20, 1989, p. 1. At the same time, these are changes for specific Medicare procedures and would not have that kind of impact on the typical physician's total income. That overall impact would depend on the Medicare procedures performed by the particular physician (which could include both winners and losers under the RBRVS) and on the proportion of a physician's income derived from Medicare.

94. *Annual Report* (1989), pp. xvi, xvii.

95. The two service types are (1) evaluation and management and (2) services and tests and procedures, including surgery. Site of care are (1) office, (2) hospital inpatient, and (3) other. Ibid (1990), pp. 63–65.

96. Even for the RVS, there were a number of additional issues, such as how to factor in malpractice costs and what to include in the surgical global fees.

97. For most of its history, the Commission has had only one surgeon among its members. At present, it has one. Most of the rest of the Commissioners could be counted as either themselves representing a primary care or beneficiary point of view or strongly sympathetic to one or both of these orientations.

98. Whether self-defined, determined by board eligibility, by board certification, etc.

99. Interview with John Eisenberg, PPRC, July 10, 1989.

100. Omnibus Budget Reconciliation Act of 1986 (P.L. 99-509, October 21, 1986), Sec. 9331.

101. Ibid., Sec. 9331(c).

102. Cf. *Annual Report* (1988), Ch. 7.

103. In this case, metropolitan statistical areas, as with PPS.

104. *Annual Report* (1989), pp. 122–123.

105. Supported, for instance, by Rep. Henry Waxman (D., Ca.) and included on a limited basis in the ultimate legislation.

106. Tying the physician component to the medical profession would have been circular. Also, one objective of the Commission was to build in an upward adjustment for rural areas.

107. *Annual Report* (1989), p. 126.

108. *Annual Report* (1988), p. 100.

109. The official explanation was that the HCFA regional simulations were part of continuing work on a fee schedule and just happened to be completed at that time. Rather than having the figures "leaked," DHHS published them. There were various speculations: that some within DHHS thought fee schedules a bad idea and were trying to scuttle them; or that the HCFA was letting Congress and the PPRC know that they could still be significant players. Whatever the motivation, the report was a surprise to PPRC and taken as a hostile gesture. "Impact Analysis of a Resource-Based Relative Value Scale," DHHS, May 22,

1989; *Medicine and Health,* June 5, 1989, p. 1; Interviews with John Eisenberg, PPRC, June 10, 1989; and with George Greenberg, Office of the Secretary, DHHS, August 14, 1989.

110. MAACs would be abolished.

111. The American Academy of Family Physicians was one of the very few that endorsed mandatory assignment.

112. Interview with John Eisenberg, PPRC, June 10, 1989.

113. *Annual Report* (1989), p. 137.

114. Mostly because of office visits, which would receive increased payment and are heavily used by Medicare beneficiaries.

115. *Annual Report* (1989), p. 161.

116. Perhaps true given the separation of powers and the pluralism that obtains in policy-making in the U.S. *Annual Report* (1989), p. 174 ff.

117. Interviews with Philip R. Lee, Chairman of PPRC, October 20, 1989; and with Lauren B. LeRoy, Deputy Director of PPRC, October 21, 1989.

118. Interview with Paul Ginsburg, Executive Director, PPRC, January 18, 1990.

119. Interview with Philip Lee, October 26, 1989.

120. *Annual Report* (1989), Ch. 13; Interview with Anthony Tirone, Office of the Attorney Adviser, HCFA, May 10, 1988.

121. *Annual Report* (1989), pp. 217 ff.

122. *Annual Report* (1990), Ch. 3.

123. Ibid., Ch. 3.

124. Interview with Philip Lee, October 26, 1989.

125. A fact noted by Philip Lee. At a later stage, during the actual passage of the legislation, inquiries were made about the Administration's position or proposals—without eliciting any response.

126. Interview with Rep. Henry A. Waxman (D., Ca.), May 30, 1990.

127. Interview with Peter Bouxsein, House Energy and Commerce Committee staff, January 17, 1990.

128. Interview with Jamie Reuter, staff, Health Subcommittee, House Ways and Means Committee, May 30, 1990. As he put it, "It would be too easy to hang this bill up if it became politically controversial . . . think of the opportunities to poke holes in it, to argue it to death if it ever got to the floor."

129. Roper left the HCFA early in 1989, to become the Deputy for Domestic Policy. He was also Director of the White House Office of Policy Development.

130. Roper speaks modestly of his own role. Those close to the legislative process, though, describe his contribution as vital. Interview with William L. Roper, M.D., Director, Centers for Disease Control, July 2, 1990.

131. *American Medical News,* August 18, 1989, p. 38.

132. Ibid., pp. 38–39.

133. Paul Ginsburg thinks this to be a misinterpretation of the data—in particular, a failure to allow for the small numbers of primary care physicians within the comparatively large areal subdivisions of Texas. Interview with Paul B. Ginsburg, Executive Director, PPRC, January 19, 1990.

134. One reaction to the practice guidelines proposal was, "Do both," i.e., include the practice guideline and the ETs. Interview with George D. Greenberg, Senior Medicare Program Analyst, Office of the Secretary, DHHS, January 18, 1990.

135. When Mitchell became Senate Majority Leader, the Health Subcommittee was divided, with Rockefeller becoming chairman of the Subcommittee on Medicare and Long-Term Care.

136.   Including both research and practice guidelines.
137.   Update not less than zero nor more than MEI + 2%.
138.   Interview with Jamie Reuter, staff for Health Subcommittee, House Ways and Means, May 30, 1990.
139.   As events transpired, the Gramm–Rudman sequester did go into effect, but the budget reconciliation still passed, after the deadline, and included the MFS in it.
140.   *Congressional Quarterly,* September 23, 1990, pp. 2444–2445.
141.   Which would have left the Gramm–Rudman sequester in place.
142.   Ibid., November 18, 1989, p. 3137.
143.   Largely working from the House reconciliation proposals and adding their own amendments to that. Interview with George Greenberg, May 30, 1990.
144.   Interview with Rep. Henry A. Waxman, May 30, 1990.
145.   Ibid.
146.   *Congressional Quarterly,* November 25, 1989, p. 3240.
147.   Interview with George Greenberg, January 3, 1990.
148.   *Congressional Quarterly,* Ibid., p. 3240.
149.   The Senate language of "volume performance standard" was adopted though the substance of the provisions continued to be much in dispute.
150.   "Linking" meant that the update would be increased and decreased depending on how much actual physician performance, i.e., volume, deviated from the performance standard that was set. Partial linkage could have taken various forms. In this case, the update differential was linked on the "up side" or for favorable performance but limited on the "down side" and dependent on a Congressional "default" or failure to set the update itself.
151.   Interview with Rep. Henry A. Waxman, May 30, 1990; and with George D. Greenberg, May 30, 1990.
152.   Interview with Jamie Reuter, staff, Health subcommittee, House Ways and Means, May 30, 1990.
153.   Ibid.
154.   Primus is chief economist for the Ways and Means Committee. According to report, he often acts as a special emissary for Rostenkowski.
155.   By way of illustration, the Senate draft had been done in great haste. On the other hand, the House Legislative Counsel, Edward Grossman, was an expert and experienced draftsman. As a consequence, House versions often prevailed where it was an issue of specific language. Interview with George Greenberg, January 19, 1990.
156.   Interview with Peter Bouxsein, staff, Health Subcommittee of House Energy and Commerce, January 17, 1990.
157.   Interview with George Greenberg, May 30, 1990.
158.   *Congressional Quarterly,* November 25, 1989, pp. 3217–3218.
159.   Interview, May 30, 1990.
160.   Waxman's argument was that it cost more to live and practice medicine in high cost areas (such as Los Angeles, New York, or Hawaii). Others, and especially those from rural and small town districts, thought that people who liked the life-style should expect to pay the price for it. Peter Bouxsein, then on the Energy and Commerce staff, said that this was, for him, the most troublesome and time-consuming issue of the entire Conference, and recalled "going one-on-one for three hours" with Rep. Mike Synar (D., Okla.) in the course of negotiations. Interviews with Peter Bouxsein, January 17, 1990.

161. A list developed with the help of the PPRC. Henry Waxman was particular strong for this approach, believing the length of the transition was less important than getting an early start.

162. Initially, the non-PAR physicians are even more harshly treated. Until the fee schedule limits go into effect in 1992, these percentage limits are added to the non-PAR prevailing charge limits, already reduced by 5% below those for Medicare participating physicians.

163. Interview with George Greenberg, January 19, 1990; and with Peter Bouxsein, January 17, 1990.

164. The terminology was sufficiently reassuring, for instance, for the AMA to claim that ETs had been defeated, cf. *American Medical News*, December 1, 1989, p. 30. Rep. Gradison also reported that "ET has gone home."

165. The "carve out groups" (COGs) were urged on Congress by William Roper. In his view, these and other managed care options were essential to give physicians ways to meet the ETs or VPSs. This was, taken by itself, a cogent proposition, but no one could figure out how such COGs would be defined, paid, or monitored.

166. PPRC, *Annual Report* (1990), p. 192.

167. The Commission was categorically opposed to additional specialty VPSs. On subnational ones, it recommended that the national VPS be tried and that experience evaluated before considering a move to subnational ones. Ibid., p. 183.

168. A view expressed particularly by Rep. Henry Waxman. Interview, May 30, 1990.

169. Energy and Commerce has jurisdiction over the Public Health Service. Peter Bouxsein, who played a major role in developing this part of the legislation, said that one of its purposes, in addition to providing for effectiveness research and practice guidelines, was to upgrade health care research and reassure some of the health policy research community that the Federal government continued to take seriously its commitment to this endeavor. Accordingly, the National Center for Health Services Research/Health Care Technology Assessment was abolished and its functions incorporated into this larger enterprise.

170. Limited Licence Practitioners: dentists, podiatrists, optometrists, chiropracters.

171. For particulars, see the Proposed Rule of June 5, 1991. *Federal Register*, Vol. 56, No. 108 (Washington, D.C.: Government Printing Office, 1991).

172. Interview with Jamie Reuter: staff of the Health Subcommittee, House Ways and Means, May 30, 1990.

173. A move that led many, including the Congress and the physician community, to wonder whether or how long the five-year deficit reduction pact would last. *Medicine and Health*, June 3, 1991, p. 2.

174. The "behavioral offset" is intended to compensate for volume increases as fees are reduced. Fifty percent (added to the fee reductions) was an amount historically employed and seemed justified by experience with fee freezes. PPRC objected that this figure made no adjustment for volume reductions where fees were increased; but little was known about this kind of situation and the HCFA stuck to the 50% figure. Because the fee schedule would be phased in, moreover, the offset was multiplied by three to achieve budget neutrality.

175. Glaser (1989) "Commentary: The Politics of Paying American Physicians," *Health Affairs*, Vol. 8, pp. 129–146 (Fall 1989); and see the response, Ginsburg et al. (1989).

176.   There is, of course, the Volume Performance Standard; but not only does it punish collectively for individual excesses, its penalties take effect long after the event, i.e., they impose reductions in year three for behavior that occurred in year one. It seems almost deliberately calculated to stir resentment.

177.   Sec. 6102.

178.   See note 87, *supra*.

179.   OBRA 1989, Sec. 6102; OBRA 1990, Sec. 4118 (j).

180.   Otherwise, as one civil servant said, "We will have wasted five years of effort to get minor changes in the way we pay fee-for-services." William Roper and others in the Reagan Administration shared this skeptical appraisal of MFS prospects. Interview with George Greenberg, Office of the Secretary, DHHS, June 20, 1991.

6

Conclusion

The Prospective Payment System and the Medicare Fee Schedule are both impressive accomplishments, bringing together enormous amounts of data, technical expertise, and clear-headed analysis of policy options. In this respect, they fit with a certain American style of policy-making, depending as they do on vast data collections and their manipulation with the high-speed computer; collaborative endeavors of government, business, and academia; and a shared faith in technical problem solving. It remains to be seen what problems have been solved. But both the DRG-based prospective payment system and the resource-based Medicare fee schedule are monumental in scope and complexity, and worth a moment of respectful silence on that account alone.

Together, the two payment reforms are, arguably at least, the most important changes in health policy since the passage of Medicare–Medicaid in 1965. Each in effect cut through a multitude of regulations and incremental changes—the layered accretions of a generation—to establish new, technically sound, and demonstrably fair bases of payment. PPS changed not just the payment mechanism, but transformed the incentives of the hospital industry and the relations between it, as recipient, and the government, as payer. Where PPS was radical in concept, the MFS was sweeping in scope, putting over 6000 procedures on a new resource-based value scale, deliberately redistributing income between geographic regions and medical specialties, and encouraging a continuing and fundamental appraisal by physicians of their daily practice decisions. How effective these schemes will prove to be is for some future audit, but the underlying conceptions and the ultimate aims were not paltry in their vision nor timid in their reach.

For changes that are so far reaching, both hospital and physician payment reform are remarkable for the lack of intense or visible controversy accompanying them. They were not quite done "in a fit of absence of mind,"[1] like Britain's acquisition of empire; but neither was any great attention paid them in Congress. Nor did they kindle much passion among providers, beneficiaries, or the wider public. As noted earlier, PPS went through Congress in what was then record time, as a tacked on section of the Social Security Amendments of 1983; and the MFS was one relatively short part of OBRA 1989. Both were closely held and low-profile policy events, accorded only a few sticks of newsprint in national newspapers such as the *New York Time*, the *Wall Street Journal*, or the *Washington Post*.

The antagonism between Congress and the President with respect to domestic policy and the continuing budget deficits were the great, supervening influences driving events and shaping the eventual outcomes for Medicare payment reform during the entire decade of the 1980s. This was especially true after the elections of 1982, when domestic policy became increasingly a matter of Congress vs. the President. While the Administration successfully maintained some budget parameters and anti-regulatory priorities, the substance of health policy was made through subcommittee micro-management and the budget reconciliation process. There were important historic influences, such as the earlier failures of hospital cost containment and the timing of both the Prospective Payment System and Medicare Fee Schedule in the presidential electoral cycle. But the substance of policy was shaped largely by the strategic maneuvering of Congress and the executive agencies and the immediate politics of the budget and deficit reduction.

With the prevailing budget deficits and divisions over policy, an approach to Medicare payment reform that entailed a great debate, or even a peaking of the more controversial issues, would almost certainly have doomed either PPS or the MFS to defeat, much as National Health Insurance or Hospital Cost Containment had failed earlier in the Carter Administration. Though the process differed, a non-controversial and low profile strategy may have been essential to success for either of these payments reforms. PPS was developed within DHHS, almost in secret, and then passed through Congress with great speed and a minimum of visibility—almost like a forced march in the dark of night. MFS was more incremental, a case of numerous, small amendments by Congressional subcommittees that were incorporated in successive budget reconciliation acts. It could be compared to a gradual investment followed by a peaceful surrender—or perhaps to a death of a thousand cuts, depending on the point of view. In either event, major controversy over the grand design was avoided.

Both PPS and the MFS were, in differing ways, based on payment formulas that were intended to be fair and technically sound. They were put forward by their proponents and supported by the physicians and the hospitals as a way of establishing a "level playing field," evened out by equitable initial calculations that could be subsequently "updated" or amended by means of an impartial and largely non-political method. As a conflict-minimizing device, this approach had obvious merits. Furthermore, had either PPS or the MFS been seriously chargeable with unfairness or provoked general criticism on this account they would have bogged down in political controversy. Yet it is also important to note the policy burden that is put on this notion of technically sound and fair calculations of payment amounts. Each of these payment systems represents virtuoso technical achievements. Yet, each could be viewed, more pessimistically, as high-tech gimmicks that lend plausibility to particular payment or update formulas but that are, at the same time, prone to political manipulation and bury important issues of principle or conflicting interest under these formulas.

These two studies illustrate a characteristic failing of American government: that institutional weakness in policymaking leads to a deferring of difficult issues. The initial Medicare legislation (and Medicaid, for that matter) was a historic instance of this tendency on a grand scale: important issues of hospital and physician reimbursement were deferred by adopting the traditional payment methods and delegating administration to the established payment intermediaries. PPS and the MFS are long-delayed addenda to this early history. Yet they are hardly concluding chapters. Furthermore, each, in a different way, continues this national predilection for resolving difficulty with some variety of problem-solving that avoids conflict and makes too little of remote consequence. PPS would, in principle, displace or avoid controversy by means of a technically driven system. The MFS combined incremental problem-solving with a resource-based fee schedule. Both of these approaches are good ways to postpone conflict, but they leave unresolved some important non-technical and non-incremental political issues: for instance, how Part A and Part B of Medicare should relate to each other, how Medicare payment policy affects the private sector, and what to do if either providers or the government flagrantly or persistently violate the implied contracts underlying each of these payment reforms.

The history of each of these payment systems is different and each is, in its own way, unique. They developed at different phases in the presidential electoral cycle as well as in the unfolding evolution of Congressional–Executive relations. A natural question, then, is "What is to be learned from this set of two differing case studies, other than a familiarity with the historic issues and actors?" Possibly, several kinds of results or conclusions can be developed. One is a judgment about which decisions in the development or implementation of these payment reforms seem warranted by circumstance and the available weight of opinion. Another result is more anticipatory: seeking to identify unresolved issues that are likely to occasion future difficulty. Finally, there is the broader, systemic concern of how well the American Federal government manages a sector of its health policy in this strange, possibly transitional, period of perennial budget deficits and troubled relations between the President and the Congress.

I. TWO PAYMENT REFORMS: ALIKE AND NOT ALIKE

At a high level of abstraction or generality, both PPS and the MFS can be described as similar approaches to different aspects of Medicare payment reform. They both entailed the development of an administered pricing system based on technical calculations of resource use. And they both rely on Congressionally created commissions to advise about annual updates and specific modifications. Although this approach to rate-setting is novel,[2] it has seemed promising enough for Congress to follow the precedent by providing for a Drug Payment Review Commission in the legislation on catastrophic health insurance. There have also been suggestions for combining ProPAC and PPRC into one Medicare commission, that might review Part A and Part B payment issues together and serve as a technical advisory body for future schemes, such as National Health Insurance. As an approach to policymaking, this experiment seems to have substantial appeal. At the same time, PPS and the MFS provide not one example but two: their history, modes of action, and their likely courses of development differ substantially—and in ways that can be important for assessing their own future prospects or for adapting this method of policy development to other substantive areas. Consequently, a brief comparison and contrast will be helpful to support some conclusions.

Prospective Payment System

The development and initial implementation of PPS were close to a textbook example of the policy process. There was a generally acknowledged problem and a devised solution. The wastefulness and inappropriate incentives of the existing cost reimbursement approach had been extensively documented. There were researches and demonstrations exploring alternate payment mechanisms, most of which promised little to mitigate the difficulties. Congress and the DHHS sought a technically sound and systematic answer and PPS was that. The DRG methodology was compared with and evaluated against the other available options. Moreover, it was chosen in the light of explicit policy criteria and designed to meet those criteria. The preparations for initial implementation were meticulous and thorough, with checks and rechecks of regulations, the running of simulations and impact studies, prepping the regions, the fiscal intermediaries, and the hospitals, and designing the methods for monitoring and evaluating PPS once it began operations. Finally, for a number of years, the HCFA and ProPAC have managed to sustain the systemic, analytic, and data driven aspects of the System substantially intact, despite the political buffeting it has received.

As compared with physician payment reform, PPS began much earlier chronologically and at a different point in the presidential electoral cycle. Hospital expenditures had been targeted for some time as needing urgent attention, so that preceding PPS was a history of frustrating attempts including the Carter Administration's bloody battles over hospital cost containment and two failed "voluntary efforts," sponsored by the industry.

These developments helped create awareness in the hospital industry, as well as within the government, that fundamental changes would have to be made. The hospitals and their associations also got accustomed to new ways of dealing with the government, increasingly developing action proposals of their own and "coming to the table" ready to deal. By 1981, the industry was expecting a major legislative initiative. For the leadership echelons of the American Hospital Industry, the Catholic Health Association, and the Federation of American Hospitals, change in some form was accepted as a parameter for political negotiation. Furthermore, the big three had learned to function as "peak associations" for their members: unified, informed, able to carry their membership, and prepared to negotiate.

One appeal of the DRG-based Prospective Payment System was that it provided a technical solution to the problem of how to pay hospitals. In other words, there was a "right" answer that also seemed fair or equitable. This belief increased the conviction of proponents and helped providers gain the confidence needed to risk their economic future on this scheme. For providers, PPS provided a sound and equitable basis for initial payments: a "level playing field,"[3] in the current metaphor. It also provided a method whereby changes—updating or amendment—could be decided on by means of technical analysis and numbers rather than politically, an important assurance for the future. The zero-sum and budget neutral features of PPS were additional features that helped to encourage decision by analysis and computation and to resist preferential advantage, "mindless incrementalism," or politically inspired exceptionalism. Time will tell how strong or "tamper-proof" these technical–rational properties will prove to be; but they *have* been important in setting parameters for debate, providing terms of argument largely accepted by the parties as legitimate, and giving the industry, Congress, and even the Administration important incentives to play the game as originally intended.

The Prospective Payment System had the benefit of substantial agreement on the part of Congress, the Administration, and the hospital industry about the design and purposes of the system. True, each of these parties differed about their top priorities as between cost containment, regional and industry protectiveness, deregulation and management incentives, and earning profits or hospital "margins." But there was a consensus that this was, in the phrase popular at the time, "the only game in town." There was shared support for the critical zero-sum, budget neutral,[4] and formula driven norms of PPS. These factors were especially important in structuring controversy, in focusing debate on commonly acknowledged technical issues, and in translating much of the dispute over hospital payment into issues of technology and data.

The implementation of PPS has been a success or not, depending on how "success" and "implementation" are defined. So far as organizing to achieve assigned tasks and acting effectively to achieve them, both the HCFA and ProPAC have done that. But there remains a more difficult question of whether the program can itself continue to be effectively implemented and whether the task still makes sense or needs to be redefined.

The initial implementation, now part of a fading memory, still deserves recalling. Not only was it a technical feat of heroic proportion, but as one participant said, they "got it right." There were, of course, some initial overpayments and unaudited cost reports, but the system worked with remarkable precision. This technical accuracy contributed significantly to the hospitals' early acceptance of PPS and to its durability as a system. At the same time, this appreciation prompts a sobering question of whether the HCFA could perform such a feat today.[5]

Since 1983, in the course of year-by-year implementation, one notable fact is that PPS has survived the budget and deficit reduction politics of a Congress and Administration divided politically and over policy aims. On several occasions, moreover, Congress and ProPAC have taken steps that worked to strengthen and tighten the system. As the tension between system integrity and special concession played out, some issues got resolved analytically and by the numbers and others were dealt with politically. Continuing budget reconciliation imperatives led to a growing danger that PPS would be eventually "exceptioned to death" through a ratcheting-down on aggregate hospital payments while providing special relief to particular hospitals. Yet after the disreputable OBRA of 1987 there was a respite, a relenting on the update, and a number of steps taken to improve the analytic base and strengthen the systemic features of PPS.

A major problem with PPS and its commission, ProPAC, is a kind of technological obsolescence. It is not that PPS was badly designed or inappropriately implemented, but that the task assignment has proved to be too limited in scope. The DRGs, on which PPS is based, capture only the hospital operating costs associated with inpatient stays. But the cost-shifting within hospital walls and the shifting of patient care to sites outside them have meant that, over time, PPS was becoming less and less effective, either to contain costs or to change incentives. Without increasing the Commission's jurisdiction and the scope of the task, moreover, efforts to tighten and improve PPS were likely to yield modest returns and could even be perverse in their impact. And, finally, both ProPAC and the Congress perceived that the megatrends within the hospital economy were only a part of even larger problems affecting the health care industry as a whole, private business and insurance, and the individual American citizen.

Imaginative steps taken by ProPAC, with the acquiescence and encouragement of Congress, have addressed the necessity for a broadening of initial mission. But to propose a worthy enterprise is not to bring it off. Furthermore, there is an unreconciled difficulty, that of bringing together the technical role of the Commission with its increased policy responsibilities. None of these initiatives makes PPS any more effective or adaptable as a regulatory device for controlling aggregate hospital costs or affecting their institutional behavior. PPS may or may not prove adaptable to new institutional settings. But a jurisdiction expanded to new institutional sites will increase the complexity of the technical activities and political stakes involved. And the new activities of ProPAC will be more advisory in nature and with respect to policies about which there are sharp political differences. In time, ProPAC will probably grow increasingly to resemble PPRC, but without resolving this underlying contradiction between the technical and the political. To that extent, the initial conception of PPS will have been compromised.

The Medicare Fee Schedule

In broad outline, the Medicare Fee Schedule developed in ways similar to PPS, and especially in the sense that it, too, was a technically devised solution to an issue that policymakers *chose* to constrain within such a framework. In this respect it, too, reflected an abiding American faith in technical gimmicks, boldly imaginative though they may be. At the same time, the Medicare Fee Schedule was developed in ways that differed substantially from PPS and that may be significant for its future development.

One important difference between the two systems is that for the Medicare Fee Schedule there was no equivalent of the "TEFRA experience." Before TEFRA and leading up to it, there had been a history of policy arguments and political conflict that changed peoples' perspectives in government and out of it. There had been the fights over hospital cost containment in the Carter Administration, a lengthy national debate over cost containment alternatives, two failed "voluntary efforts," and a growing recognition in the government and within the hospital industry that "something" had to be done, and most likely would be done in the near term. During this period of time, the "big three" of the hospital industry—the American Hospital Association, the Catholic Health Association, and the Federation of American Hospitals[6]—had come to act pretty much as peak associations for the industry, prepared to deal on its behalf with the government. The recession of the early 1980s, a mounting budget deficit, and threats to the hospital trust fund added a sense of urgency, even of crisis. A consequence was that Congress, the Administration, and the hospital industry were all prepared for fundamental change.

For the physician community, perhaps the closest parallel to TEFRA was the experience with the fee freeze of 1984–1986 and the MAACs that succeeded it. Yet this was surely a more ambiguous and dubious experience. For the fee freeze and the MAACS may have alerted physicians that Congress meant business and could, like the Internal Revenue Service, make them miserable. Yet neither of these initiatives did much to educate the physician community in responsible collective behavior or increase their confidence in the efficacy or the equity of government regulation of their fees. In other words, where TEFRA may have had a salutary impact on the hospitals, the fee freeze and the MAACs would seem to have done about as much to educate physicians in *incivisme* as to encourage responsible leadership in the Part B community of providers.

Hospital payment got addressed first and independently of physician reimbursement. Money was an important reason, for Medicare hospital expenditures were running $34.3 billion in FY 1982, while Part B payments were only $14.8 billion, an important difference at a time when the deficit was regarded as a grave threat and hospitals were seen as a major contributor to that deficit. Lack of experience with or knowledge about alternative payment systems was another reason that physician payment was not addressed earlier.[7] Also, the Reagan Administration had its policy: vouchers, tax caps, and co-pays. Fee schedules or similar regulative devices went against Administration priorities and would also have irritated the physicians, generally regarded as Reagan allies.

For such reasons, physician payment reform was, early on, a stepchild of national policy. Attention shifted to the physicians only after PPS had been enacted, the regulations written, and bills were being paid. One major difference, then, is that Part B reforms came late in the cycle of presidential politics, long after the first initiatives of the new Administration had succeeded or failed. In 1983, the Democrats regained working control of the House.[8] By 1984, when serious consideration of changes in physician payment began, Congress and the President had settled into the trench warfare of budgetary politics and many high officials within the DHHS and the HCFA had left or were making travel plans. So, within the executive branch there was little will or capability to provide the kind of leadership that had been effective with respect to PPS.

It also appeared, after canvassing the alternatives, that physician payment reform was not likely to make up into a neat package: there was no elegant solution, as there had been for hospital payment. For PPS, although there was disagreement along the way, the DRG option represented a kind of closure. It provided an acceptable methodology for *both* calculation and control: a formula for payment and leverage to control costs. Not so with physician payment, where each of the alternatives seemed, by contrast, to represent only partial solutions. Capitation, physician DRGs, or a fee schedule—each came up short in some vital respect. Capitation lacked an adequate methodology for calculating a payment. Physician DRGs suffered in this respect and raised additional issues of provider acceptability and of whom to pay. And a physician fee schedule, while providing a technically adequate, even elegant, solution for calculating payment, was weak on the control side, especially with respect to the "volume" issue.

While PPS had involved a large contribution by the Administration, especially the HCFA and DHHS, because of a different historic background Congress and the Administration tended to go their separate ways on physician payment. The Administration never really developed a proposal of its own, unless its ritualistic invocation of "vouchers" or capitation could be counted as that. As a consequence, physician payment reform lacked, in substantial measure, a contribution the bureaucracy could have made: a systematic canvassing of the alternatives; evaluating options in the light of cumulated administrative expertise and R&D; and planning in advance for implementation and monitoring. This difference is a matter of degree, for much of the work that was once performed by the executive bureaucracy got done by the PPRC, other

Congressional agencies, and the committee staffs. But there was, and remains, a distinctive contrast between the two payment reform initiatives and a point of continuing interest will be to see what practical consequences flow from this difference.

Lacking a proposal from the Administration, at least one to be taken seriously, Congress acted on its own, legislating with respect to fees, balance billing, overvalued procedures, and the annual update, and using the budget reconciliation process to make incremental changes in ways familiar to Congressional subcommittees. To inform itself about where it might be heading as well as about what ought to be done, Congress set up its own advisory commission, the PPRC. One consequence of this mode of policy development is that the parameters of physician payment reform were largely determined before they were evaluated. Moreover, the analytical foundation for the Medicare Fee Schedule was completed and installed after these parameters had been implicitly established. With PPS, the analytical foundation was developed first and was, indeed, an important reason for choosing this particular DRG-based option. With physician payment, it was the other way around: Congress was already strongly inclined toward a fee schedule, and the role of the PPRC was largely to advise how to do that and help develop an analytic base to support that option. Stating these contrasts is not intended to detract from the magnitude of the achievement represented by the development of a national fee schedule; but the difference is of some significance. For it meant that much the greater part of the design effort was directed toward developing the analytic base and the multipliers, and comparatively little spent on considering alternatives to a fee schedule or ways in which total costs would be constrained.

The terminology itself conveys an important difference: a Prospective Payment *System* as opposed to a Medicare Fee *Schedule*. Where PPS was designed to be a relatively "tight," zero-sum system, the development of the fee schedule was a more open-ended process. The approach was to build consensus by tackling first the technical and noncontroversial issues, such as the relative value scale, and to move then to more politically charged and divisive topics, such as balance billing and expenditure targets. An element of this strategy was the calculation that a relative value scale or fee schedule could be subsequently adapted to other cost-constraining strategies, such as lowering overvalued procedures, bundling of services, or the use of physician DRGs or capitation. Pursued effectively by the PPRC, this approach of beginning with the technical and noncontroversial made the most of existing political realities. It also facilitated the development and legislative enactment of a fee schedule in a relatively short period of time. And yet, in the course of this development, there was little exploration by the Commission, the

Congress, or the Administration of what lay ahead in the process: of how practicable a strategy of increasingly global fees or an eventual capitation option might be, of how effective expenditure targets or volume performance standards would be or how the physician community would respond to them, of how soon practice guidelines or outcome assessments could be developed and whether they would, indeed, win the hearts and minds of the physicians.

This distinction between system and process points to another difference in the two programs: in particular, the relation between design and implementation. For PPS, until recently at least, the role for ProPAC has been largely to advise in the implementation of a completed system and to propose some amendments or further embellishments, such as DRG modifiers or a formula for the inclusion of capital. With respect to physician payment, by contrast, the role of the PPRC was, and continues to be, one of helping create the design and, furthermore, participate as a major partner not just in the early, critical stages of implementation but also in some of the most important and politically charged decisions yet to be made in completing the final design. Invoking the traditional "policy–administration" dichotomy, the boundary is much less distinct or significant in physician payment reform.

System vs. process helps identify some additional particulars with respect to these different approaches to reform. In the case of PPS, its system-like qualities have been an important strength, especially in encouraging all parties to go by technical analysis and the numbers. A common interest in substantive and procedural fairness has helped significantly in winning the acquiescence of the hospital industry and restraining Congress and the Administration. These system-like qualities have created incentives for reforms that can tighten the system and help preserve it. But at the same time that these modifications help to perfect and institutionalize the system, they can work against bigger changes. PPS is systemic and zero-sum; but almost every variable in the equation builds in proxies, historic formulas, or special adjustments that would be affected by any major reform, such as new DRG modifiers. Consequently, the systemic quality of PPS may work against any reforms that go farther than tinkering. But tinkering is what Congress loves to do, and that activity, long continued, gradually "loosens" the system and robs it of its technical rationality and acceptability. As previously noted, there are counter-indications: a move in Congress and the Commission to accelerate the inclusion of capital and DRG reform. Some are hopeful and others are skeptical about the likely outcomes. But this is an example of systemic reform—important for the long-term viability of PPS—that may entail more political upset and controversy than Congress or the Commission can or will endure.

For physician payment reform, the emphasis is on process. There is a five year phase-in and a number of transitions, including the establishment of an initial "hit-list" of overvalued procedures and schedules for introducing geographic adjustments, balance billing limits, and the volume performance standards. Much is left to the future and to an expectation that practice guidelines and effectiveness research might help with the "volume" issue. For the PPRC, the health subcommittees in Congress, and the HCFA, getting the Medicare Fee Schedule fully operative will require close attention and relatively continuous intervention for at least the next six years. The problems to be identified and resolved and the decisions yet to be made are full of intellectual challenge and will demand the kind of skillful negotiation and political maneuvering that have, fortunately, largely characterized the work of the Commission and of the Congress from the beginning of this process. Once the fee schedule is in place, there will continue to be major policy issues about the update, how to implement the volume performance standards, what to do about more global, techniques of bundling services or redressing geographic and specialty inequities, and how to institutionalize the amendment procedures.

Need for continuing intervention has a virtue, in that it will require a monitoring of the process and keep it lively and progressive. But the payment reform scheme has built in a rather serious conflict between a long-term strategy and the likely realities of politics in the short-run. Great hope rests on the prospect of cooperating with the Medicare physicians and gradually persuading them to practice a better and more cost-effective brand of medicine through the use of practice guidelines and research into therapeutic outcomes. These are attempts at persuasion over the long-term. Meanwhile, the new legislation emphasizes cost containment and a reduction of overvalued procedures and geographic and specialty differentials.[9] A part of the subtext is that, with and beyond the advice of PPRC, Congress will itself be heavily and peremptorily engaged in micro-managing the details: setting rates and establishing specific mandates, categories, and exceptions. But more is involved than tinkering, for some of the important and politically contentious features of the Medicare Fee Schedule remain to be determined, such as the details of the volume performance standards and the geographic modifiers. And the regulatory process for physician payment lacks the same kind of zero-sum, "tamper-resistant" features that characterizes PPS. A danger is that Congress will overstep, in seeking cost savings or in redressing putative inequities, so that the long-term result will be not winning the hearts and minds of the physicians, but vexing them and creating a sense of grievance that encourages angry and perverse responses that increase the volume or intensity of services provided or violate the spirit of the Medicare Fee Schedule in other ways.

Congress and the Executive are only one kind of political problem. For the MFS involves not just thousands of codes, but 32 specialty societies in addition to the AMA and 7 categories of non-physician providers. Prudence bids us recognize that the MFS will involve regulation of a sort never before undertaken in the United States or elsewhere: challenging—to say the least—in both its technical difficulty and in the byzantine complexity of the public-private transactions to be negotiated. A grave risk, both in the initial implementation and the continuing adaptation of the MFS, is a surrendering of control over the minutia of decisions and a gradual compromising of program integrity.

Both the Prospective Payment System and the Medicare Fee Schedule are remarkable in part as acts of faith. They are based on the belief that an objective and fair basis of payment for Medicare hospitals could be created through calculation of work and resource use and that providers would, by and large, accept payments so determined because they were rationally grounded and equitable. Each of these payment reforms represents technical feats of impressive magnitude; and they were endorsed as acceptable by the providers themselves. Moreover, PPS has survived and the MFS was largely developed during a period of ideological politics and strong policy differences between Congress and the President. As noted previously, there is in each case a danger that technical rationality and an initially fair calculus of payments will prove inadequate as a sustaining influence, especially when subjected to the stresses of American national politics. Each payment reform also represents a partial and a technical solution to problems of health care costs, equity, and access that are systemic in nature and politically divisive. As previously noted, there is a "policy gap" with each system: for PPS it is how to connect its technically rational features with changing industry behavior and an expanded mission; and for the MFS, it is how to ensure a growing compliance despite the fee schedule's redistributive and punitive features. What the future holds remains to be seen. But an understanding of the strengths and weaknesses of these two experiments in payment reform may help to preserve them or guide steps toward a next phase.

II. MEDICARE AND THE AMERICAN POLITICAL SYSTEM

The development and implementation of health policy in the United States have been characterized historically by two salient features. One is "professional dominance" (cf. Freidson 1970): the status and power of health professionals, physicians especially, that enables them not only to exert authority over patients but to set their own norms of conduct and fend off attempts by outsiders to regulate their behavior. The other is "institutional weakness" in the making of health policy, especially resulting from constitutional arrangements such as separation of powers and federalism and political features such as weak party systems and interest group politics. The wealth, power, and alternate resources of the medical profession, giving it the capacity to block change, was matched in the public sector by an institutional weakness and inability to develop sustained and coherent health policies at the level of national government.

As a consequence of these two characteristic features of professional dominance and institutional weakness, health policy concerns are often addressed in ways that reduce the scope or intensity of political conflict (or both). This can be achieved by dealing with part of an issue rather than the whole: for instance, cost containment for Medicare hospitals only rather than an all payers approach. Another method is by delegating or devolving part of a program: by leaving Medicaid eligibility to the states, or by providing that the carriers and fiscal intermediaries rather than the Federal government would process Medicare claims and pay the bills. And yet another way, familiar to the American scene, is to sublimate conflict, either through some form of subsidy or additional payment or by finding a technical resolution for the differences of interest or opinion—methods that have especially characterized both PPS and the MFS.

The Medicare–Medicaid program was from its inception an instance of policy development and implementation characterized by professional dominance and institutional weakness. Largely because of professional dominance a national program of health insurance comes late in America and in a diminished and constrained form. It was a partial program, dealing with the elderly and the medically indigent rather than the entire population. It was fragmented, in the sense that it was both a national and a state program and that it began with two schemes of payment, one for the hospitals and another for the physicians. It contained, as well, numerous subsidies for and concessions to providers, designed to secure their support for the program or, at least, to buy a grudging acquiescence.

From the beginning of the Medicare–Medicaid program, Congress and the Administration, the state governments, health care providers, and beneficiaries were confronted with the shortcomings of this constrained and partial solution and the dilemmas of how to cope with the unresolved issues. There was cost escalation, especially on the hospital side. There were problems of coverage and out-of-pocket expense for the Medicare beneficiaries and of access and quality of care for the poor. There was cost-shifting among the providers and hunting for deep pockets. The Federal government responded to one partial solution with other partial solutions: hospital utilization review, health planning, categorical programs for the poor, and so forth. Indeed, much of the largest part of national health policy since 1966 has been directed at an attempt to remedy or deal with the compromised program structure established by the Medicare–Medicaid legislation in 1966.

The Prospective Payment System and the Medicare Fee Schedule can be seen as a continuation of this history of partial remedies, even though they represent well-crafted and ambitious attempts to deal with cost containment and to address, in lesser measure, some of the issues of access, equity, and quality of care. It is worth recalling that both PPS and the MFS are based on research begun under Section 223 authority as part of early efforts to design a technically adequate method of cost containment. And it was the failure of more comprehensive approaches toward health insurance or hospital cost containment that helped set the agenda for PPS and, after that, for physician payment reform.

The Reagan and Bush administrations, though, represent an important discontinuity and the introduction of a new policy variables: most importantly, the semi-permanent partisan division of Congress and the President and the perennial impetus supplied by the annual deficit and the felt necessity for reducing it. This is another version of institutional weakness which, as such, expresses itself in the inability of Congress and the President to collaborate effectively on health policy, with a brief exception of the actual passage of PPS. And yet, sometimes, less is more. Mounting government outlays for Medicare, which are a major contribution to the deficit, provided a visible and well-defined target. And powerful legislative committees with Social Security jurisdiction, utilizing the budget reconciliation process, could push through payment reforms with a minimum of cooperation from the executive branch. Paradoxically, sweeping changes in Medicare payment were achieved, despite the organized power of health providers and their political ploys, in a period when Congress and the President were mostly at odds over domestic policy.

At the same time that PPS and the MFS should be acclaimed for the boldness of the conception and the technical and political skills that helped create them, it is important to recognize ways in which they, like the initial Medicare program, fall short of a comprehensive or adequate solution. These limitations are significant both for the future of the programs as such as well as, more globally, for the American economy and polity. Three items merit particular comment.

These payments reforms were, first of all, primarily cost containment measures directed at Medicare. As programs to limit Federal government outlays, they may or may not succeed. But they do nothing, directly, to constrain rising health care costs for Medicaid or for the private sector. Constraint in one area and lack of it in another encourages internal cross-subsidies and cost-shifting. And today, the private sector faces not only its own unconstrained and rising health care costs but the shifting to it of some unknown quantum of Medicare expense, along with other unpaid bills arising from Medicaid, AIDS, "crack" cocaine, and the uninsured, who wind up in the emergency rooms and urban hospitals and must be paid for in some way. Once again, a "crisis" is on us, one that has helped create a truly formidable alliance of providers, "Fortune 500" corporations, trade unions, insurance companies, and health policy activists, all demanding a program of National Health Insurance—an industry "bail-out" at least as much as it is a benefit for individuals. Ironically, National Health Insurance may appear, in retrospect, to have been the most important legacy of a decade of action and inaction with respect to Medicare payment reform.

Like Titles XVIII and XIX of the original Medicare–Medicaid legislation, these two payments reforms developed independently, at different times, and with their own distinctive constituencies of supporters and affected providers. They were designed to achieve different objectives: ProPAC more for implementation and PPRC to be more advisory and programmatically innovative. As with any dedicated or purpose-built piece of equipment, each Commission and each payment reform is limited, to an extent, by prescribed objective and a separate evolution. This specialism may prove to be a serious limitation. As recent signals from ProPAC have indicated, hospital costs are increasingly difficult to constrain without more effective controls on physicians' decisions. These pressures on hospital costs are symptomatic, in turn, of cost-shifting incentives and opportunities that may make physician behavior especially difficult to affect without a coordinated attack and new payment methodologies. Yet the specialized and dedicated character of each regulatory system militates against combining them, for instance, into a single Medicare commission. It also makes the two commissions limited resources for developing comprehensive proposals that would facilitate a coordinated attack on Part A and Part B expenditures simultaneously.

Both Medicare itself and the Medicare payment reforms were responses, in part, to institutional weakness in policy development. With Medicare and Medicaid, the characteristic responses or strategies were delegation and devolution: the delegation of decisions, explicitly and implicitly, to intermediaries and the providers; and the devolution of Medicaid, in large measures, to the states. There was an element of implicit delegation in payment reform, in that both PPS and the MFS were provider approved solutions. But these reforms relied particularly on the rational authority of expert and technical calculations as a way to deal with institutional weakness. Each system was based on payments generally accepted as equitable because warranted by data and analysis. There is about this strategy a fundamental question of whether statistics can indeed prevail against despotism: of how well a technocratic strategy can survive the stresses of the budget cycle and deficit reduction politics. As to this outcome, much depends on the vagaries of politics. But the underlying strategy of sublimating conflict by translating it into calculations of resource use or "work," however valuable or necessary it may have been for developing these separate payment reforms, specifically fails to address a vital question. That question is how to combine technical expertise with *future* changes of policy involving major political or policy issues and hard conflicts of interest—such as a generic reform of the DRGs, a major adaptation of policy for the volume and intensity program, or some version of bundling or capitation that would combine both the hospitals and the physicians in a coordinated reform proposal.

The Prospective Payment System and the Medicare Fee Schedule are elegant but partial solutions to the problems of rising health care costs, equity of payment, and beneficiary protection. They are skillfully contrived systems and represent much of the best wisdom we have. They are likely, for these reasons as well as simply because they are in place, to be important parts of a payment system and cost-containment strategy should some version of all-payers legislation, mandated benefits, or national health insurance be on the national agenda in the near future. But for any of these programs, a technically elegant but partial solution is not likely to suffice; and ways in which to bring into play the larger coordinative and conflict-resolving capabilities of other institutions will be essential. Stated in a rather obscure fashion, this is but another version of the policy-administration dilemma, and, of course, one of the ways in which this policy-administration dichotomy got resolved, traditionally, was through the mediating role of the administrative department and the "neutral competence" of such staff agencies as the Office of Management and Budget. In this respect, it is worth recalling the devising and implementation of PPS, for that is the last time we witnessed Medicare policy being developed in something like the classic model: with a comprehensive assessment of alternatives, a deliberate program design, and a detailed and closely monitored strategy of implementation. It is further worth remembering that both the Prospective Payment System and the Medicare Fee Schedule were built on research begun years in advance and with the encouragement of bureaucrats in the DHEW, under the authority of the Social Security Amendments of 1972. But all of that was a lifetime ago and before the political developments of the last decade changed the traditional roles of the Congress, the White House Office, and the administrative departments in the development of domestic policy. Indeed, this change may prove to be the biggest and, as yet, uncounted cost of the new separation of powers. For one item, it makes difficult, if not virtually impossible, any revision of health policy that is both technically sound and comprehensive so that we may, for instance, lurch toward National Health Insurance, but lack the capacity to design it well. Yet, this kind of policy-making threatens even more limited initiatives, such as these two separate efforts at Medicare payment reform, for we use such partial reforms not as a way to address the larger problems but as a way to escape pressing difficulty.

And yet a gloomy perspective is not the worst, for to acknowledge difficulty is to begin to confront it. For Medicare, more than most programs or areas of domestic policy, the past is prelude to the future. And this account of Medicare payment reform may help, both in thinking about the next steps as well as in understanding and making allowance for the formidable obstacles to progress imposed by our own system of self-government.

NOTES

1. Sir John Seeley (1834–1895), British historian.

2. An earlier institution that was similar was the Postal Rate Commission, established by the Postal Reorganization Act of 1970, which created the U.S. Postal Service. This heritage may not augur well for the Medicare commission, even though they could in no way be said to derive from the Postal Rate Commission. Cf. *U.S. Postal Service—Reorganization Proposals* (Washington, D.C.: American Enterprise Institute, 1976). I am indebted to Bruce L. R. Smith, Brookings Institution, for calling my attention to this historic antecedent.

3. A metaphor that obscures some issues, such as what assessments to make of initial price levels and their components, whether to level the field down or up, who the players are, what represents equality or justice between them, who referees, and who keeps score.

4. PPS was "budget neutral" with respect to TEFRA for two years; but budget and deficit reduction exercised a similar kind of constraint, instilling a consciousness that increments had to be "instead ofs" rather than "add ons."

5. Charles Booth, the Director of the Office of Reimbursement Policy, has observed that the HCFA faces a similarly challenging task in getting the Medicare Fee Schedule in place by January 1, 1992. But PPS involved not just implementation but designing a zero-sum system as well.

6. Now called the "Federation of American Health Systems," a change in terminology that calls attention to changes taking place within the industry.

7. Research in the field had lagged. Aside from formidable data problems, provider groups, and especially the AMA refused to cooperate. There was also comparatively little interest within the health policy research community or in Congress, partly because of these factors.

8. And in 1986 they regained control of the Senate.

9. These will, of course, be phased in, but so also will some of the benefits, like increased payments for visit codes. How the overall satisfaction nets out will be interesting to see.

Glossary

AAPCC	Adjusted Average per Capita Cost
ACP	American College of Physicians
ACS	American College of Surgeons
ACR	American College of Radiology
AARP	American Association of Retired Persons
APGs	Ambulatory Patient Groups
ASPE	Assistant Secretary for Planning and Evaluation, DHHS
BERC	Bureau of Eligibility, Reimbursement and Coverage, HCFA
BMAD	Part B Medicare Annual Data Files
BPO	Bureau of Program Operations, HCFA
CBO	Congressional Budget Office
CPR	Customary, Prevailing, and Reasonable
CPT	Current Procedural Terminology
DAF	Discretionary Adjustment Factor
DRG	Diagnosis-Related Group
DHHS	Department of Health and Human Services
EOMB	Executive Office of Management and Budget
EM	Evaluation and Management (services)
ET	Expenditure Target
FFS	Fee-for-Service

FI	Fiscal Intermediary
GAO	General Accounting Office
HCFA	Health Care Financing Administration
HCPCS	HCFA Common Procedure Coding System
HMO	Health Maintenance Organization
LOS	Length of Stay
MAAC	Maximum Allowable Actual Charge
MCR	Medicare Cost Report
MEI	Medicare Economic Index
MFS	Medicare Fee Schedule
OBRA	Omnibus Budget Reconciliation Act
OMB	Office of Management and Budget
PAR	Participating Physician Program
PPRC (PhysPRC)	Physician Payment Review Commission
ProPAC	Prospective Payment Assessment Commission
PRO	Peer Review Organization
RAP	Radiology, Anesthesiology, Pathology
RoE	Return on Equity
RBRVS	Resource-Based Relative Value Scale
RWV	Relative Work Value
RVS	Relative Value Scale
SMI	Supplementary Medical Insurance Program (Medicare Part B)
SOI	Severity of Illness
UCR	Usual, Customary, and Reasonable
UR	Utilization Review
VPS	Volume Performance Standard

TERMS

Adjusted Average per Capita Cost (AAPCC):   An actuarial estimate of the amount required to serve a Medicare population within a geographic area (county), adjusted for age, sex, institutional, and disability status.

Agency for Health Care, Policy, and Research: Agency created as part of the Medicare Fee Schedule legislation with special responsibility for research into effectiveness and appropriateness of medical services and procedures and for recommending and helping implement practice guidelines.

Assignment (or, "taking assignment"):   Agreement by a physician to accept the Medicare allowed charge as payment in full, i.e., to forego balance billing.

Balance Bill/Extra Bill: Physician charges that exceed those allowed by Medicare or other third party payer.

Blue Cross/Blue Shield: The largest association of health care insurance companies, first begun in 1929. Plans vary by state. Blue Cross pays for hospital stays; Blue Shield covers physician charges.

Bundling: Combining an array of services into a single package for coding, billing, or payment. Unbundling: Separating the items in a package, especially in order to increase the total amount billed.

Capitation: Payment of a fixed amount per person, rather than by salary or fees for specific services.

Carrier: Under Medicare, a private contractor (typically an insurance company) that processes claims for physician services paid under Part B.

Carve-out Group (COG):   A group, such as an HMO, that may be entitled to a separate Volume Performance Standard under the Medicare Fee Schedule legislation.

Case-Mix Index: An index (number) that measures the severity of cases experienced by a provider.

Certificate-of-Need (CON):   Certification that health care facilities or services meet certain criteria of public need.

Code: A number assigned to identify a physician service. Upcoding is claiming a higher, sometimes unjustified, level of payment for a particular service; Code creep refers to a gradual upcoding.

Common Working File (CWF):   A new HCFA file combining Part A and Part B claims data.

Competitive Medical Plan (CMP):   An option created by TEFRA 1982, allowing health plans that did not meet Federal HMO qualifications to enter into Medicare risk contracts.

Conversion Factor (CF):   In a fee schedule, a multiplier that includes various up-dates and adjustments and is used to convert the relative value scale into dollar amounts.

Co-pay (co-insurance):   The amount an insurance beneficiary must pay after an initial deductible (if any) is met.

Cost Reimbursement: Payment on the basis of audited costs, especially for Medicare hospital providers prior to PPS. Payment was typically made on the basis of a "per diem" (room and board) and "ancillaries" (other hospital inpatient costs for nursing care, medication, etc.).

Current Procedural Terminology (CPT):   A coding system developed by the American Medical Association and widely used as a basis for payment. It also formed the basis for the HCFA Common Procedures Coding System used for Medicare.

Customary, Prevailing, and Reasonable Charge (CPR):   Terminology for the charge limits under Medicare prior to the Medicare Fee Schedule. Medicare would pay the lesser of a physician's actual charge or the charge prevailing in the Carrier locality. Usual, Customary, and Reasonable (UCR) was a similar system followed by private third party payers, such as Blue Shield or Aetna.

Deductible: The amount of medical expense a beneficiary must pay before receiving benefits under an insurance scheme.

Diagnosis-Related Groups (DRGs):   A methodology developed for classifying cases by diagnosis (or procedure). Used as a basis for payment under the Medicare Prospective Payment System for in-patient hospital stays. Physician DRGs or MD DRGs: A similar methodology applied to a related bundle of medical derives. RAP DRGs: A proposed application of the DRG methodology to services provided by radiologists, anesthesiologists, and pathologists.

DRG Amendment (Reclassification):   Reassigning diagnoses or including different procedures under a particular DRG.

DRG Recalibration: A periodic readjustment of all DRG weights to reflect more accurately the relative costs under existing practice patterns.

Discretionary Adjustment Factor (DAF):   A factor in computing the annual update for the Prospective Payment System that takes account of technical and scientific advances and changes in site and productivity. Termed the "Policy Target Adjustment Factor" (PTAF) by the HCFA.

Disproportionare Share (hospital):   Hospitals that serve a disproportionate share of poor patients or experience heavy (30%) losses from indigent care qualify for a disproportionate share adjustment under the Prospective Payment System.

Effectiveness: Benefit from a particular medical service or procedure, as distinguished from its cost or its appropriateness relative to another service or procedure.

Exempted hospitals: Hospitals not included under the Prospective Payment System, sometimes called TEFRA hospitals, because they come under the earlier legislation. The most important categories are psychiatric, long-term care, childrens', and rehabilitation hospitals.

Expenditure Target (ET): An overall cap or target figure for total expenditures, used to adjust future payments in accord with actual performance in relation to the target.

Fee-for-Service: Payment of physicians by individual fees for specific services, as opposed to capitation or salary.

Fee Freeze: A "freeze" on Medicare physician charges, in force from July 1984 until January 1987.

Fee Schedule: A schedule of payments for specific medical services or procedures.

Fiscal Intermediary (FI): Private contractor that processes and pays claims for Medicare hospital services.

Geographic Multiplier: A multiplier used to make geographic adjustments in the Medicare Economic Index.

Geographic Practice Cost Index: An index adopted in the Medicare Fee Schedule designed to make regional adjustments in practice costs.

Global Serve: A bundle of related services treated as a unit for coding, billing, or payment. Especially important for surgery.

Gramm–Rudman–Hollings: The Balanced Budget and Emergency Deficit Control Act of 1985. An act providing for reductions in the budget deficit, targeting Medicare among other programs.

Grouper: The computerized system designed by the HCFA to classify PPS claims for payment.

Health Care Financing Administration (HCFA): Unit within the U.S. Department of Health and Human Services with primary responsibility for Medicare and Medicaid.

HCFA Common Procedure Coding System (HCPCS): A coding system based on the AMA Current Procedural Terminology and used by Medicare carriers.

Health Maintenance Organization (HMO): An organization that provides comprehensive health services to a member for a prepaid amount.

Hospital Market Basket: An index of hospital inputs, similar to the Consumer Price Index, that helps to determine the Update Factor under the Prospective Payment System. The other important index in the update is the Discretionary Adjustment Factor (DAF).

Inherent Reasonableness (limits):   A procedure established in OBRA 1986 for limiting physician charges for selected procedures.

Indirect Teaching Adjustment or Indirect Medical Expense Adjustment: Payment made to hospitals under the Prospective Payment System for the indirect costs of medical education.

International Classification of Diseases, 9th Edition, Clinical Modification (ICD-9-CM):   A classification of diseases published by the World Health Organization in 1979 that figured prominently in the design of the Diagnosis-Related Groups (DRGs).

Maximum Allowable Actual Charge (MAAC):   A limit on Medicare charges by nonparticipating physicians. The MAACs replaced the "fee freeze" of 1984 and remained in force until the phase-in for the Medicare Fee Schedule began.

Medicaid: A program of health insurance for the poor and "medically indigent," jointly financed by the Federal government and the states.

Medicare Cost Report (MCR):   A report filed be each Medicare hospital to determine reimbursable costs for services rendered to Medicare patients during the fiscal year.

Medicare Economic Index (MEI):   An index of physician inputs and expenses constructed by the Federal government and used since 1975 to limit prevailing charges for Medicare services.

Medicare Fee Schedule (MFS):   Fee schedule for Medicare physician payments mandated to go into effect January 1, 1992.

Medicare Provider Analysis and Review File (MED-PAR file):   An HCFA file of Medicare claims data submitted by hospitals.

Notice and Comment: A stage in the (informal) rulemaking process during which comments from interested parties are invited.

Omnibus Budget Reconciliation Act (OBRA):   An act concluding the congressional budget process, reconciling anticipated budget outlays with negotiated targets.

Outlier: Under the Prospective Payment System, an atypical case deviating statistically from the norm, either in cost or length of stay.

Overvalued Procedure: Procedures designated for reduction because determined to be substantially overpriced relative to other CPR procedures. PPRC uses "overvalued"; OBRA 1987 refers to "overpriced."

Part B Medicare Annual Data System (BMAD):   One of the important data files.

Participating Physician and Supplier Program (PAR):   A program, established in 1984, that offered financial and other inducement to physicians who would take assignment.

Peer Review: A review of the work of providers by other health care professionals, especially with respect to its quality and necessity.

Peer Review Organization (PRO):   An organization under contract with the HCFA to review the medical care provided to Medicare beneficiaries.

Physicians' Advisory Group (technically, Physicians' Discussion Group): A group formed by the HCFA in 1983 to consider alternatives for Medicare physician payment reform.

Policy Target Adjustment Factor (PTAF):   See Discretionary Adjustment Factor (DAF).

Practice Costs: "Office" costs and other nonphysician inputs associated with the medical services provided by a physician.

Practice Guidelines: Specific clinical recommendations for patient care based on medical lore or research.

Pricer: The computerized system designed by the HCFA to compute payments for hospitals under the Prospective Payment System.

Prospective Payment System (PPS):   A system for payment of Medicare hospital claims on a prospective, per case basis, effective October 1, 1983.

Reasonable Costs: Providers' direct and indirect costs determined to be necessary and proper for the efficient delivery of health care services to Medicare beneficiaries.

Regional (or Rural) Referral Center: A large, rural or semirural hospital qualifying for higher urban rates under the Prospective Payment System. Initially, the lower limit was 500 beds, later changed to 275 beds.

Relative Value Scale (RVS):   An index that assigns relative weights to medical services that are used as a basis for payment. A resource-based relative value scale (RBRVS) estimates resource inputs. A charge-based RVS bases payments on a proportion of actual or allowed charges.

Return on Equity (RoE):   An amount allowed to compensate investors, especially applicable to for-profit hospitals.

Risk Contracts: Under Medicare, an arrangement made in 1972 that allows HMOs to be compensated on a "risk" or "incentive" basis, i.e., through periodic capitation payments, with some subsequent allowable cost adjustments.

Rulemaking: A process by which implementing regulations are developed within the executive departments or by regulatory agencies.

Severity of Illness (SOI) Index: One of a variety of adjustments considered as a modification of the DRGs, intended especially to take account of severe, costly cases.

Sole Community Hospital: A hospital that is, practically speaking, the sole source of inpatient care for an area. Such hospitals qualify for special treatment under the Prospective Payment System.

Specialty Differential: A difference paid under a fee schedule for a service when it is performed by specialists.

Standardized Amount: Under the Prospective Payment System, an average payment for a Medicare hospital discharge. There are separate standardized amounts for rural, urban, and large urban areas. Once this basic unit is established, other adjustments are made to it, for case-mix, teaching status, annual update, etc., to determine an individual discharge payment for a specific case.

Supplementary Medical Insurance Program (SMI):   Covers Part B, or physicians' services under Medicare. Unlike the Part A or Hospital Insurance program, SMI membership is at the option of the beneficiary and requires the payment of an annual premium.

Update Factor: Under the Prospective Payment System, the annual percentage change in payments for hospital charges.

Utilization Review: An internal or outside review to determine whether services performed were medically necessary and appropriate.

Volume: The amount of physicians' services supplied under a payment system.

Volume Performance Standard: A modified version of an expenditure target that appears in the Medicare Fee Schedule legislation. Initially intended as "advisory," it ultimately incorporated a weak sanction for failing to meet annual targets.

Voucher: A fixed subsidy or grant, typically made to an individual or family head, and limited to the purchase of a specific good, such as food, education, or health care.

MAJOR LEGISLATION

Social Security Amendments of 1965, P.L. 89-97 (July 20, 1965). Medicare and Medicaid.

Social Security Amendments of 1972, P.L. 92-60 (October 30,

1972). Title II contained many innovative provisions affecting Medicare and Medicaid, including authority for research and demonstrations to develop alternate payment systems.

TEFRA

Tax Equity and Fiscal Responsibility Act of 1982, P.L. 97-248 (September 3, 1982). Created a payment system for the TEFRA or "exempted" hospitals; mandated the development of a Prospective Payment System; included various other provisions dealing with HMOs, CMPs, and PROs.

DEFRA

Deficit Reduction Act of 1984, P.L. 98-369 (July 18, 1984). Congressional reduction of the PPS update; legislated the physician "fee freeze."

COBRA

Consolidated Omnibus Budget Reconciliation Act of 1985, P.L. 99-272 (April 7, 1986). Various cost-saving amendments of PPS; established the Physician Payment Review Commission; mandated the development of a relative value scale.

OBRA 1986 (SOBRA)

Omnibus Budget Reconciliation Act of 1986, P.L. 99-509 (October 21, 1986). More cost-saving amendments of PPS; legislation on "inherent reasonableness" procedures and the MAACs.

OBRA 1987

Omnibus Budget Reconciliation Act of 1987, P.L. 100-203 (December 22, 1987). Especially radical PPS amendments; Congress begins directly

	legislating cuts in "overvalued" procedures; mandates development of Medicare Fee Schedule by January 1, 1990.
MCCA	Medicare Catastrophic Coverage Act of 1988, P.L. 100-360 (July 1, 1988), repealed December 13, 1989.
OBRA 1989	Omnibus Budget Reconciliation Act of 1989, P.L. 101-239 (December 19, 1989). Medicare Fee Schedule passed.
OBRA 1990	Omnibus Budget Reconciliation Act of 1990, P.L. 101-508 (November 5, 1990). Additional responsibilities assigned to ProPAC and PPRC; discretionary caps and 5-year pact for deficit reduction.

Selected Bibliography

Altenstetter, Christa, "An End to a Consensus on Health Care in the Federal Republic of Germany," *Journal of Health Politics, Policy and Law,* Vol. 12(3): 505–536, 1987.

Ashby, John, and Carolyn Parmer, "The Impact of Medicare Prospective Payment on Central City and Suburban Hospitals, *Health Affairs,* Vol. 4(4): 99–107, 1985.

Averill, Richard F., et al. Design and Evaluation of a Prospective Payment System for Ambulatory Care, Final Report (Wallingford, Conn.: 3M Health Information Systems, 1991).

Bardach, Eugene, *The Implementation Game: What Happens After a Bill Becomes a Law* (Cambridge, MA: MIT Press, 1977).

Becker, Edmund R., et al., "Relative Cost Differences Among Physicians' Specialty Practices," *Journal of the American Medical Associations,* Vol. 260(16): 2397–2402, 1988.

Benda, Peter M., and Charles H. Levine, "Reagan and the Bureaucracy: The Bequest, the Promise, and the Legacy," in Charles O. Jones (ed.), *The Reagan Legacy: Promise and Performance* (Chatham, NJ: Chatham House Publishers, 1988).

Bentley, James D., and Peter W. Butler, *Describing and Paying Hospitals—Developments in Patient Case Mix* (Washington, D.C.: American Association of Medical Colleges, 1980).

Braun, Peter, et al., "Cross-Specialty Linkage of Resource-Based Relative Value Scales," *Journal of the American Medical Association,* Vol. 260(16): 2390–2396, 1988.

Brown, Lawrence D., *Politics and Health Care Organization—HMOs as Federal Policy* (Washington, D.C.: Brookings Institution, 1983).

Burney, Ira, and Julia Paradise, "Medicare Physician Participation and Assignment," *Health Affairs,* Vol. 6(2): 107–120, 1987.

Burney, Ira, and George Schieber, "Medicare Physicians' Services: The Composition of Spending and Assignment Rates," *Health Care Financing Review,* Vol. 7(1): 81–96, 1985.

Dobson, Allen, "Prospective Payment System Construction Issues" (unpublished), May 1983.

Dobson, Allen, and Elizabeth W. Hoy, "Hospital PPS Profits: Past and Perspective," *Health Affairs*, Vol. 7(1): 126–129, 1988.

Dunn, Daniel, et al., "A Method for Estimating the Preservice and Postservice Work of Physicians' Services," *Journal of American Medical Association*, Vol. 260(16): 2371–2378, 1988.

Dutton, Benson L., Jr., and Peter McMenamin, "The Medicare Economic Index: Its Background and Beginnings," *Health Care Financing Review*, Vol. 3(1): 137–139, 1981.

Eddy, David M., "Variations in Physician Practice: The Role of Uncertainty," *Health Affairs*, Vol. 3(2): 74–89, 1984.

Eddy, David, and John Billing, "The Quality of Medical Evidence: Implications for Quality of Care," *Health Affairs*, Vol. 7(1): 19–32 (1988).

Eisenberg, John M., *Doctor's Decisions and the Cost of Medical Care* (Ann Arbor, MI: Health Administration Press, 1986).

Enthoven, Alain C., *Theory and Practice of Managed Competition in Health Care Financing* (Amsterdam: North-Holland, 1988). Distributed in the U.S. by Elsevier Science Publishing Co., Inc.

———. "Managed Competition: An Agenda for Action," *Health Affairs*, Vol. 7(3): 25–47, 1988.

Etheredge, Lynn, "Negotiating National Health Insurance," *Journal of Health Politics, Policy and Law*, Vol. 16(1): 157–167, 1991.

———. "A Pro-Competition Regulatory Structure for the American Health Care System" (unpublished), February 1991.

Etheredge, Lynn, and Allen Dobson, "Review of the Resource-Based Relative-Value Scale Study" (Washington, D.C.: Consulting Group, 1989).

Evans, Robert G., *Strained Mercy—The Economics of Canadian Health Care* (Toronto: Butterworths, 1984).

Feder, Judith M., *Medicare: The Politics of Federal Hospital Insurance* (Lexington, MA: D. C. Heath, 1977).

Feder, Judith M., John Holahan, and Theodore Marmor, eds., *National Health Insurance: Conflicting Goals and Policy Choices* (Washington, D.C.: Urban Institute, 1980).

Feder, Judith M., Jack Hadley, and Stephen Zuckerman, "How Did Medicare's Prospective Payment System Affect Hospitals," *New England Journal of Medicine*, Vol. 317(14): 867–873, 1987.

Federal Register, Vol. 48, No. 171, *Prospective Payments for Medicare Impatient Hospital Services*, September 1, 1983.

———. Vol. 55, No. 171, *Model Fee Schedule for Physicians' Services*, September 4, 1990.

———. Vol. 56, No. 108, *Medicare Program; Fee Schedule for Physicians' Services; Proposed Rule*, June 5, 1991.

Feldstein, Martin S., *Economic Analysis for Health Service Efficiency* (Amsterdam: North-Holland Publ. Co., 1967).

Feldstein, Martin S., *Health Care Economics*, 3d ed. (Albany, NY: Delmar Publishers, 1988).

———. *Hospital Costs and Health Insurance* (Cambridge, MA: Harvard University Press, 1981).

Frech, H.E., and Richard Zeckhauser, eds., *Health Care in America* (San Francisco: Institute for Public Policy, 1988).

Freddi, Giorgio, and James W. Bjorkman, eds., *Controlling Medical Professionals: The Comparative Politics of Health Governance* (Newbury Park, CA: Sage Publications, 1989).

Freidson, Eliot, *Professional Dominance: The Social Structure of Medical Care* (New York: Atherton Press, 1970).

Fuchs, Victor R., *The Health Economy* (Cambridge, MA: Harvard University Press, 1986).

———. *Who Shall Live? Health, Economics, and Social Choice* (New York: Basic Books, 1974).

Ginsberg, Paul B., "Medicare Vouchers and the Procompetition Strategy," *Health Affairs*, Vol. 1(1): 39–52 1982.

Ginsberg, Paul B., Philip R. Lee, William C. Hsiao, et al., "Perspectives on Physician Payment Reform," *Health Affairs*, Vol. 8(4): 67–96, 1989.

Ginsburg, Eli, "Procompetition in Health Care: Policy or Fantasy," *Milbank Memorial Fund Quarterly*, Vol. 60: 386–398, 1982.

Glaser, William A., *Paying the Hospital: The Organization, Dynamics, and Effects of Differing Financial Arrangements* (San Francisco: Jossey-Bass, 1987).

———. "Commentary: The Politics of Paying American Physicians," *Health Affairs*, Vol. 8(3): 129–146, 1989.

Goldsmith, Jeff C., *Can Hospitals Survive? The New Competitive Health Care Market* (Homewood, IL: Dow Jones-Irwin, 1984).

———. "Death of a Paradigm: The Challenge of Competition," *Health Affairs*, Vol. 3(3): 5–19, 1984.

Gray, Bradford H., ed., *For-Profit Enterprise in Health Care* (Washington, D.C.: National Academy Press, 1986).

Gray, Bradford H., and Marilyn J., Fields, eds., *Controlling Costs and Changing Patient Care? The Role of Utilization Management* (Washington, D.C.: National Academy Press, 1989).

Greenberg, Warren, ed., "Competition in the Health Care Sector: Ten Years Later," *Journal of Health; Politics, Policy and Law*, Vol. 13(2): 223–363, 1988.

Hager, George, "New Rules on Taxes, Spending May Mean Budget Standoff", *Congressional Quarterly*, Vol. 49(4): 232–237, January 26, 1991.

Hammons, Glenn T., Robert H. Brook, and Joseph P. Newhouse, *Selected Alternatives for Paying Physicians under the Medicare Program* (Santa Monica, CA: Rand Corporation, 1986).

Heclo, Hugh, "Issue Networks and the Executive Establishment," in Anthony King, ed., *The New American Political System* (Washington, D.C.: American Enterprise Institute, 1978).

Holahan, John F., and Lynn M. Etheredge, eds., *Medicare Physician Payment Reform: Issues and Options* (Washington, D.C.: Urban Institute, 1986).

Hsiao, William C., and William B. Stason, "Toward Developing a Relative Value Scale for Medical and Surgical Services," *Health Care Financing Review*, Vol. 1(2): 23–38, 1979.

Hsiao, William C., Harvey M. Sapolsky, Daniel L. Dunn, and Sanford L. Wiener,

"Lessons of the New Jersey DRG Payment System," *Health Affairs*, Vol. 5(2): 32–45, 1986.

Hsiao, William C., et al., "Resource-Based Relative Values," *Journal of the American Medical Association*, Vol. 260(16): 2347–2438, 1988. Nine articles on various aspects of the RBRVS.

Hsiao, William C., et al., *A National Study of Resource-Based Relative Value Scales for Physician Services: Final Report* (Boston: Harvard School of Public Health, 1988).

Hsiao, William C., et al. *A National Study of Resource-Based Relative Value Scales for Physician Services: Phase II Final Report* (Boston: Harvard School of Public Health, 1990).

Iglehart, John K., "Medicare Begins Prospective Payment of Hospitals," *New England Journal of Medicine*, Vol. 308(23): 1428–1432, 1983.

———. "Health Policy Report—Payment of Physicians under Medicare," *New England Journal of Medicine*, Vol. 318(13): 863–868, 1988.

———. "Medicare's New Benefits: Catastrophic Health Insurance," *New England Journal of Medicine*, Vol. 320(5): 329–335, 1989.

Jencks, Stephen F., and Allen Dobson, "Strategies for Reforming Medicare's Physician Payment—Physician Diagnosis-Related Groups and Other Approaches," *New England Journal of Medicine*, Vol. 312(23): 1492–1499, 1985.

Jonas, Steven (ed.), *Health Care Delivery in the United States*, 3d. ed. (New York: Springer Publishing Co., 1986).

Kaufman, Bruce E. "Education, Training, and Earnings Differentials: The Theory of Human Capital," in *The Economics of Labor Markets and Labor Relations*, 2nd ed. (Hinsdale, IL: Dryden Press, 1988).

King, Anthony, *The New American Political System* (Washington, D.C.: American Enterprise Institute, 1978).

Kinney, Eleanor D., "The Medicare Appeals System for Coverage and Payment Disputes: Achieving Fairness in a Time of Constraint," *Administrative Law Journal*, Vol. 1(1): 1–103, 1987.

Kirschten, Dick, "Reagan to Congress: It's Your Move Now," *National Journal*, Vol. 15: 264–278, 1983.

Kusserow, Richard, *Hospital Closures* (Washington, D.C.: Office of the Inspector-General, Department of Health and Human Services, 1990).

Landsberger, Henry A., *The Control of Cost in the Federal Republic of Germany: Lessons for America?* (Hyattsville, MD: Public Health Service, 1981).

Lave, Judith and Lester, "The Extent of Role Differentiation among Hospitals," *Health Services Research*, Vol. 6(1): 15–38, 1971.

Lee, Philip R., Paul B. Ginsberg, et al., "The Physician Payment Review Commission Report to Congress," *Journal of the American Medical Association*, Vol. 261(16): 2382–2388, 1989.

Levit, Katherine R., Mark S. Freeland, and Daniel R. Waldo, "Health Spending and Ability to Pay: Business, Individuals, and Government," *Health Care Financing Review*, Vol. 10(3): 1–11, 1989.

Lewin, Marion Ein (ed.), *From Research into Policy—Improving the Link for Health Services* (Washington, D.C.: American Enterprise Institute, 1986).

Lewis, Thomas, *The Youngest Science—Notes of a Medicine Watcher* (New York: Viking Press, 1983).

Lomas, Jonathan, and Catherine Fooks, et al., "Paying Physicians in Canada: Minding our P's and Q's," *Health Affairs*, Vol. 8(1): 80–101, 1989.

Marmor, Theodore R., *The Politics of Medicare*, 2d ed. (Hawthorne, NY: Aldine, 1992).

Marmor, Theodore R., ed., *Political Analysis and American Medical Care* (New York: Cambridge University Press, 1983).

Mathematical Policy Research Inc., *National Medicare Competition Evaluation Final Analysis Report: The Structure of Quality Assurance Programs in HMOs and CMPs Enrolling Medicare Beneficiaries* (Washington, D.C.: 1987).

McMenanin, Peter, "A Crime Story from Medicare Part B," *Health Affairs*, Vol. 7(5): 94–101, 1988.

Mitchell, Janet B., "Packaging Physician Services: Alternative Approaches to Medicare Part B Reimbursement (unpublished), August 1987.

Mitchell, Janet B., and William B. Stason, et al., "Are Some Surgical Procedures Overpaid?," *Health Affairs*, Vol. 6(2): 121–131, 1987.

Mitchell, Janet B., Gerard Wedig, and Jerry Cromwell, "The Medicare Physician Fee Freeze—What Really Happened?," *Health Affairs*, Vol. 8(1): 21–33, 1989.

Meyer, Jack A., ed., *Incentives vs. Controls in Health Policy—Broadening the Debate* (Washington, D.C.: American Enterprise Institute, 1985).

———. *Market Reforms in Health Care: Current Issues, Directions, Strategic Decisions* (Washington, D.C.: American Enterprise Institute, 1983).

Myers, Robert J., *Medicare* (Homewood, IL: Irwin, 1970).

Mullner, Ross M., and David McNeil, "Rural and Urban Hospital Closures," *Health Affairs*, Vol. 5(3): 131–141, 1986.

Nathan, Richard P., *The Administrative Presidency* (New York: Wiley, 1983).

Nathanson, Michael, et al., "Modern Hospitals Turn to SOI's, But Experts Question Their Usefulness," *Modern Health Care*, Vol. 15(4): 63–66, 1985.

National Health Service, *Working for Patients* (London: HMSO, 1989).

National Leadership Commission on Health Care, *For the Health of a Nation* (Washington, D.C., 1989).

Newhouse, Joseph P., *The Economy of Medical Care* (Reading, MA: Addison-Wesley Publishing Co., 1978).

Newhouse, Joseph P., et al., "Some Interim Results from a Controlled Trial of Cost Sharing in Health Insurance," Rand Corporation Publication No. R-2847-HHS, January, 1982. Reprinted in Linda H. Aiken and Barbara H. Kehrer, eds., *Evaluation Studies Review Annual*, Vol. 10, 1985.

Oday, Larry A., "Development of PPS" (unpublished). 1984.

Pauly, Mark V., and William L. Kissick, eds., *Lessons from the First Twenty Years of Medicare: Research Implications for Public and Private Sector Policy* (Philadelphia: University of Pennsylvania Press, 1988).

Payer, Lynn, *Medicine and Culture: Varieties of Treatment in the United States, England, West Germany and France* (New York: Henry Holt, 1988).

Pettingill, Julian, and James Vertrees, "Reliability and Validity in Hospital Case-Mix Measurement," *Health Care Financing Review*, Vol. 4(2): 101–126, 1982.

Phelps, Charles E., *Health Economics* (New York: Harper Collins, 1991).

Physician Payment Review Commission, *Medicare Physician Payment: An Agenda for Reform* (Washington, D.C.: PPRC, 1987).

———. *Annual Report to Congress, 1988* (Washington, D.C.: PPRC, 1988).

———. *Annual Report to Congress, 1989* (Washington, D.C.: PPRC, 1989).

———. *Annual Report to Congress, 1990* (Washington, D.C.: PPRC, 1990).

———. *Annual Report to Congress, 1991* (Washington, D.C.: PPRC, 1991).

———. *Pre- and Postoperative Visits Associated with Surgical Global Services* (Washington, D.C.: PPRC, 1991).

Pope, Gregory, W. Pete Welch, et al., "Cost of Practice and Geographic Variation in Fees," *Health Affairs*, Vol. 8(3): 117–128, 1989.

Pressman, Jeffrey L., and Aaron B. Wildavsky, *Implementation* (Berkeley, CA: University of California Press, 1973).

Prospective Payment Assessment Commission, *Hospital Outpatient Services: Background Report* (Washington, D.C.: ProPAC, 1990).

Prospective Payment Assessment Commission, *Medicare Prospective Payment and the American Health Care System—Report to Congress, June, 1989* (Washington, D.C.: ProPAC, 1989).

———. *Medicare Prospective Payment and the American Health Care System—Report to Congress, June, 1990* (Washington, D.C.: ProPAC, 1990).

———. *Medicare's Capital Payment Policy* (Washington, D.C.: ProPAC, 1991).

———. *Technical Appendixes to the Report and Recommendations to the Secretary, U.S. Department of Health and Human Services, April 1, 1985* (Washington, D.C.: ProPAC, 1985).

———. *Technical Appendixes to the Report and Recommendations to the Secretary of Health and Human Services, April 1, 1986* (Washington, D.C.: ProPAC, 1986).

———. *Technical Appendixes to the Report and Recommendations to the Secretary to Health and Human Services, April 1, 1987* (Washington, D.C.: ProPAC, 1987).

Rachlis, Michael, and Carol Kishner, *Second Opinion: What's Wrong with Canada's Health Care System and How to Fix it* (Toronto: Collins Publishers, 1989).

Rivlin, Alice, *Systematic Thinking for Social Action* (Washington, D.C.: Brooklings, 1971).

Rivlin, Alice M., and Joshua M. Wiener, *Caring for the Disabled Elderly: Who Will Pay?* (Washington, D.C.: Brookings Institution, 1988).

Rosenbach, Margo L., Janet B. Mitchell, Jerry Cromwell, et al., *The 1987 Physician's Practice Follow-up Survey, Executive Summary* (Needham, MA: Health Economic Research, Inc., 1989).

Russell, Louise B., *Medicare's New Hospital Payment System—Is it Working?* (Washington, D.C.: Brookings Institution, 1989).

Rutkow, Ira M., *Socioeconomics of Surgery* (St. Louis: C. V. Mosby, 1989).

Sheingold, Steven H., "The First Three Years of PPS: Impact on Medicare Hospitals," *Health Affairs*, Vol. 8(3): 191–204, 1989.

Sloan, Frank A., and Bruce Steinwold, *Insurance, Regulation, and Hospital Costs* (Lexington, MA: D.C. Heath, 1980).

Stevens, Carol, "Will Congress Put Canadian-Style Curbs on Medicare Fees?," *Medical Economics*, Vol. 66: 26–39, 1989.

Stevens, Rosemary, *American Medicine and the Public Interest* (New Haven: Yale University Press, 1971).

———. *In Sickness and in Wealth: American Hospitals in the Twentieth Century* (New York: Basic Books, 1989).

Sutherland, Ralph W., and M. Jane Fulton, *Health Care in Canada: A Description and Analysis of Canadian Health Services* (Ottawa: The Health Group, 1988).

Thompson, Frank J., *Health Policy and the Bureaucracy: Politics and Implementation* (Cambridge, MA: MIT Press, 1981).

Thompson, John D., et al., "Case Mix and Resource Use," *Inquiry,* Vol. 12(4): 300–312, 1975.

U.S. Congress, Congressional Budget Office, *Physician Reimbursement Under Medicare: Options for Change* (Washington, D.C.: U.S. Government Printing Office, 1986).

———. Congressional Budget Office, *Physician Payment Reform Under Medicare* (Washington, D.C.: U.S. Government Printing Office, 1990).

———. House of Representatives, Committee on Ways and Means, *Background Material and Data on Programs within the Jurisdiction of the Committee on Ways and Means,* 1988 ed., 100th Congress, 2d sess., 1988. Also, editions for 1989 and 1990.

———. House of Representatives, Subcommittee on health of the Committee on Ways and Means, *Medicare Reimbursement for Physician Services,* 99th Congress, 2d sess., April 14, 1986.

———. Office of Technology Assessment, *Health Care in Rural America* (Washington, D.C.: OTA, 1989).

———. Senate, Subcommittee on Health of the Committee on Finance, *Proposals to Modify Medicare's Physician Payment System,* 99th Congress, 2d sess., April 25, 1986.

———. Senate, Committee on Finance, *Medicare and Medicaid—Problems, Issues, and Alternatives,* Staff Report to the Committee on Finance, 91st Congress, 1st sess., February 9, 1970.

———. Senate. Subcommittee on Health of the Committee on Finance, *Reimbursement Guidelines for Medicare,* 89th Congress, 2d sess., May 25, 1966.

U.S. Department of Health, Education, and Welfare, *Forward Plan for Health* (Washington, D.C.: DHEW, 1975).

U.S. Department of Health and Human Services, *Report to Congress: Hospital Prospective Payment System* (Washington, D.C.: DHHS, 1982).

———. *Medicare Annual Report—Fiscal Year 1983* (Washington, D.C.: U.S. Government Printing Office, 1986).

———. *Reports to Congress: Medicare Physician Payment* (HCFA Publ. No. 03287) (Washington, D.C.: DHEW, 1989).

———. *Report to Congress: Studies of Urban-Rural and Related Geographical Adjustments to the Medicare Prospective Payment System* (Washington, D.C.: DHHS, 1987).

———. Health Care Financing Administration, *Model Fee Schedule for Physicians' Services* (Washington, D.C.: September, 1990).

Vogel, Morris J., and Charles E. Rosenberg, eds., *Therapeutic Revolution: Essays in the Social History of American Medicine* (Philadelphia: University of Pennsylvania Press, 1979).

Welch, W. Pete, Stephen Zuckerman, and Gregory Pope, *The Geographic Medicare Economic Index: Alternative Approaches*, Working Paper 3839-91091 (Washington, D.C.: The Urban Institute, 1989).

Wennberg, John E., "Improving the Medical Decision-Making Process," *Health Affairs*, Vol. 7(1): 99–106, 1988.

Wennberg, John E., and Alan M. Gittelsohn, "Variations in Medical Care Among Small Areas," *Scientific American*, Vol. 248: 120–126, 1982.

Zook, Christopher J., Francis D. Moore, and Richard J. Zeckhauser, "Catastrophic' Health Insurance: A Misguided Prescription?," *The Public Interest*, Vol. 62: 66–81, 1981.

Zubkoff, Michael, ed., *Health: A Victim or Cause of Inflation?* (New York: Milbank Memorial Fund, 1976).

Index